AF572497

Haller, Slovis/Pediatric Radiology

Springer
Berlin
Heidelberg
New York
Barcelona
Budapest
Hong Kong
London
Milan
Paris
Tokyo

J.O. Haller and T.L. Slovis

Pediatric Radiology

Second Edition

With 201 Figures in 473 Separate Illustrations

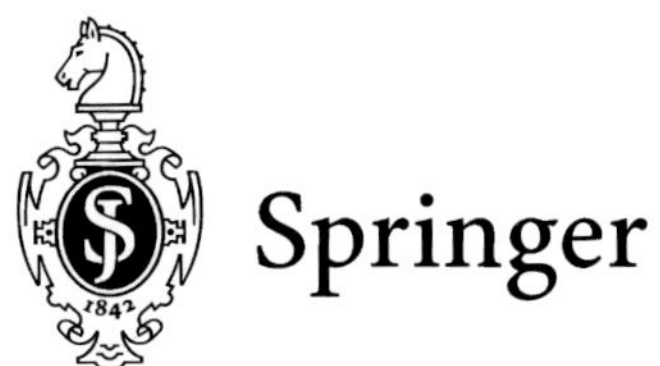

Springer

Jack O. Haller, M.D.
Professor of Radiology
State University of New York
Health Science Center at Brooklyn
Kings County Hospital
Downstate Medical Center
450 Clarkson Avenue
Brooklyn, NY 11203, USA

Thomas L. Slovis, M.D.
Professor of Radiology and Pediatrics
Wayne State University
Childrens Hospital of Michigan
3901 Beaubien Blvd.
Detroit, MI 48201, USA

Title of First Edition:
Haller, Slovis/Introduction to Radiology in Clinical Pediatrics
© 1984 by Year Book Medical Publishers, Inc. Chicago, London

ISBN 3-540-59059-5 Springer-Verlag Berlin Heidelberg New York

Library of Congress Cataloging-in-Publication Data
Haller, Jack O. (Jack Oliver), 1944- . Pediatric radiology / J.O. Haller and T. L. Slovis. - 2nd ed. p. cm. Rev. ed. of: Introduction to radiology in clinical pediatrics. © 1984. Includes bibliographical references and index. ISBN 3-540-59059-5 (hardcover: alk. paper) 1. Pediatric radiology. I. Slovis, Thomas L., 1941- . II. Haller, Jack O. (Jack Oliver), 1944- . Introduction to radiology in clinical pediatrics. III. Title. [DNLM: 1. Radiography - in infancy & childhood. WN 240 H185p 1995] RJ51.R3H34 1995 618.92'00754 - dc20 DNLM/DLC for Library of Congress 95-32581 CIP

Reproduction, dataconversion, printing, and bookbinding:
Universitätsdruckerei H. Stürtz AG, Würzburg

SPIN: 10133570 21/3135 - 5 4 3 2 1 0
Printed on acid-free paper

Dedication: First Edition

To Adolf and Frieda Haller, my mentors, my inspiration, my parents.
J.O.H

To Ellie, Michael, Debbie, Andy, and Lisa, my family, without whose love, patience, and inspiration this project could not have been completed.
T.L.S.

Dedication: Second Edition

To Walter E. Berdon, Jerome M. Levine, David H. Baker, and Joseph O. Reed whose teaching and counsel molded our careers, and whose integrity and dedication to excellence in their craft had a profound influence on our lives.
J.O.H.
T.L.S.

Preface to First Edition

The idea for this book grew out of our experience in teaching pediatric radiology to clinicians and students. Clearly, there is a strong desire on the part of those taking care of children to familiarize themselves with the rudiments of the pediatric radiograph. While radiologists have primary responsibility for the interpretation of films, clinicians bring valuable insight and information. Often they present additional important data or ask searching questions that prompt a re-evaluation of the films so that a more appropriate diagnosis may be obtained.

While primers are available in adult radiology, comparable editions in pediatrics are lacking. We have therefore adapted the teaching sessions of Joseph O. Reed, Director of Radiology at Children's Hospital of Michigan, and Professor of Radiology at Wayne State University School of Medicine, as the framework for our text. In addition, Rosalind H. Troupin has generously allowed us to use some of her ideas for this book, which is an elementary guide to common pediatric radiographic examinations and problems. It is our intent to provide an approach to these examinations to help the clinician discern the normal from the abnormal. A second goal is to help the pediatrician, house officer, and medical student learn the indications for various procedures, as well as to recognize some of the more common abnormalities. This text is by no means meant to provide an in-depth discussion of various disease entities, nor is it intended to catalog the various subtle radiographic findings in these entities.

The radiographs in this volume are often reproduced to enhance a single finding under discussion, often at the expense of other portions of the film. Also, arrows and letters have been kept to a minimum so as not to obscure the radiographs.

It is our hope that, by providing this primer for pediatric radiology, we will stimulate clinicians to visit the X-ray department, share in the interpretation of their patients' films, and continue to stimulate us so that together we can provide optimal care for children.

Jack O. Haller
Thomas L. Slovis

Preface to Second Edition

Why did we write a 2nd edition? There were several reasons. First, the popularity of the first edition demanded a repeat. Students, housestaff, clinicians, and directors of radiology, pediatric radiology, and pediatric programs across the nation were continually calling us to ask where they could obtain more copies. The first edition was simply sold out; there were no copies left.

Second, in our capacities as directors of pediatric radiology departments, we also ran out of copies; we found the first edition so helpful in acclimating our radiology and pediatric staffs to pediatric radiology, that we needed new copies for ourselves.

Third, in the ten years since publication of the first edition there have been major changes in the field of radiology. Therefore, we really needed to update it; hence, the added information on ultrasound, CT, and MRI. While it is hard to cover such complex fields in a book such as this, we have tried to give the reader at least a working practical introduction to the topics as they relate to pediatrics.

We know, based on our experience with the first edition, that this volume will be helpful to clinicians and housestaff from both radiology and pediatric departments. But we have also found that family practice and emergency physicians, nurse practitioners, and physicians' assistants profit from reading the first edition; we have also geared our new text towards these groups as well. Enjoy!

Jack O. Haller
Thomas L. Slovis

Acknowledgments: First Edition

We wish to acknowledge a number of individuals without whom this work would not have been completed. Drs. Ronald L. Poland, John K. Kelly, Harvey I. Wilner, and Alfredo Lazo offered helpful criticisms of early drafts. Drs. Alkis Zingas, Alfredo Lazo, and Lawrence R. Kuhns were kind enough to lend us computerized tomographic images and the nuclear medicine images found within the text. Virginia Newman did yeoman work in typing and retyping numerous revisions of this manuscript over a two-year period. Without her hard work, the task would have been impossible.

Albert Paglialunga and Shelley Eshelman provided the reproductions of the radiographs and the schematic diagrams, respectively. They were patient and responsive.

Dr. Joshua A. Becker, a chairman and friend, has continued to provide support and encouragement for academic pursuits and sustains a gratifying working milieu.

Drs. George B. Comerci, Lewis A. Barness, and C. Henry Kempe stimulated our interest in pediatrics and urged close rapport with our pediatric colleagues. Dr. R. Parker Allen has been responsible for first "turning out" many of this students to radiology.

Drs. David H. Baker and Walter E. Berdon, our mentors, godfathers, and friends, have always encouraged us and continue to serve as models of excellence in pediatric radiology.

Dr. Joseph O. Reed (whose Reed's Rules appear throughout this book) has helped with this guidance, teaching, and critical appraisal of the manuscript. He has provided this stimulus by emphasizing basic principles as a means to learning radiology and, in fact, medicine itself.

Acknowledgments: Second Edition

We are grateful for the efforts of many individuals who helped make this second edition possible. Particularly, we would like to thank Jennifer Handley for typing the entire manuscript with endless corrections and modifications. Michele Klein reviewed the manuscript both as a teaching tool and also as a proofreader. Her suggestions and contributions were invaluable. Cliff Roberts prepared all of the photographs in this text. He worked tirelessly to make the images perfect, and without his efforts the book would not have been possible. Lastly, we would like to thank all of those who read, corrected, or contributed to the many chapters. These include Joshua A. Becker for his continued encouragement, members of the faculty at Children's Hospital of Michigan (Gary Amundson, Cristie Becker, David Corbett, John Crowley, Daniel Eggleston, Sam Kottamasu, John Pereira, and Susan Roubal), and to the authors who allowed us to use pictures from other articles and text in this edition.

Contents

1 Diagnostic Medical Imaging: How, Why, and When

Introduction

Diagnostic medical imaging can be accomplished in many ways using various physical tools. X-rays (gamma rays) create the images seen on plain films, fluoroscopy, angiography, and routine tomography. A tomogram is an image of a thin section, a small piece of the whole organ, demonstrated with increased resolution and detail. Gamma rays are also used in nuclear medicine and positron emission tomography (PET). Sound waves create the information necessary to make an ultrasound image while magnetic fields provide the data for an image in a magnetic resonance (MR) examination. The proliferation of imaging modalities for diagnostic evaluation is predicated on the emergence of the computer. It is the vital cog for acquisition and processing of the data and/or the manipulation after processing (postprocessing). Reconstruction of images in many planes and three-dimensional rendering of the anatomy are among the most valuable options offered by postprocessing (Fig. 1.1). Use of computers for storing and moving images is rapidly evolving.

Nature of Radiographs

X-rays are short electromagnetic radiations "produced by energy conversion when fast-moving electrons from the filament of the X-ray tube interact with the tungsten anode (target)" [1] (Fig. 1.2). When an X-ray beam is directed toward a part of the body, X-rays are absorbed by the more dense tissue (e.g., bone) causing ionization within the body. X-rays that *pass through* the entire body interact with the X-ray film (intensifying screens, etc.), forming an image. The X-ray picture, or radiograph, is a recording of internal body structures in which the black areas represent regions that have allowed the X-rays to pass through and onto the film, and the white areas the regions that have absorbed all X-rays before they reach the film. Thus, the least dense body structures (i.e., lungs) appear *black*, and the more dense structures (i.e., bone), which have absorbed the X-rays, appear *white* (Fig. 1.3).

In addition to plain film radiography, there are many diagnostic X-ray methods. *Fluoroscopy* allows us to study internal body functions, for example, cardiac motion, peristalsis of bowel. In fluoroscopy the image is portrayed through an intensifier onto a television monitor. Individual static radiographs can also be taken during this procedure. *Cineradiography* is the recording of successive fluoroscopic images on videotape.

Some X-ray studies involve the use of contrast media, which are substances used to enhance, emphasize, and then visualize various structures of the body. They can be injected, swallowed, or given as enemas. Examples of contrast media are air, barium sulfate and iodine-containing solutions. The latter two are quite dense and absorb the X-ray beam – thus appearing white – hence their usefulness in demonstrating internal structures (Fig. 1.4).

Angiography is the study of blood vessels after contrast has been injected. The contrast medium flowing through the blood vessels of selected organs or masses reveals minute vascular detail (see Chap. 9). MR angiography images the blood vessels without any contrast medium but rather by computer manipulation (see below).

Radionuclide imaging – nuclear medicine – utilizes a radioisotope. It is combined with a specific compound that normally goes to a specific organ of the body, for example, the bone or liver. When injected, it accumulates in specific tissues and organs, where it emits gamma rays that can be recorded on film or on a computer. Because of specific organ-tissue binding nuclear medicine can give functional (physiological) information. The tomographic (thin-section) equivalent in nuclear medicine is single-photon emission computed tomography (SPECT), and this is gaining favor because of its increased resolution compared to routine nuclear studies. PET is also a tomographic nuclear medicine study. In this instance, however, specially created isotopes (made by a cyclotron) of high energy and very short half-life are used to bind specifically to organ receptors. A basic concept to remember is that X-rays pass through the body to hit the cassette film and blacken the film. Those X-rays stopped by the body are immediately absorbed and are seen as white

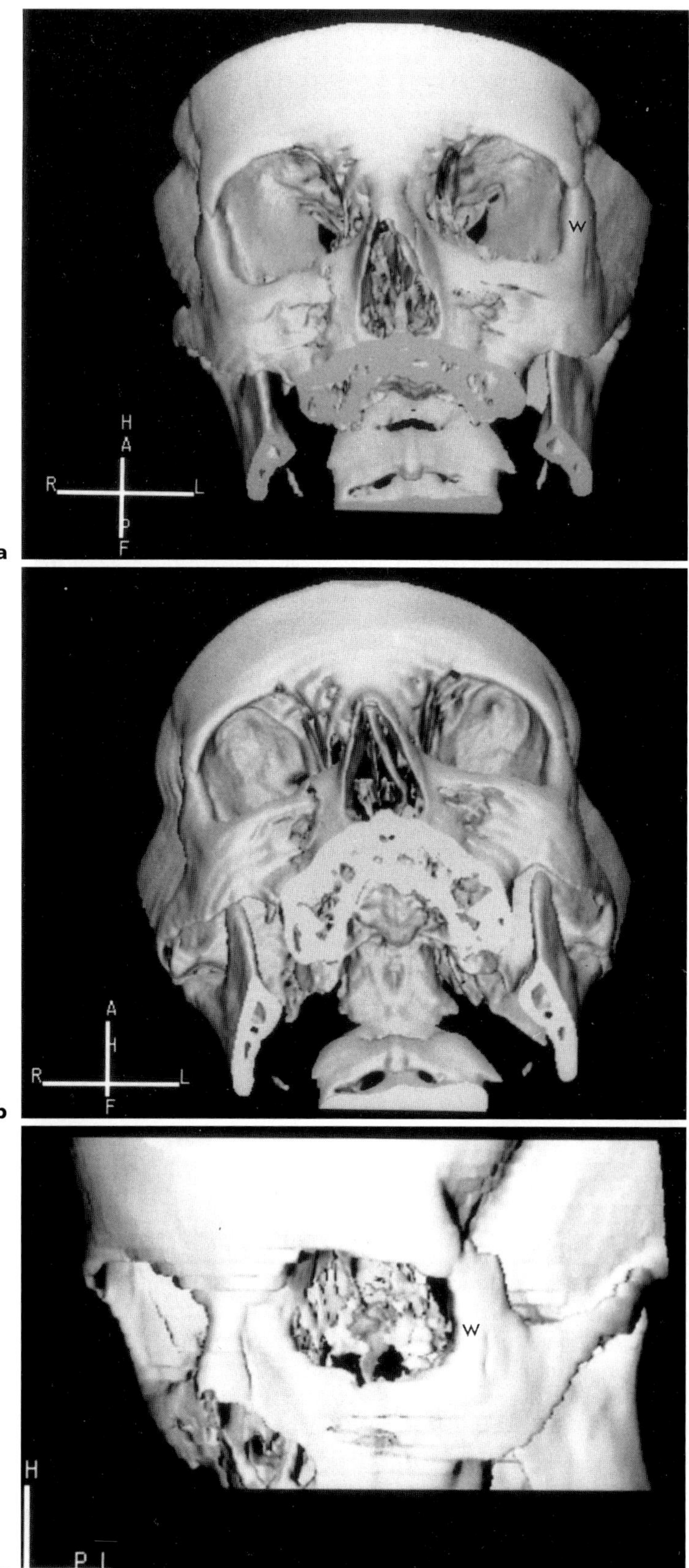

Fig. 1.1a–c. Views from a three-dimensional reconstructed CT examination of the face. **a** Straight frontal examination through the orbits. **b** The head rotated posteriorly so that we are looking up through the nose and orbits. **c** With the patient rotated to the right so that the zygoma and lateral wall of the orbit (*w*) are seen to advantage. In these reconstructions, the skull can be rotated in any plane

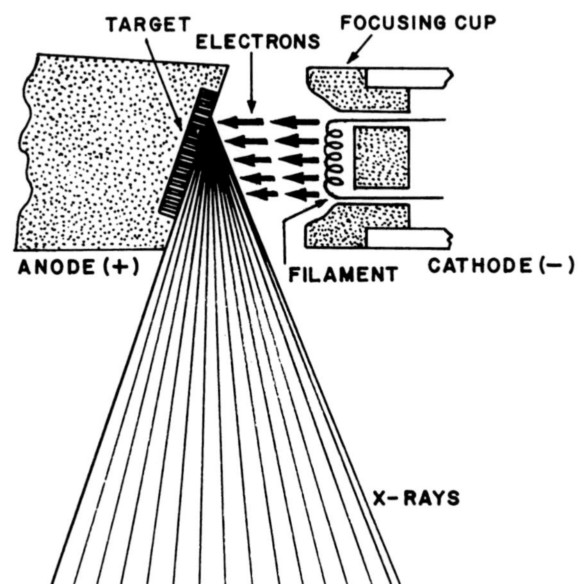

Fig 1.2. Production of X-rays

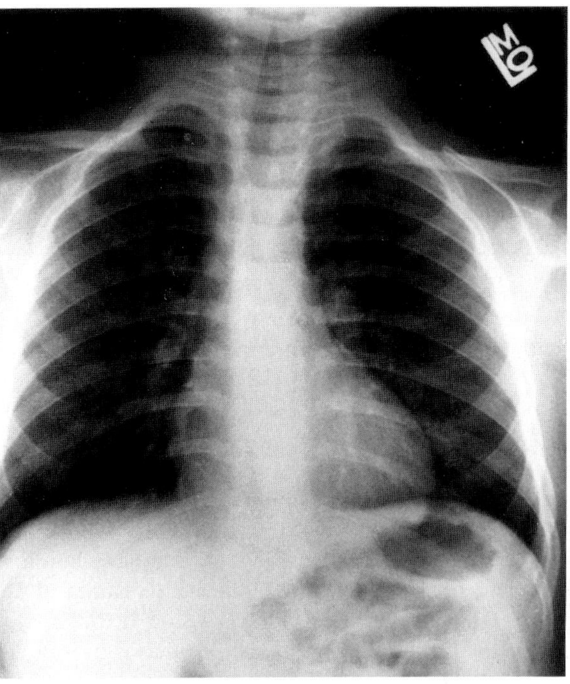

Fig. 1.3. Frontal chest radiograph shows a normal chest with the air-filled lungs being black and the soft tissues, heart and bones, appearing gray to white

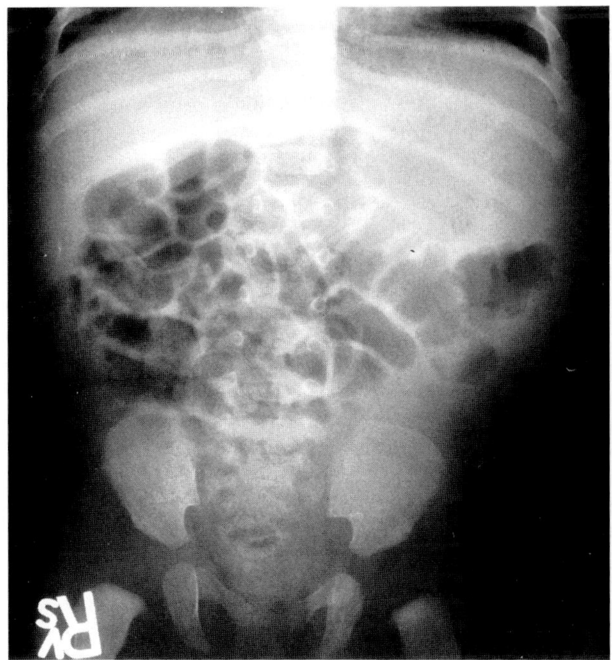

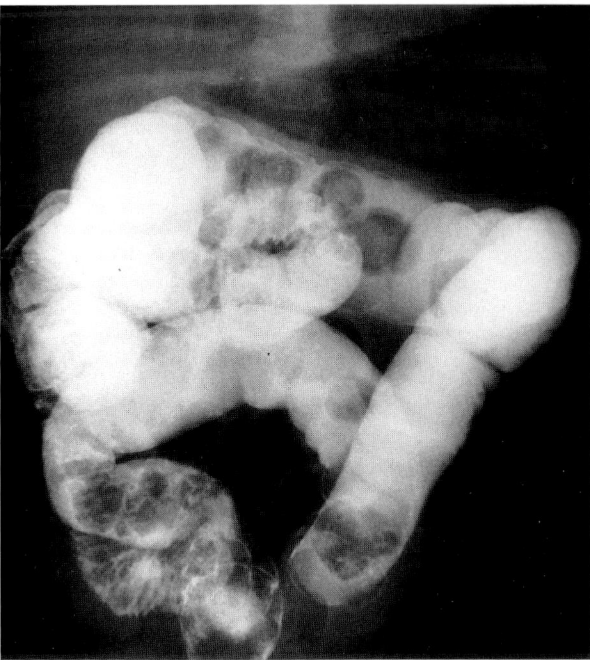

Fig. 1.4 a, b. Use of contrast. **a** Supine plain film of the abdomen shows air in bowel, but it is uncertain which is small or large bowel. **b** Barium as contrast agent was placed in the colon. Stool within the colon is outlined by barium. The X-ray beams are absorbed by the barium, and thus the colon appears white, while allowing delineation of the air-filled upper GI tract (*black*)

Table 1.1. Density and Hounsfield units as noted on CT

	Color	HU (CT Units)
Bone	Most white	750–1000
Contrast	White	75–300
Soft tissue	Gray	40–60
Water	Dark gray-black	-10 to +10
Fat	Black	-100
Air	Most black	-500

on the film (i.e., bone). In contrast, the child who is injected with a radioisotope emits the isotope until it decays – a matter of half-life of the isotope and physiological excretion. When using technetium which has a 6-h half-life in a child with normal urinary excretion, emission of radiation occurs for approximately 6 h.

Computed tomography (CT) utilizes an X-ray beam in a rotating carriage to scan a narrow cross-section of the body. In conventional CT the X-ray beam and detectors rotate about the patient, while in the newer spiral (helical) scanners there is continuous movement of the patient through the gantry while the radiographic tube and detector system rotate about the patient (continuous acquisition). When intravenous contrast is used, spiral CT can also produce angiographic images. A computer within the CT unit synthesizes the data generated by either of these processes and reconstructs them into images that can be displayed on a television monitor, recorded on film, or saved on disc or tape for later use. Table 1.1 shows the appearance of the various densities on CT. Density is measured in Hounsfield units (CT units).

Radiation Dose

The question of possibly harmful effects of X-rays is frequently raised by concerned parents. Because parents often express such concern, it is helpful to have some basic facts about radiation dosage so that parents can be reassured [2].

Each of us is exposed to approximately 100–150 mrad per year from the environment [the higher the altitude, the greater the dose (skin dose)]. A normal chest examination (two views) exposes the patient to between 10 and 20 mrad, while an intravenous urogram imparts approximately 500 mrad. Fluoroscopic studies are more radiation-producing than static studies. A barium study of the gastrointestinal tract, for example, exposes the patient to approximately 1200 mrad. How few milliradiation units cause biological damage? No one really knows. Therefore, one follows the ALARA concept – "as low as reasonably achievable" radiation dose. The best policy is to expose a patient to only the amount of radiation that a specific medical problem dictates. However, when a child's medical condition warrants taking a number of radiographs, the benefits of the diagnostic study outweigh any risks. It is extremely important to stress this fact when talking with parents. One can also help to allay anxiety by pointing out the many precautions taken to minimize dangerous ionizing radiation to both patients and staff. X-ray room walls and floors are all shielded, and machines are inspected routinely to assure continued accurate functioning. As pediatric radiologists we are specifically trained to reduce the radiation dose for children. We tailor the examination to fit a child's specific problem and use special equipment (digital radiology, last frame capture, etc.) and procedures (e.g., shielding the reproductive organs).

Nature of Other Imaging Modalities

High-frequency sound (>20 000 cycles/s) is called ultrasound and may be produced by a piezoelectric crystal. The crystal is the most important component of the ultrasound transducer (Fig. 1.5). The transducer converts an electric signal into ultrasonic energy (sound) that can be transmitted into tissues. The echoes returning from the patient are then converted back into an electrical signal and recorded on film (see [1], p.327). Color-flow Doppler imaging allows us to examine the nature of vascular flow (patency, waveform, etc.). Diagnostic ultrasound causes no known significant biological adverse effect at the frequencies

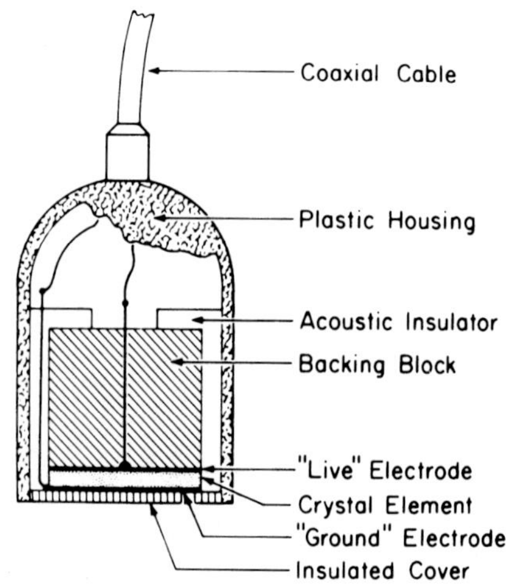

Fig. 1.5. Ultrasound transducer (with permission from [1])

that we use [3]. The ultrasonic appearance of normal body tissues is as follows:

- Without echoes: anechoic; these appear black
  - Cystic regions or fluid-filled viscera (e.g., gallbladder)
  - Blood vessels: flowing blood
- With echoes: shades of gray and white
  - Viscera (e.g., liver, spleen, brain)
  - Air: artifact behind it
  - Calcium and bone: the whitest; blocks echoes behind it (shadowing)

MR captures the rotational motion of the electrical charge on protons in the nucleus of cells of our body as they respond to a magnetic field. There is no ionizing radiation and no significant biological effects at the magnetic strengths in clinical use. As with other forms of imaging, computer manipulation of the data allows for images in multiple planes. The spin-echo concept of MR uses two basic image sequences, called T1 and T2. T1 is the anatomical sequence while T2 ("pathological sequence") shows most pathology as white. We use the different appearances of specific tissues on T1 and T2 to diagnose the nature of these entities (see Table 1.2).

Table 1.2. Appearance on MR

	T1	T2	Clues
Fat	Bright	Dark	Fat fades
Flowing blood	Dark	Dark	Blood is black
Water (fluid)	Dark	Bright	Water whitens
Bone	Black	Black	Bone is black

Everything else is variable.

MR angiography is accomplished through computer manipulation to "show" only blood vessels and to "suppress" everything else; vascular structures are beautifully visualized (MR angiography, see chapter 9).

Proper Utilization of Imaging

An imaging test should be obtained when the value of the result is greater than the cost (risk) of the test. Costs are defined in many ways – monetary, radiation, morbidity (sedation or contrast), anxiety of both patient and parents, time, and inconvenience. In the current health-care environment less is clearly better for the system but not necessarily for the patient. It is our job to make sure that every patient gets the appropriate imaging suited for his/her particular clinical need.

Once the decision is made to image, the radiologist considers the differential diagnosis and the appropriate questions asked by the pediatrician. The questions asked before ordering a test enables a proper decision among available tests. If a functional question is asked (e.g., the percentage of renal function), a nuclear study may suffice, while an anatomical study, such as ultrasound, would not (Table 1.3). The imaging study chosen should give results leading to the proper diagnosis; even a negative result may provide useful information and lead to appropriate advice or counseling.

The major problem of utilization remains *overutilization*, such as the ordering of skull films for insignificant trauma, or routine preoperative chest films, or repeating films already obtained. Proper utilization also involves choosing the correct modality to answer

Table 1.3. Comparison of modalities

Modality	Physical agent	Strength	Weakness	Comment
Plain film	X-ray	Global view of anatomy	Does not reveal fine detail of organ	Least expensive
Ultrasound	Sound waves	Good organ detail, anatomical	Operator dependent; air, bone may prevent visualization of organs	Less invasive, relatively cheap; no radiation, no sedation
CT	X-ray	Good organ detail, quick, anatomical	May need sedation, contrast	Moderately expensive
MR	Electromagnetic waves	Great tissue contrast, multiple planes; anatomical; new inroads to functional imaging	Relatively slow, needs sedation in younger children; may need contrast	Most expensive, no radiation
Nuclear	Gamma rays	Physiological (functional)	Organ specific; poor on anatomic detail	Moderate expense and invasiveness

the question. A clinician's lack of knowledge of the capabilities and limitations of an imaging procedure, overdependence on imaging rather than the clinical picture, and the use of imaging as a screening procedure all lead to many unnecessary examinations.

The pediatric radiologist alters utilization practices and helps obtain the most optimal study. Conversant with all the modalities and their pitfalls, the radiologist can diminish the number of films/examinations to decrease radiation dose and can teach the technologist the various ways to avoid repeat films or to lower the dose, for example, in CT examination, using a lower milliamperage.

The imager who examines children has a multifaceted role: (a) as a consultant determining the appropriate examination(s) and the number of films necessary, (b) as a member of the health care team interpreting films and conserving resources, and (c) as a teacher of his/her clinical colleagues.

References

1. Curry TS III, Dowdey JE, Murray RC Jr. (1990) Christensen's physics of diagnostic radiology, 4th edn. Lea and Febiger, Philadelphia, 1990
2. National Council on Radiation Protection and Measurements (1981) Radiation protection in pediatric radiology. NCRP report 68. Washington, National Council on Radiation Protection and Measurements
3. National Council on Radiation Protection and Measurements (1983) Biological effects of ultrasound: mechanisms and clinical implications. NCRP report 74. Washington, National Council on Radiation Protection and Measurements

2 Chest Examinations in Children

The chest film is the most frequently ordered pediatric radiographic examination. However, because one looks at so many chest radiographs, familiarity may create a false sense of security rather than expertise. A thorough, detailed, systematic approach to the radiographic evaluation is crucial for anyone dealing with children. In this chapter we discuss the general diagnostic principles and approach; the specifics of chest examinations for neonates and infants are reviewed in Chap. 3. This chapter also stresses those areas where the approach to the pediatric chest radiograph differs from the adult film (the 3 T's: technical factors, tubes and traps, i.e., anatomical structures unique to kids; thanks to Dr. Moira Cooper, pediatric radiologist, Izaak Walton Killam Children's Hospital, Nova Scotia, Canada) as well as the different pathological conditions.

Technical Factors

Technical problems in pediatric radiology are caused largely by uncooperative children. The young patients are not feeling well, the environment is strange, and may as a result be quite frightened. Preliminary evaluation of the chest radiograph should assess these technical factors:

- The degree of inspiration: lung volume
- The position of the patient: extent of rotation and posture of the patient
- How the exposure was made: erect or supine with the difference in tube-film distance (72 in. in erect and 40 in. in supine).
- Adequacy of the exposure

Lung Volume

The radiographic examination of the chest begins with frontal and lateral roentgenograms taken after deep inspiration. The degree of inspiration, i.e., the lung volume, generally determines what is seen on the film. The answers to the questions in Table 2.1 determine whether or not adequate lung volume is obtained.

If the child has taken a shallow breath, the heart may appear enlarged, the vessels may coalesce to give a false impression of an infiltrate, especially in the region of the bases and hila, and sometimes the radiograph has a hazy quality due to the influx of blood and lack of aerated lung.

Hyperexpansion of the lungs - pathological increase in lung volume or air trapping - is involuntary, and the changes of hyperexpansion listed in Table 2.1 should be visible on both frontal and lateral films. Figures 2.1–2.4 demonstrate the differences between the normal radiograph and those in which inspiration is either pathologically increased or suboptimal. Can you pick out the optimal radiograph?

Position of the Patient

The position of the patient is determined by rotation and posture (lying, sitting, or standing).

The child's posture is important. When the patient is supine, the vascular supply to the upper and lower lobes is equal since gravity has no effect. When the child is sitting or standing, gravity plays a significant role, and the upper-lobe vessels are less distended than the lower-lobe vessels (one-third to two-thirds size). One can determine an erect film by looking at the air fluid level in the stomach and at changes in the pulmonary vasculature (see Fig. 2.1).

Rotation of a child is determined by the answers to the questions in Table 2.2. Figures 2.5 and 2.6 show the parameters that determine rotation, while Figure 2.7 exemplifies the posture of the patient, showing supine and erect films. Compare these figures with Fig. 2.1.

Methods of Film Exposure

The third major technical factor to keep in mind is how the film was obtained. Greater magnification occurs when structures, such as the heart, are farther from the film. When the X-ray beam passes through the patient from back to front [a posterior-anterior

Table 2.1. Determining lung volume: questions and answers

Question	Answer
How much of the heart projects below the dome of the diaphragm on the frontal view?	More than 1/3: expiratory effort; not enough air in the lungs Less than 1/3: good inspiratory effort; normal amount of air None: may be hyperexpanded; too much air
On the frontal view, are the domes of the diaphragm flat?	No: very domed; expiratory effort Rounded: good inspiratory effort Yes: flat; good or may be too great a lung volume
Are the hemidiaphragms flat or vertically oriented on the lateral?	No: horizontally oriented; expiratory effort Yes: vertically oriented; good or possibly increased lung volume
Which anterior rib crosses the diaphragm on the frontal film? (Remember that the anterior ribs move more than the posterior ribs on good inspiration.)	3rd or 4th: expiratory effort 5th or 6th: inspiratory effort 7th or lower: good or possibly too great a lung volume
On the lateral view, is there a triangle of air behind the heart?	No: expiratory effort (except if large heart) Yes: inspiratory effort
Are the lungs black or white on the frontal film?[a]	Black: air filled, inspiratory White or gray[b]: not air filled; expiratory

[a] Lung density is influenced by exposure.
[b] At times there may be a good lung volume, but the lungs are "white." This white appearance is caused when the child holds its breath while simultaneously pushing against the closed glottis, thus increasing intrathoracic pressure.

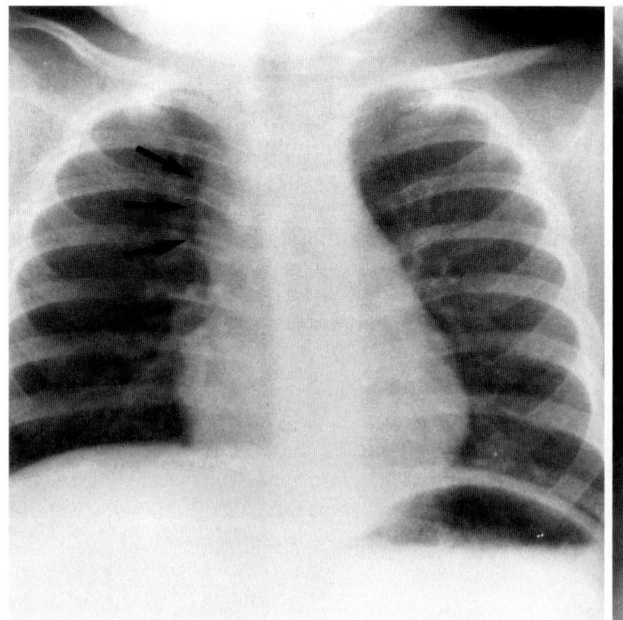

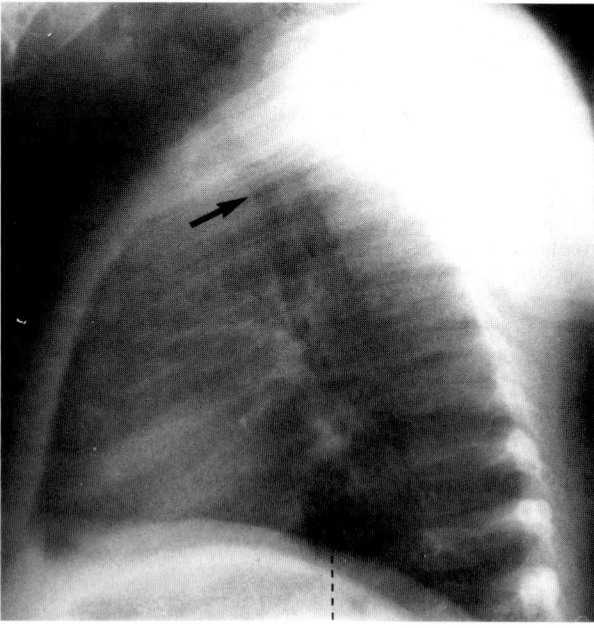

Fig. 2.1 a, b. Inspiratory chest. **a** Frontal examination reveals a normal lung volume. The criteria for a normal lung volume are: (a) less than one third of the heart is projected below the hemidiaphragm; (b) the diaphragm is rounded, and the seventh anterior rib intersects the diaphragm; and (c) the lungs are air filled (*black*). This is a properly positioned, nonrotated film as evidenced by (a) comparative anterior ribs equidistant from the pedicles, (b) medial aspects of the clavicles symmetrically positioned, (c) the carina approximates the right pedicles, and (d) no difference in aeration between the two sides. The film was taken with the patient erect, as shown by the air fluid level in the stomach. The right lobe of the thymus is prominent (*arrows*) but entirely within normal limits. **b** Lateral examination confirms normal aeration of the lungs.

Fig. 2.2 a, b. Expiratory chest. **a** Normal frontal film taken during expiration, i.e, (a) more than one-third of the heart projects below the diaphragmatic margins, (b) hemidiaphragms are domed, and the fourth anterior rib crosses the diaphragmatic margin, and (c) the lungs are not as well aerated. The patient is rotated, as shown by (a) asymmetric comparable ribs in relationship to the pedicles and (b) asymmetric position of the clavicles. The end of the right clavicle (*c*) is well to the right of the spine, and (c) the right lung does not appear as well aerated (*black*) as the left. **b** Expiratory lateral film shows the loss of air space behind the heart. The ribs (*arrows*) are seen but not the spinous processes of the vertebrae, indicating rotation

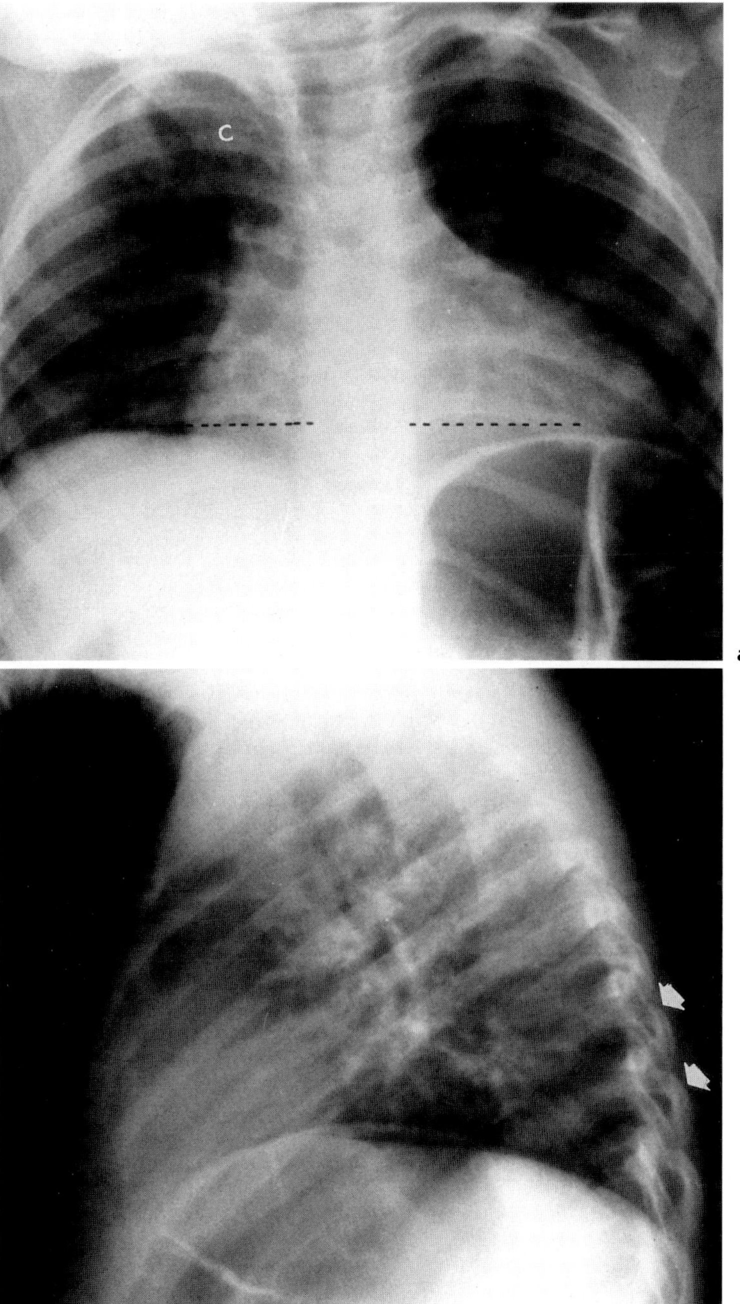

(Fig. 2.1: continued)
The normal triangular air space is seen behind the heart, bounded by the heart anteriorly, the diaphragm inferiorly and the vertebrae posteriorly. The patient is not rotated, as the spinous processes of the vertebrae are seen. An air fluid level in the stomach attests to the erect position of the patient. The airway can be seen from the oropharynx to the carina and is not bowed forward. Note the normal indentation at the thoracic inlet (*black arrow*). The anterior mediastinal space above the heart contains normal thymic tissue. The heart does not project behind an imaginary line extending from the carina inferiorly

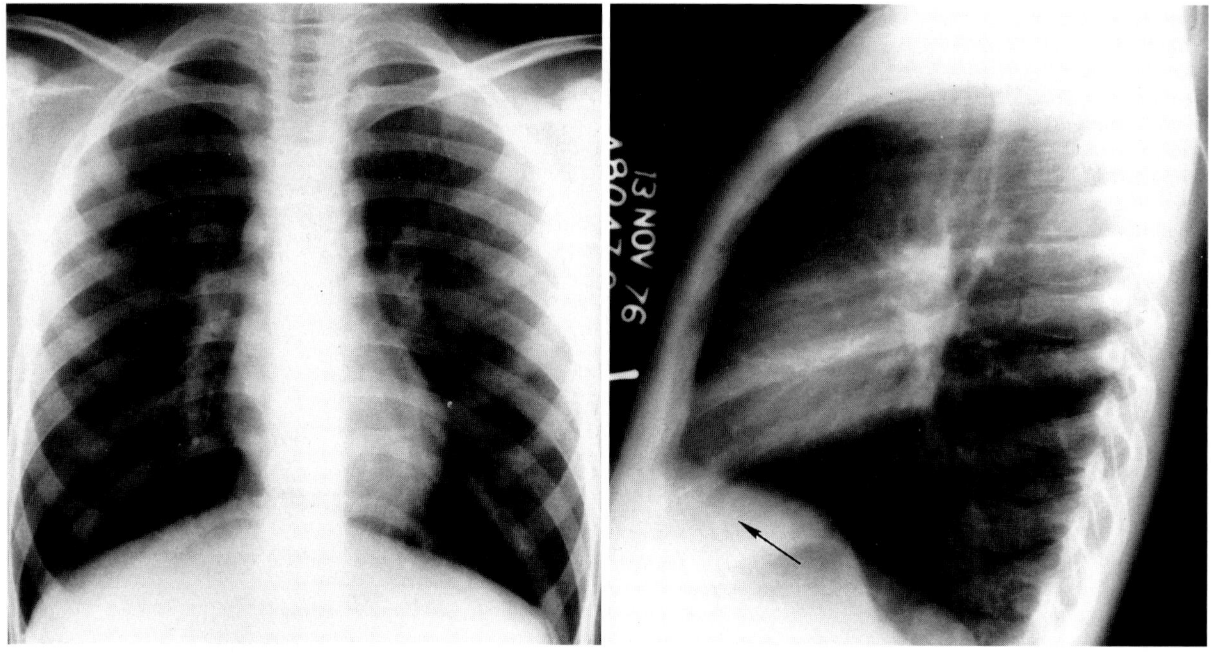

Fig. 2.3 a, b. Hyperexpanded frontal and lateral radiographs. **a** Frontal view. The entire heart is projected above the diaphragm, the hemidiaphragms are flattened, and the lungs are quite black – yet the film is not overexposed. **b** Lateral view. The hemidiaphragms are vertically oriented (*arrow*), and there is a very large air space both behind and in front of the heart. Remember: hyperexpansion is involuntary and is caused by air trapping. It must be seen on both frontal and lateral projections

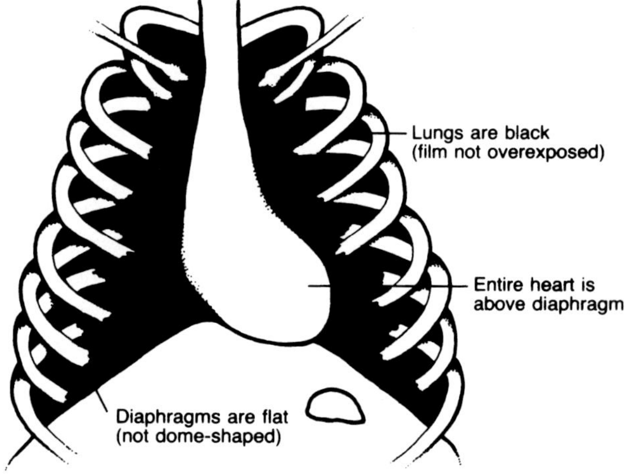

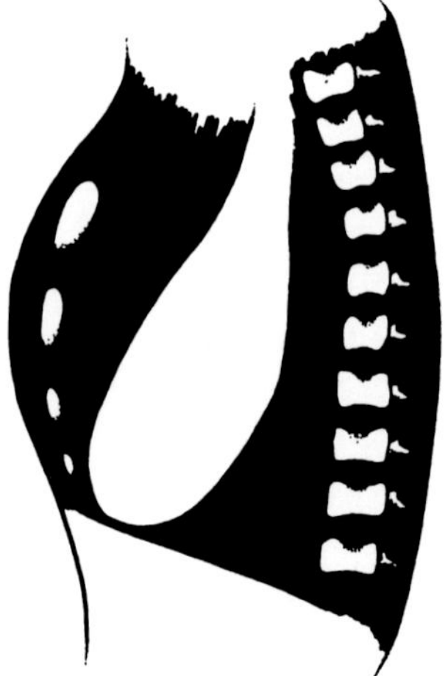

Fig. 2.4. The hyperexpanded chest ▶

Table 2.2. Determining rotation: answers and questions

Answer	Question
On the frontal film, are the anterior ribs equidistant from ipsilateral pedicles?	No: rotated patient Yes: straight patient
Are the medial aspects of the clavicles symmetrical in relation to the midline on the frontal view?	No: rotated patient Yes: straight patient
What is the position of the carina in relation to the right pedicles on the frontal film?	To the left of the right pedicles: patient is rotated, or another abnormality is present Approximates the right pedicles: patient is straight
Is one lung blacker than the other on the frontal view?	Yes: patient is rotated, or abnormality is causing localized difference in aeration No: straight patient
On the lateral view, are the ribs seen posteriorly?	Yes: rotated patient No: straight patient

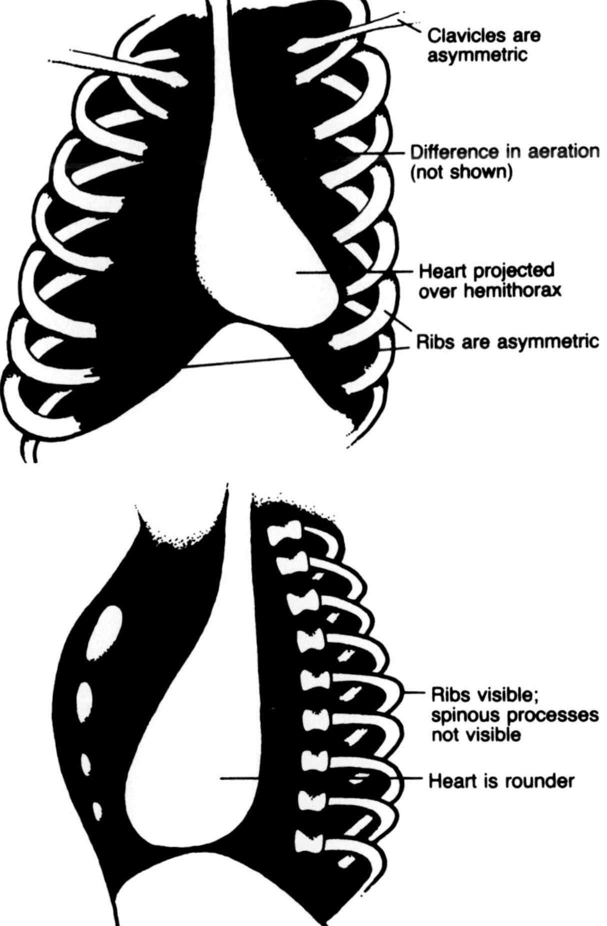

Fig. 2.5. The rotated chest film ►

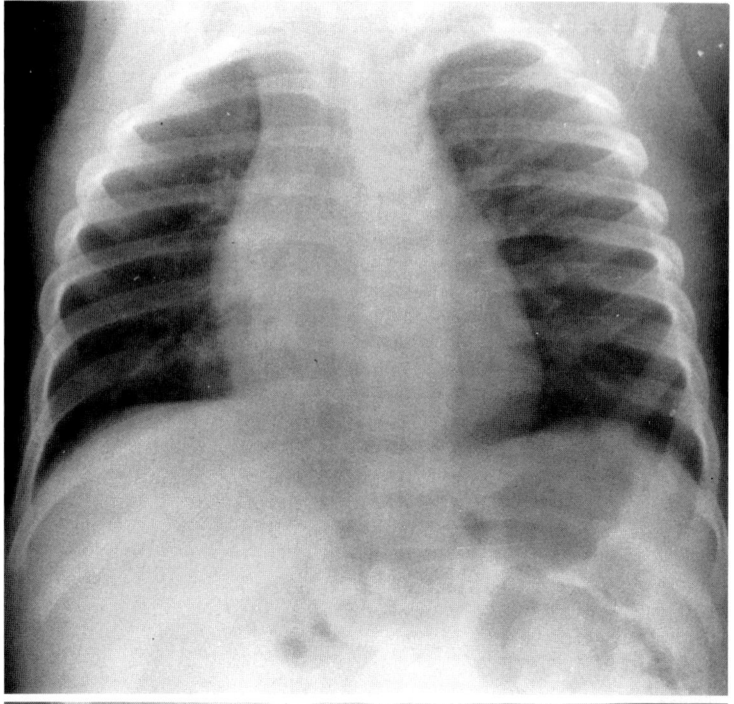

a

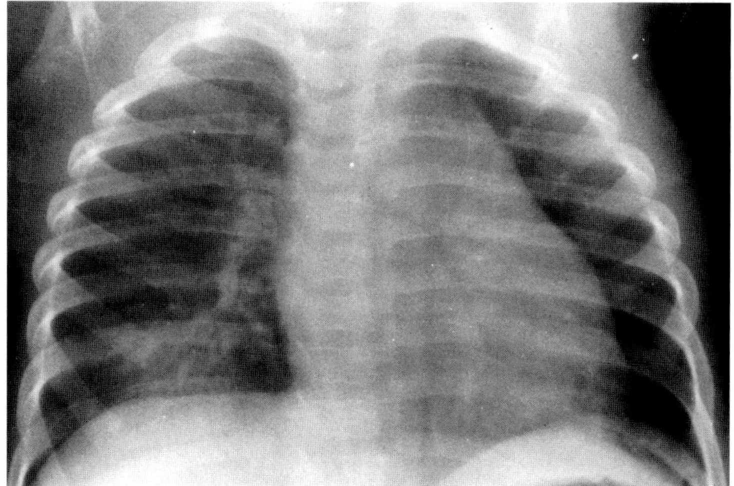

b

Fig. 2.6 a, b. Examples of rotated films. The two panels are films of two different children rotated in opposite directions. In each, can you find the parameters for estimating rotation? **a** To which side is the patient rotated? **b** To which side is the patient rotated? (Answers in "Appendix 2")

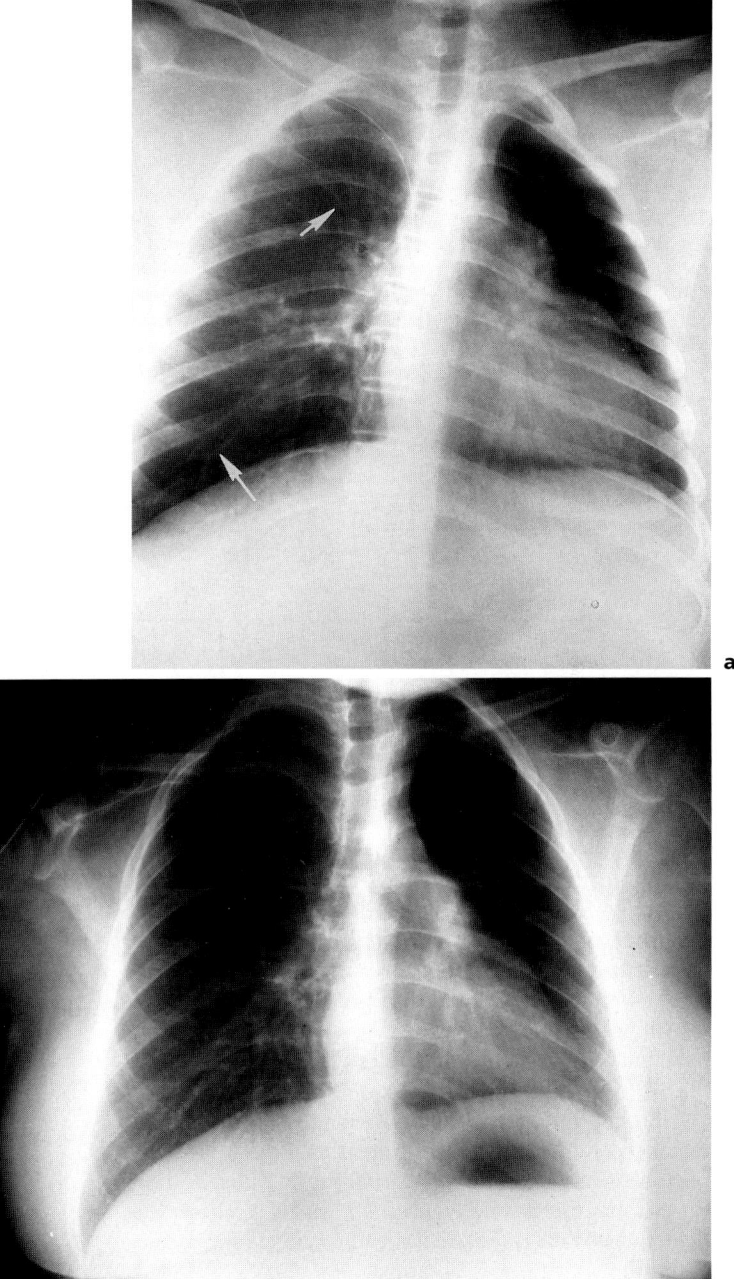

Fig. 2.7 a, b. Effect of patient position and the tube target distance. **a** Patient in supine position, with approximately 46 in. between the X-ray tube and the film. Upper-lobe vessels (*arrows*) are equal in size to those of the lower lobe (*arrows*). The heart is magnified. **b** Patient is erect and 6 ft from the X-ray tube

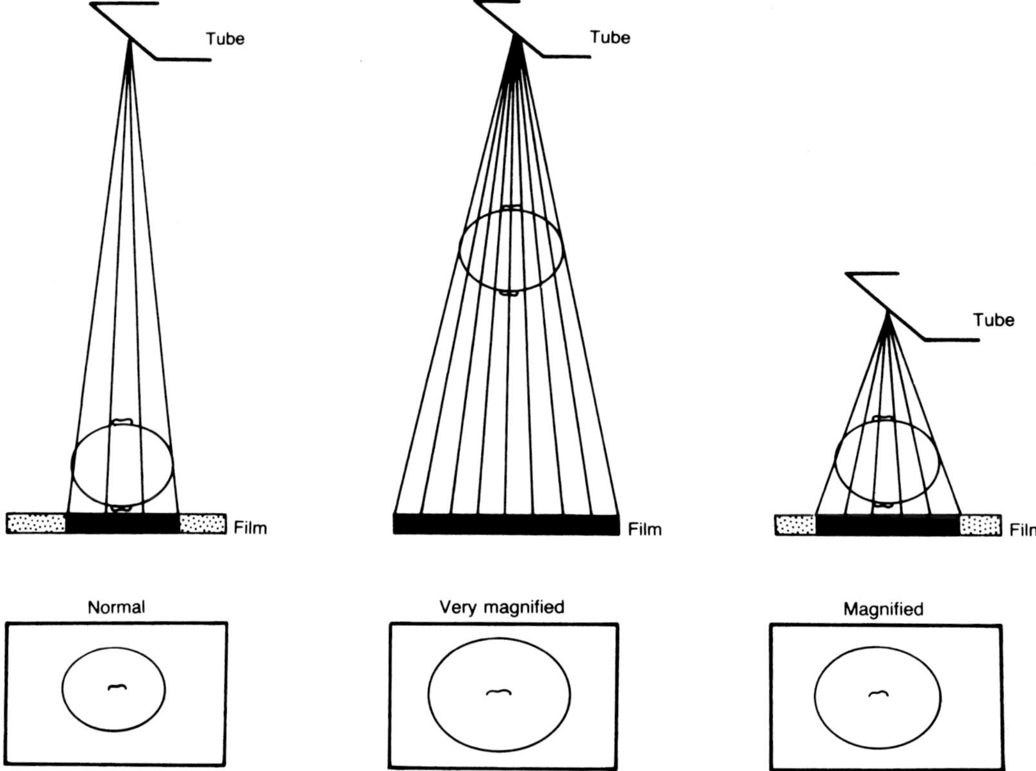

Fig. 2.8. Tube-film distance and magnification

(PA) projection], the heart is closer to the film and is less magnified. Conversely, if the X-ray beam enters the front of patient's chest, passes through the back and onto the film [an anterior-posterior (AP) projection], the magnified heart and great vessels may give the impression of cardiomegaly. This is a common problem with portable chest films, which are taken in the AP direction.

Another important factor in magnification is the distance of the X-ray tube from the film. Routinely, portable films are exposed 40 in. from the tube, adding to the magnification. Figures 2.7 and 2.8 show the principles of magnification and the criteria for recognizing how a film was obtained.

Adequacy of Exposure

Be sure that the film is properly exposed. You can tell this on the frontal film by examining the vertebral column *behind the heart*. If you can see the detailed spine through the heart and can also see the pulmonary vessels in the lung peripherally, the exposure is correct. If you see *only* the spine but not the pulmonary vessels, the film is too dark (overexposed).

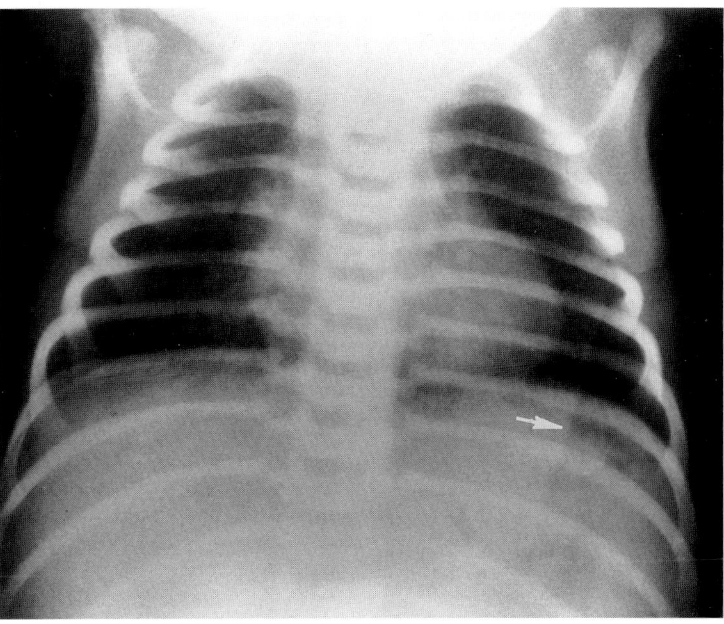

Fig. 2.9. Skin fold. This infant was lying supine and had a vertical opacity (*arrow*) along the left chest. This is a skin fold because there are markings lateral to this opacity (markings not seen on this reproduction), and the orientation of this skin fold does not follow any known orientation of lung collapse or pneumothorax

Traps: Unique Anatomical Normal Variants and Positions of Tubes

The chest radiograph accounts for at least 50% of all pediatric imaging, and therefore you must be aware of the normal variants. The thymus gland may dominate the mediastinal silhouette (see below). Normal skin folds are frequently seen in young infants and must be differentiated from pneumothoraces (the presence of pulmonary vessels extend into the "black area" when there is a skin fold; there are no markings when there is a pneumothorax; Fig. 2.9).

The central cleft of the two posterior neural arches which have not fused is often noted (Fig. 2.10). These spinous processes of the spine usually fuse between the ages of 3 and 5 years.

It is important to note the position of the tubes, clips, sutures, and monitoring devices. If the child who is intubated is having unexplained respiratory distress, two views (frontal and lateral) may help define tube position (Fig. 2.11).

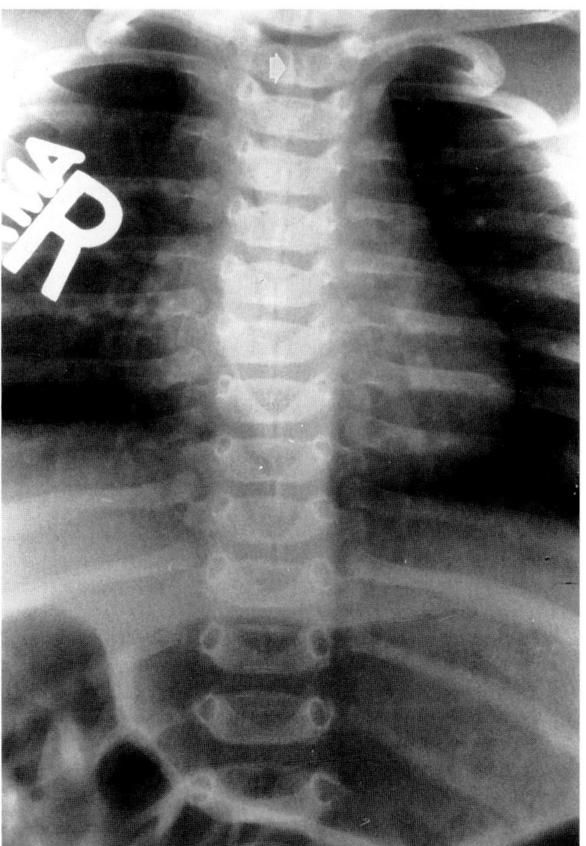

Fig. 2.10. Nonfusion of spinous process. On this supine film in an infant the thoracic vertebra spinous processes (*arrow*) are not fused

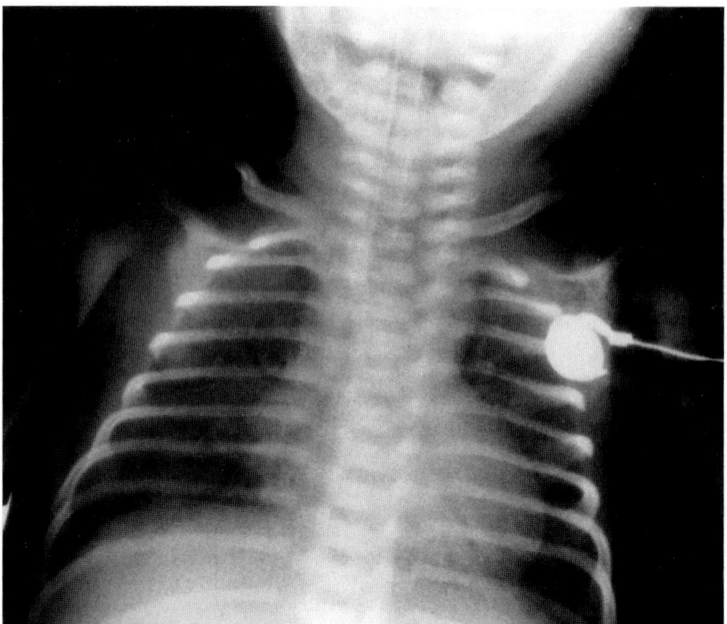

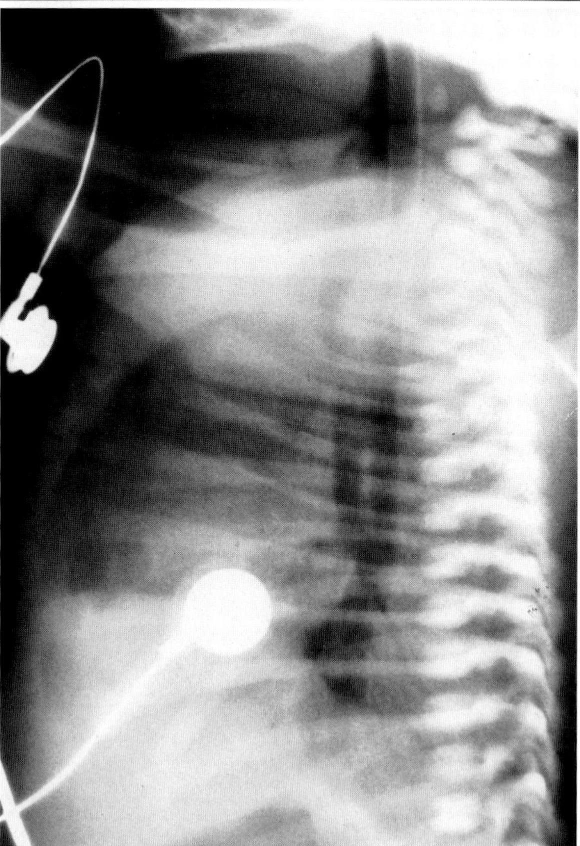

Fig. 2.11 a, b. This neonate had respiratory distress. **a** Frontal radiograph shows the endotracheal tube in the appropriate position. However, see the lateral film. **b** On this lateral radiograph, the endotracheal tube is noted in the esophagus. Whenever there is a question of unexplained respiratory distress, a lateral film may be helpful, particularly in an intubated patient

Interpreting the Film: The Radiologist's Circle

Anyone can glance at a pediatric chest film, and with very little training identify obvious abnormalities – right? Wrong! It takes most radiologists years to get into the habit of reading a chest radiograph properly. Let's face it: anyone ordering a chest film is going to look at the heart and lungs, but radiologists look first at the nonpulmonary areas, i.e., the abdomen, bones, soft tissues, and airway, to be sure that they do not miss any abnormality. Only then does one go to the cardiopulmonary anatomy.

A good habit to develop is to make an imaginary circle on the film so as to dispense with all the noncardiopulmonary areas. Begin at the corner where the patient information is. Check the name, date, and especially the left or right marker. Nothing is more embarrassing than missing dextrocardia with abdominal situs inversus because one did not look for the marker and therefore put the film up wrong. An easy way to complete the circle is to go from the name tag, to the markers, to the ABC's of the film: A = abdomen, B = bones and soft tissues, C = chest (airway, mediastinum, lungs, and diaphragm).

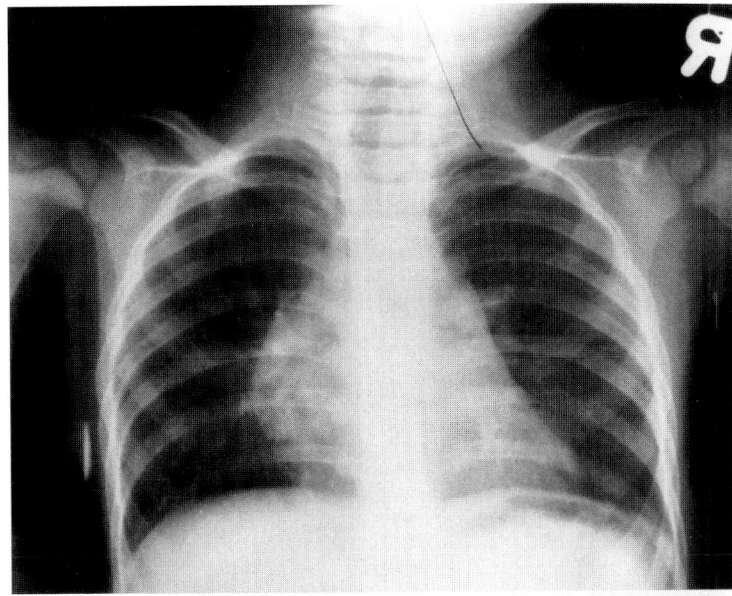

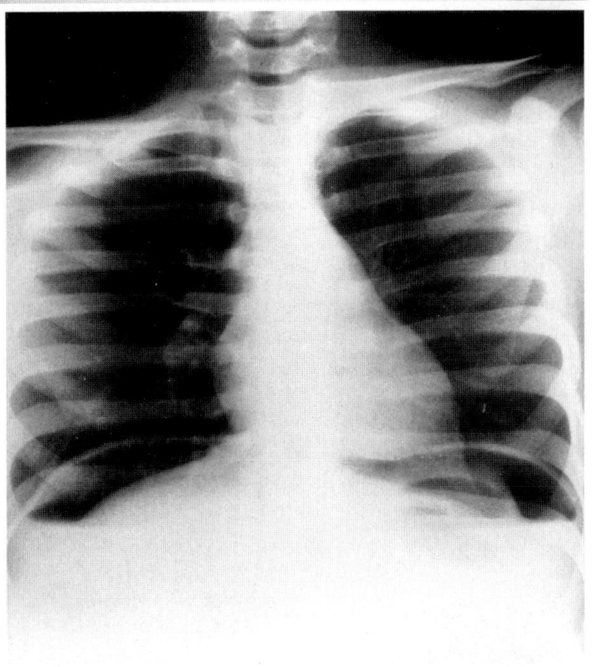

Fig. 2.12 a, b. Can you find the abnormality? (Look at the films; then read on.) **a** Film of a 12-month-old boy. No, the film is not labeled incorrectly. The patient has dextrocardia and abdominal situs inversus. **b** A 9-year-old girl with abdominal pain. Free air is seen beneath the diaphragm. (Note how you see both sides.) The patient has a perforated viscus

Abdomen

► *Reed's Rule No. 1:* On every chest film, read the abdominal portion as you would read an abdominal film. (Throughout this text, we include these fundamental concepts, which are used daily in the teaching sessions of Joseph O. Reed, M.D. See "Appendix 1.")

Evaluate the abdomen (regardless of how little of it can be seen) on every chest film, and note whether the stomach bubble is on the left and the liver on the right. Look specifically for calcifications, such as gallstones or pancreatic stones. Is the bowel distended? Are there air fluid levels? (Is this an erect film?) Can you see free intraperitoneal air or fluid? Now look at Fig. 2.12 with these clues in mind; on every chest film, look at the abdomen as if you were reading an abdominal film.

Bones and Soft Tissues

One can often scan portions of the arms, shoulders, ribs, sternum, and mandible, as well as cervical, thoracic, and lumbar vertebrae. Be alert for fractures, congenital abnormalities, bone destruction, or other signs of disease. It is very embarrassing to miss absent clavicles on a chest film because the bones were not viewed systematically. This is also a good time to examine the soft tissues of the neck, thorax, and abdomen to detect any swelling, foreign body, calcifica-

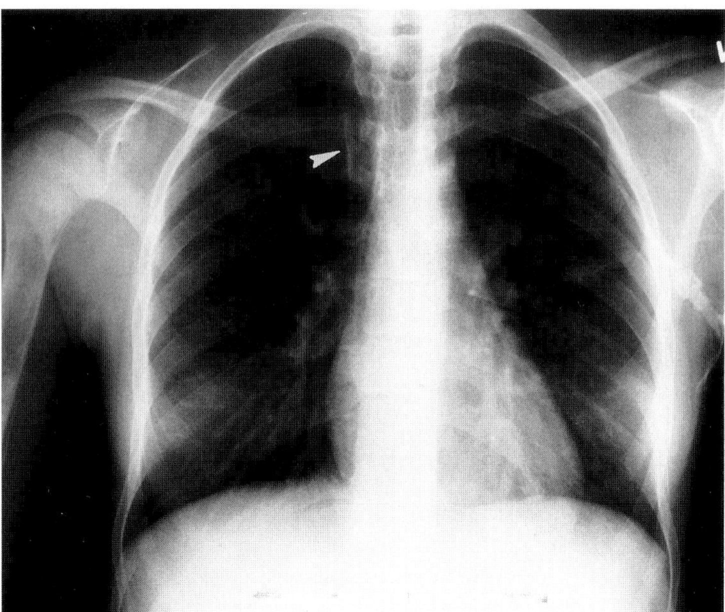

Fig. 2.13. This 13-year-old girl presented with fever and pain. Can you detect the abnormality on this chest film? Did you look at the bones? There is destructive process of the right humerus consistent with osteomyelitis in this sickle cell patient. Note also that there is an azygous lobe fissure (*arrowhead*) and a catheter in the right atrium for intravenous therapy

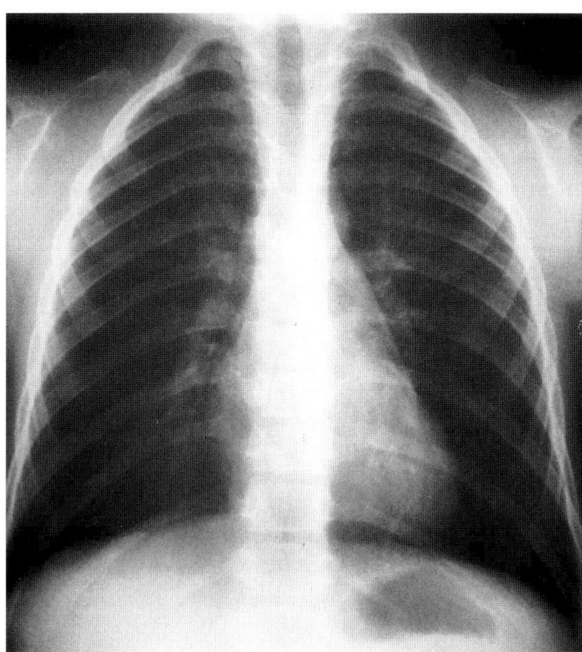

Fig. 2.14. A 9-year-old boy with a cough. (Look at the film; then read on.) Frontal chest film reveals the heart and lungs to be normal, but there is something missing – the clavicles. This patient has cleidocranial dysostosis

tions, etc. The soft tissues may reveal multiple artifacts, such as hair braids, buttons, bandages, or redundant skin folds. Soft tissue swelling or subcutaneous calcifications can be clues to systemic disease. By now you have returned, via your imaginary circle, to the cervical area, and you are ready to inspect the vertebrae. What abnormalities do you see in Figs. 2.13–2.17? Look at the films and try to make the diagnosis, then read the captions.

Chest (Airway, Mediastinum, Lungs, Diaphragm)

► *Reed's Rule No. 2:* Knowledge of anatomy is the key to correct radiographic diagnosis.

Airway

The cephalic-most portion of the airway is the nose and choanal air space. These structures are seen best on CT (Fig. 2.18), but the rest of the airway is best and most conveniently seen on the plain film.

The lateral view of the neck is optimal for evaluating the supraglottic (*supra*, above; *glottis*, vocal cords) airway (Figs. 2.19, 2.20). A proper study is obtained by aligning the top of the film with the top of the patient's

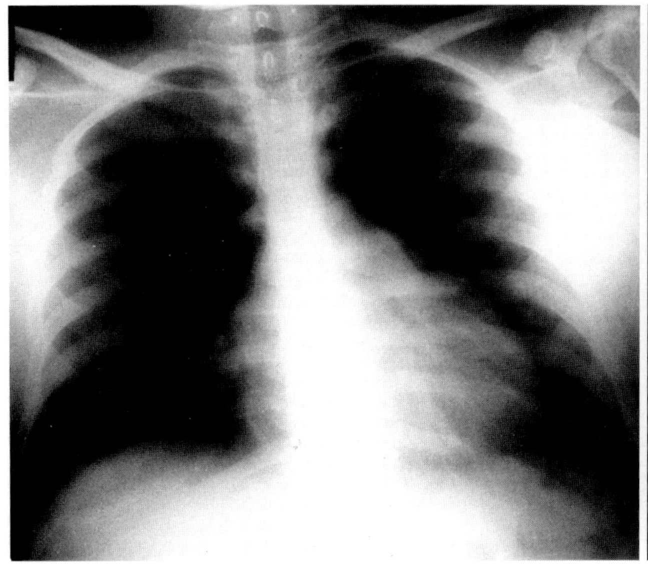

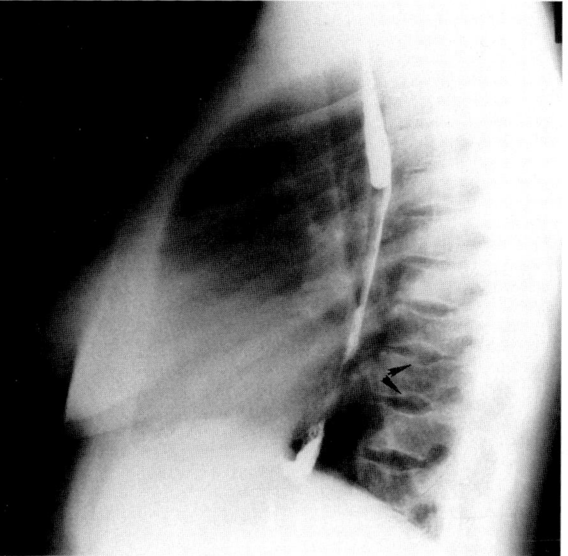

Fig. 2.15 a, b. A 17-year-old boy with a cough. **a** The heart is large on the frontal film. **b** On the lateral view, the cortical end plates of most of the thoracic vertebrae are depressed. This patient has sickle cell anemia, and the depressed end plates (*arrowheads*) are due to infarctions. These are called "H" vertebrae and are typical of sickle cell disease

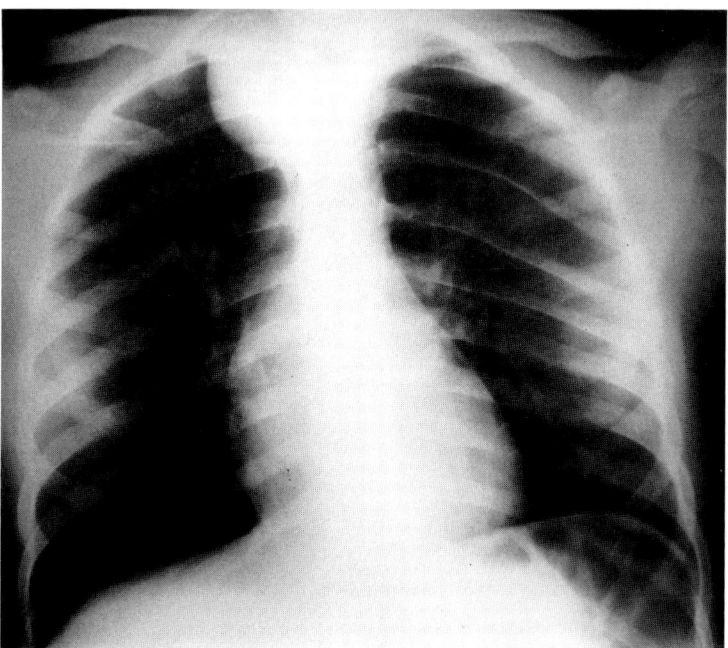

Fig. 2.16. This 12-year-old presented with café au lait spots and scoliosis. Aside from the obvious large mediastinal mass superiorly there are ribbonlike irregularities of the left fourth through sixth ribs. The combination of the mediastinal mass, rib changes, and café au lait spots suggests a diagnosis of neurofibromatosis. The chest mass is either an anterior meningocele or a neurofibroma. The ribs are wavy secondary to dystrophic bone and hypertrophied neural tissue in the subcostal groove

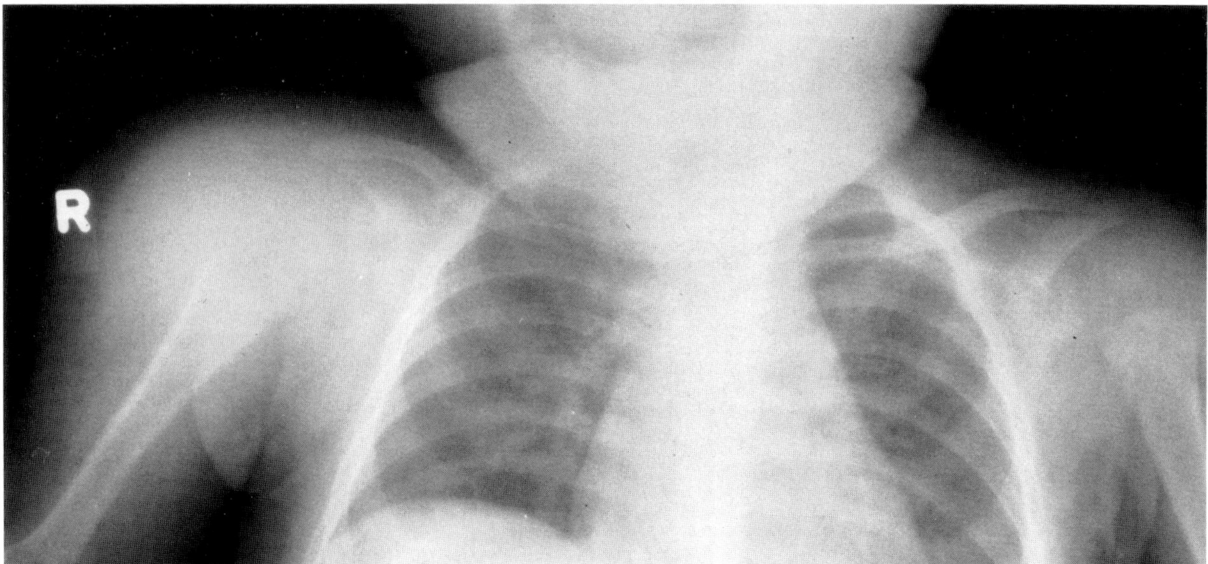

Fig. 2.17. A 6-month-old infant with fever of unknown origin. The frontal chest film shows a soft-tissue swelling of the right shoulder. This patient has osteomyelitis of the right humerus

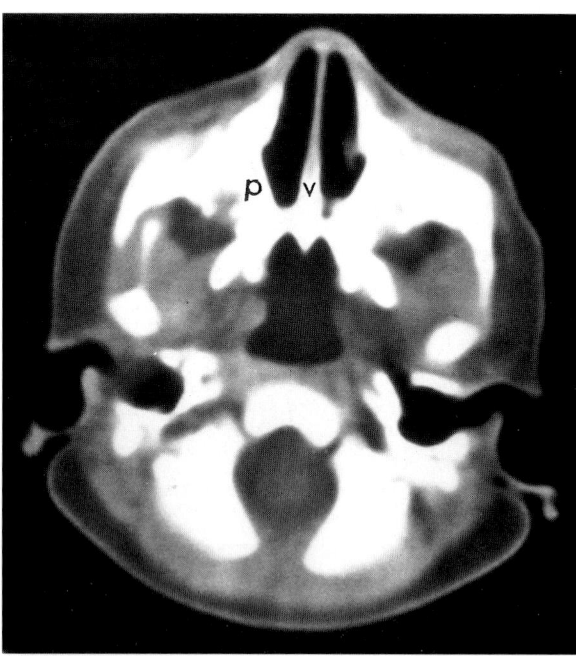

Fig. 2.18. Choanal atresia. In this newborn baby there is bony connection between the volmar (*v*) and the lateral palatine bone (*p*). All these bones have fused and this is bony choanal atresia

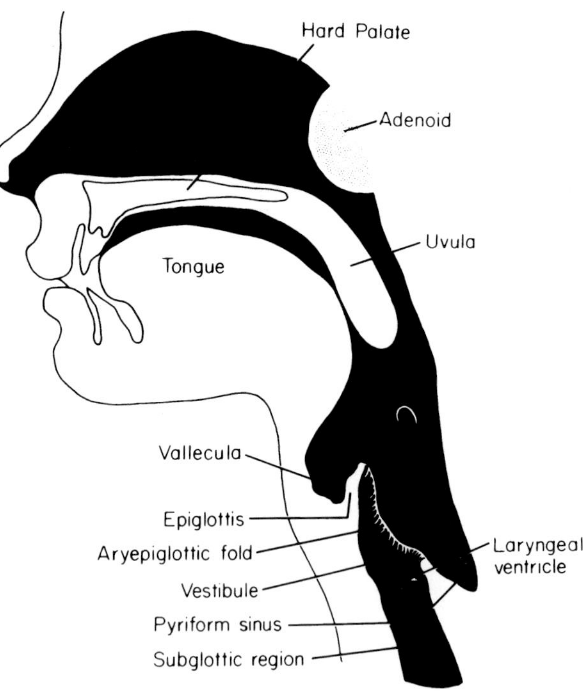

Fig. 2.19. The normal airway, lateral view. (From [5] with permission)

ear. The cephalic-most portion of the airway is the nasopharynx, which communicates anteriorly with the nares and merges posteriorly to form the hypopharynx. For all practical purposes, the borders of the nasopharynx are the soft palate, the uvula, and the adenoid closure. The oropharynx (below the hard and soft palate) leads to the air spaces at the base of the tongue, which are the valleculae. Immediately behind the valleculae is the epiglottis. The hyoid bone is inferior and anterior to the valleculae. The oropharynx also merges posteriorly with the nasopharynx to form the hypopharynx. One can see the palatine tonsils in the lateral walls of the hypopharynx. Anteriorly, the hypopharynx leads to the larynx and becomes the esophagus inferiorly and medially. The pyriform sinuses are the most lateral and inferior aspects of the hypopharynx; their inferior margins provide a handy landmark for the level of the vocal cords. It is important when obtaining a lateral neck examination to slightly hyperextend the patient's head and neck. This flattens the redundant soft tissues in the retropharyngeal area against the cervical spine.

The frontal radiograph is best for viewing the subglottic airway. The true vocal cords are at the same level as the tip of the pyriform sinuses. Immediately below the glottis is the subglottic region, which is only several millimeters long and merges inferiorly into the proximal trachea (Figs. 2.21, 2.22). Note that the airway is a dynamic system, and that an isolated, single film may be quite misleading. Nonetheless, an abnormal configuration of the airway should be pursued in

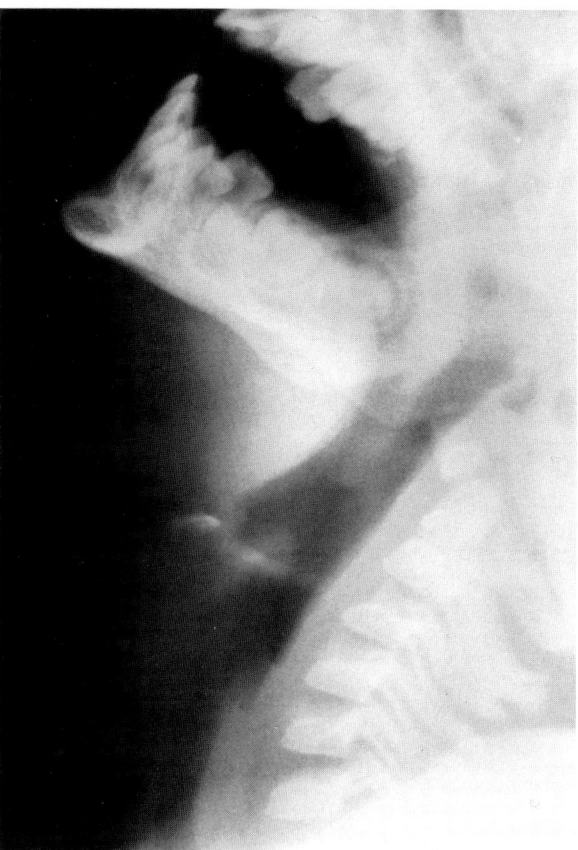

Fig. 2.20. Lateral roentgenogram corresponding to the schematic view in Fig. 2.19

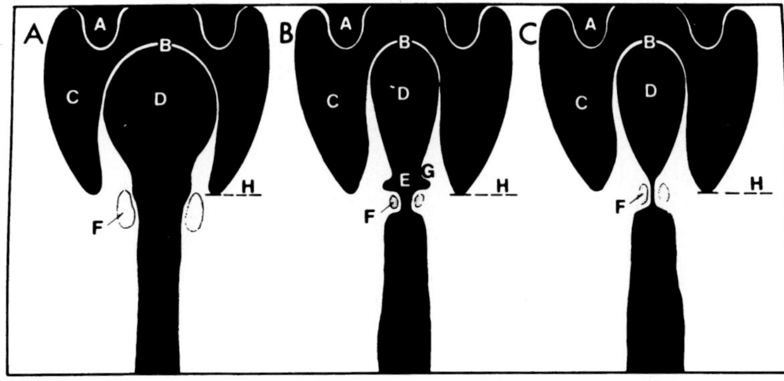

A. Vallecula
B. Epiglottis
C. Pyriform Sinuses
D. Vestibule
E. Larygeal Ventricle
F. True Cords
G. False Cords
H. Tip of Pyriform Sinus - Level of True Cords

Fig. 2.21. Schematic drawings of the frontal airway during various phases of respiration and phonation. *A*, Quiet breathing; *B,C*, phonation. (From [5] with permission)

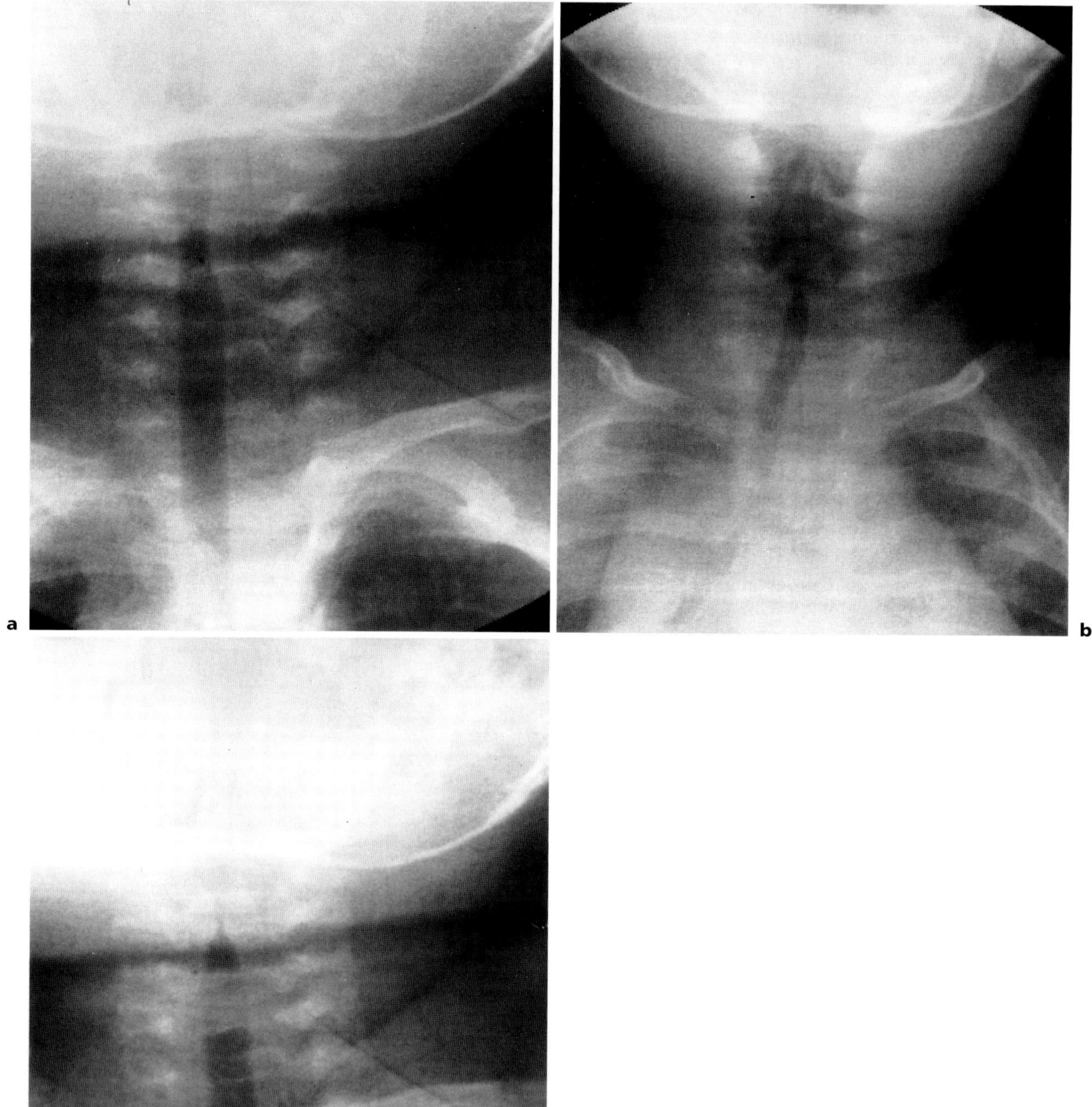

Fig. 2.22 a–c. Three frontal radiographs corresponding to the schematic view in Fig. 2.21

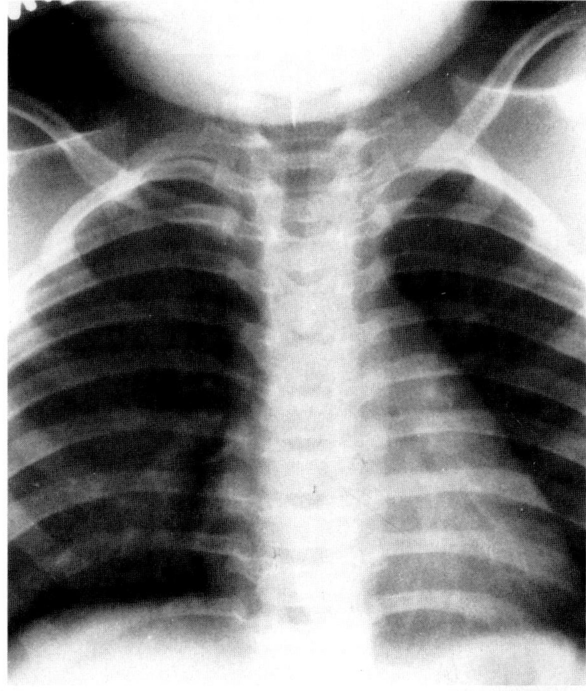

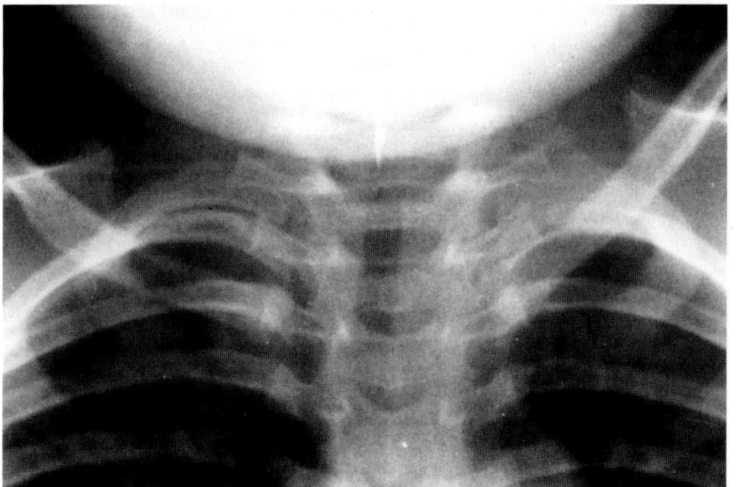

Fig. 2.23 a, b. A 1-year-old boy with stridor. **a** Frontal radiograph shows the lungs to be of normal volume and the heart of normal size. The thoracic airway is clearly demonstrated, but there is a density overlying the airway in the cervical region. **b** Close up of this region. A piece of eggshell was later removed. (From [6] with permission)

the light of the clinical history. What is the abnormality in Fig. 2.23?

▶ *Reed's Rule No. 3:* The airway should be visible on all normal chest films.

Figure 2.24 depicts a common pathological state of the airway diagnosed by radiographs of the chest or neck. What is the anatomical abnormality, and what is the disease?

The parameters to evaluate the airway, be it extra or intrathoracic, are *patency, position,* and *size.* One should see the entire airway, from the oral and nasal pharynges to the right and left main-stem bronchi. The walls should be parallel and smooth. However, buckling of the trachea to the right in the lower neck and upper thorax is normal in an infant. The intrathoracic airway is not a midline structure (the carina overlies the right pedicles). What abnormality can you detect in Fig. 2.25?

The size of the airway is difficult to ascertain, as it is a dynamic structure that changes in caliber. However, an airway or a portion of the airway that is consistently narrow demands further investigation.

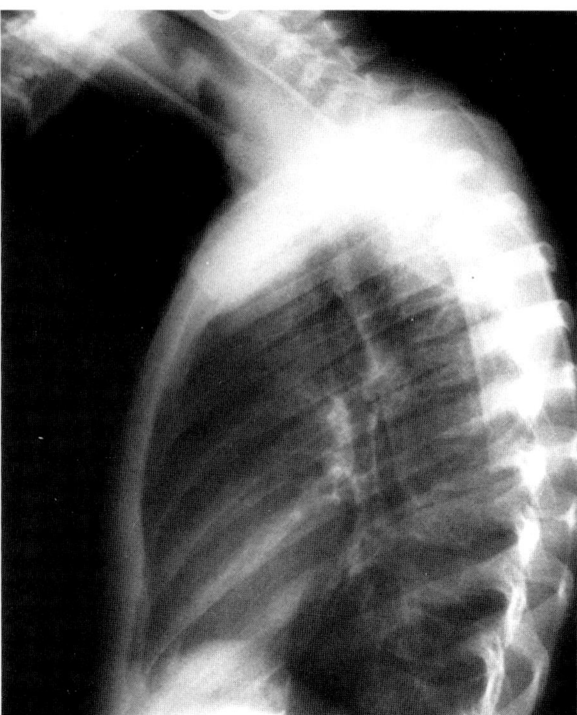

Fig. 2.24. What anatomical abnormality can you see in this examination? (Answer in "Appendix 2")

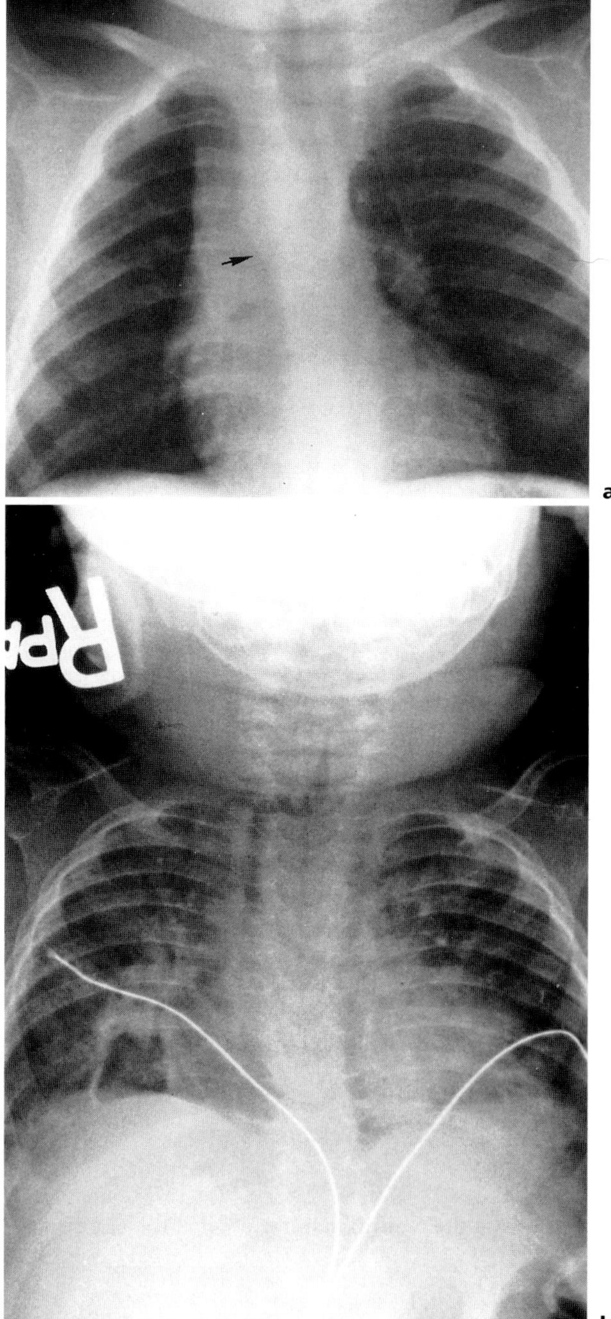

Fig. 2.25 a, b. A 6-month-old infant with cough. **a** Frontal radiograph shows the carina pushed to the left. There is a bulge on the right side of the airway. Can you see a normal aortic arch on the left? This is a right aortic arch to the right of the trachea with a right descending aorta (*arrow*) to the right of the spine. This child had congenital heart disease, tetralogy of Fallot. Many children with this disease have a right aortic arch. **b** Normal buckling of the airway in another child. This patient has chronic lung disease

Mediastinum

The mediastinum is composed of the thymus, trachea, heart, great vessels, esophagus, lymph nodes, and neural elements. Graphically, it is separated into the anterior, middle, and posterior compartments (Fig. 2.26). In examining the mediastinum, remember:

▶ *Reed's Rule No. 2:* Knowledge of anatomy is the key to correct radiographic diagnosis.

In the mediastinum, look for *position, size,* and *contour* of the individual components. The initial examination of the mediastinum is best accomplished by the plain film. However, for most abnormalities or question of abnormality, MR or CT is utilized. Therefore in this discussion of the mediastinum plain film findings are followed by cross-sectional imaging.

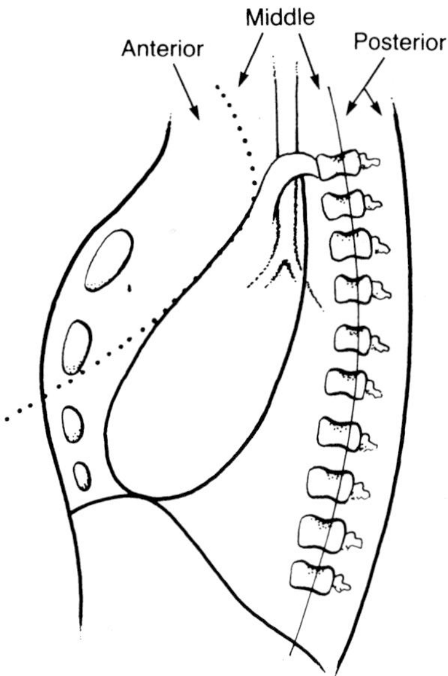

Fig. 2.26. Mediastinum. *Anterior,* the space in front of the heart and great vessels; *middle*, the space between the anterior and posterior mediastinal components, including heart, airway, esophagus, and lymph nodes; *posterior*, everything *behind* a line connecting the midportion aspects of the vertebrae, including the vertebrae, neural elements, and paraspinal lymph tissue. (See "Masses and Pseudomasses" for masses typical of these areas)

Thymus

One of the major factors that makes pediatric chest X-rays difficult to evaluate is the thymus. It is said that he who masters the thymus has mastered 90% of pediatric chest films, because this gland can simulate cardiac enlargement, lobar collapse, pulmonary infiltrates, and mediastinal masses. The thymus is prominent in many children until 4–5 years of age. It starts to become a problem when it is still prominent in children over the age of 5.

The thymus is always anterior in position, which is why it is difficult to diagnose right heart enlargement in a younger child based on fullness of the anterior mediastinum. Since it is such an anterior structure, it is subject to wide variations in position on the frontal chest radiograph: even with the slightest degree of rotation, the thymus may obscure almost the entire right or left lung. To avoid errors in interpretation, check the degree of inspiration and the position of the patient before deciding about unusual densities (Fig. 2.27) (see "Technical Factors," above).

Thymic size is a major area of concern. The thymus may occupy the entire anterior thorax, extending down to the diaphragm and out to the lateral thoracic wall. It usually shrinks as the child gets older, but thymic remnants can remain even into adulthood. It is a unique organ which also shrinks during periods of stress. The contour of the thymus is "wavy" because it insinuates itself between anterior ribs. It is a "soft" organ and does not push other mediastinal structures aside. Occasionally, fluoroscopy is necessary to decide whether the contour of a "mediastinal mass" is indeed wavy and anterior, consistent with a thymus.

More often, however, if an abnormality is suspected in the mediastinum, cross-sectional imaging (CT or MR) is performed. Both tests require the young patient to be sedated. CT, of course, entails radiation exposure, and the patient also receives intravenous contrast, but it has the advantage of showing calcium and, if pertinent, the lung parenchyma (see below). For proper evaluation of the mediastinum with CT, contrast is essential. With contrast, the vessels and heart "light up" (turn white – enhance). Thus, anything not enhanced must be explained by normal anatomical structures or else it is abnormal. MR has the advantage of presenting images in multiple planes (coronal, sagittal, axial, and oblique) and most precisely shows extension of tumor into the spinal canal. MR differentiates tissue characteristics to a greater extent than CT, but it is poor for calcium and lung parenchyma.

Since either test may be better depending on the pathology, images of both modalities are presented (Figs. 2.28, 2.29). These images help define masses, lymph nodes, and aberrant vessels between and around normal structures.

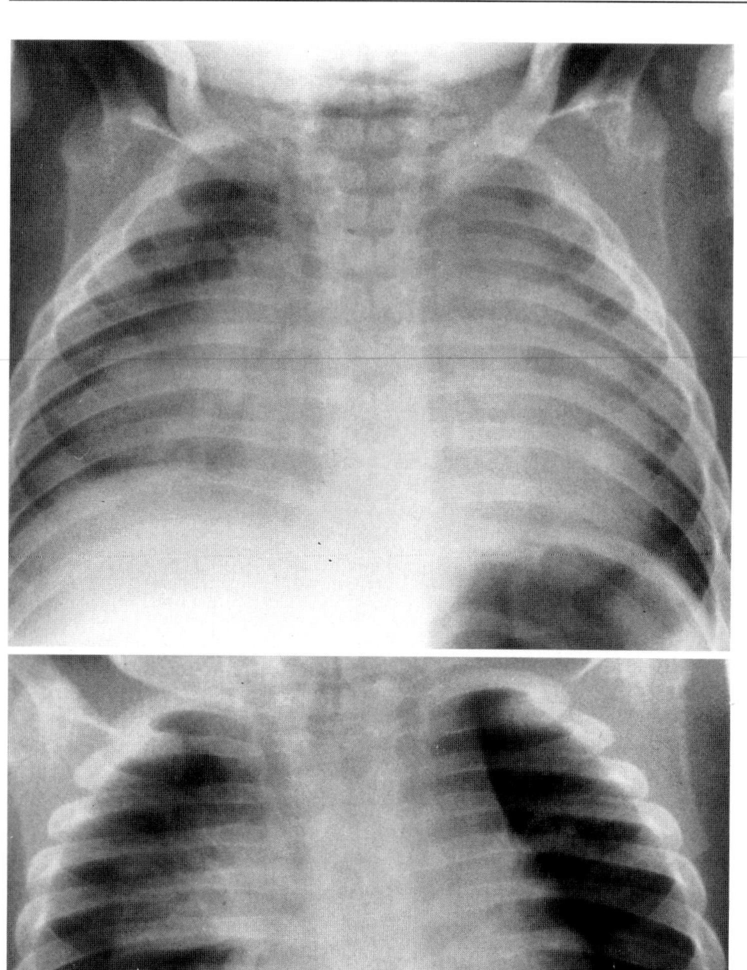

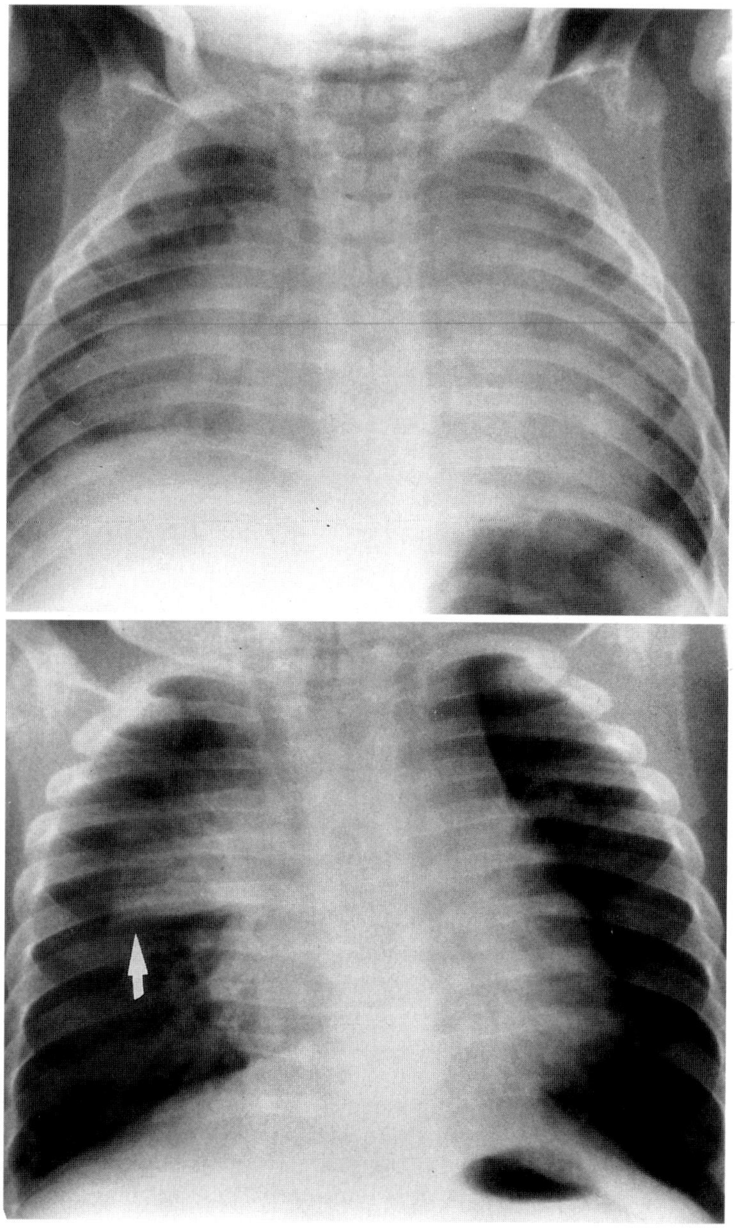

Fig. 2.27 a, b. A 6-month-old infant with cough. **a** Frontal radiograph shows all the parameters of a film taken during expiration. If you are not acquainted with these criteria, you may interpret this film as showing an infiltrate in both lungs. (See Fig. 2.2 for criteria establishing that the film is taken during expiration.) Note that the spinous processes are not fused. **b** With a good inspiratory effort, same child shows that the major component of these " infiltrates " was really thymus which is quite prominent on the right. Notice the thymic sail sign (*arrows*)

Fig. 2.28 a–d. Normal contrast enhanced CT of the mediastinum (axial projection). Remember: vessels and heart " light up." **a** The cephalic-most section reveals the rectangular, homogenous thymus anteriorly beneath the sternum and in front of vessels. The vertebral body and dural sac are seen posteriorly on all the sections. **b** The next section is at the level of the aortic arch (*a*) with the superior vena cava on the right and trachea and esophagus behind. **c** The third section is at the level of the main pulmonary artery (*p*). The ascending and descending aorta (*a*), as well as the right and left pulmonary arteries are demonstrated. **d** The next caudad plane is at the level of the left atrium (*l*) ▶

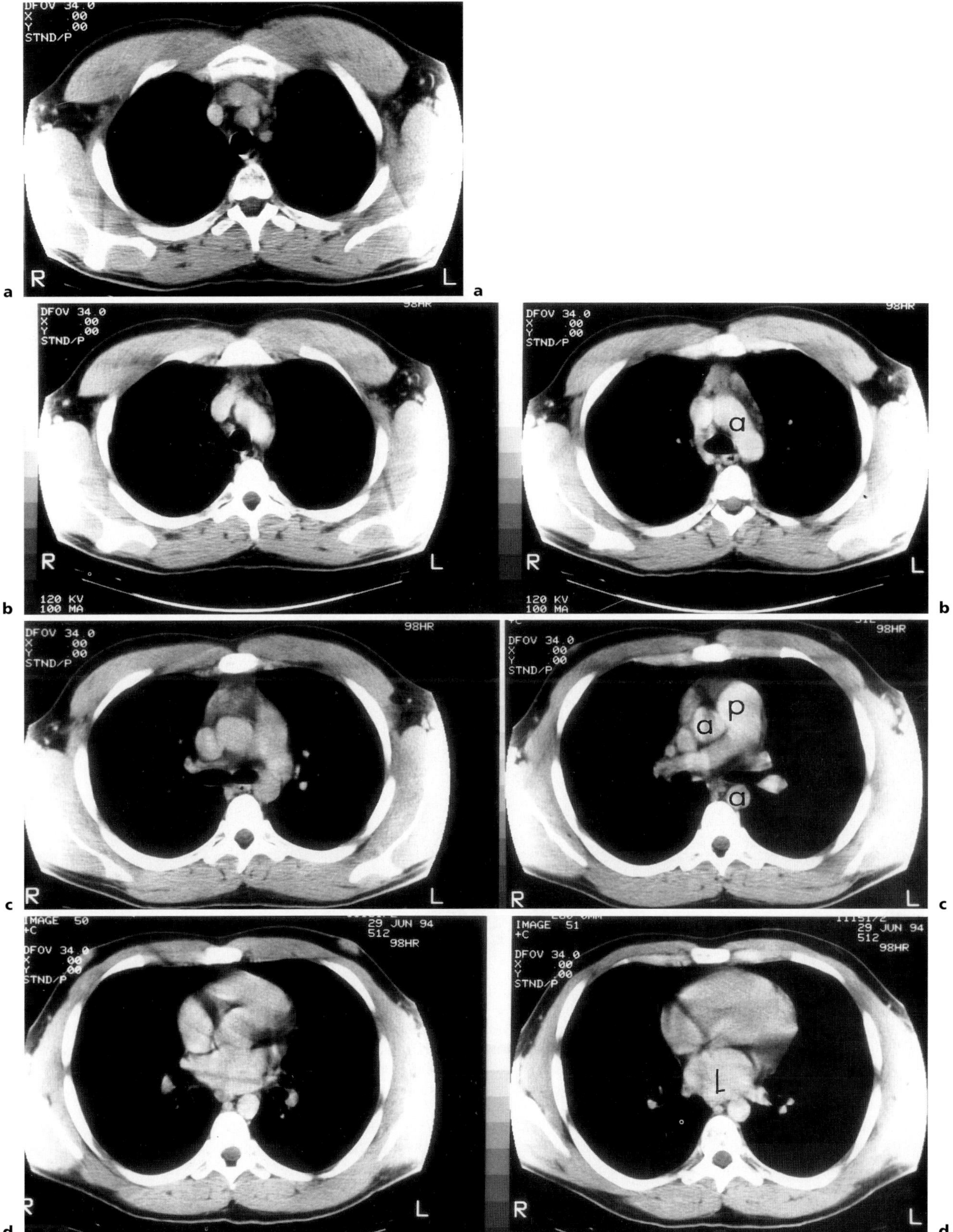
a
DFOV 34.0
X .00
Y .00
STND/P
R
L
a
b
DFOV 34.0
X .00
Y .00
STND/P
98HR
R
L
120 KV
100 MA
a
b
c
DFOV 34.0
X .00
Y .00
STND/P
98HR
R
L
p
a
a
c
d
IMAGE 50
+C
29 JUN 94
512
98HR
DFOV 34.0
X .00
Y .00
STND/P
R
L
IMAGE 51
+C
29 JUN 94
512
98HR
L
d

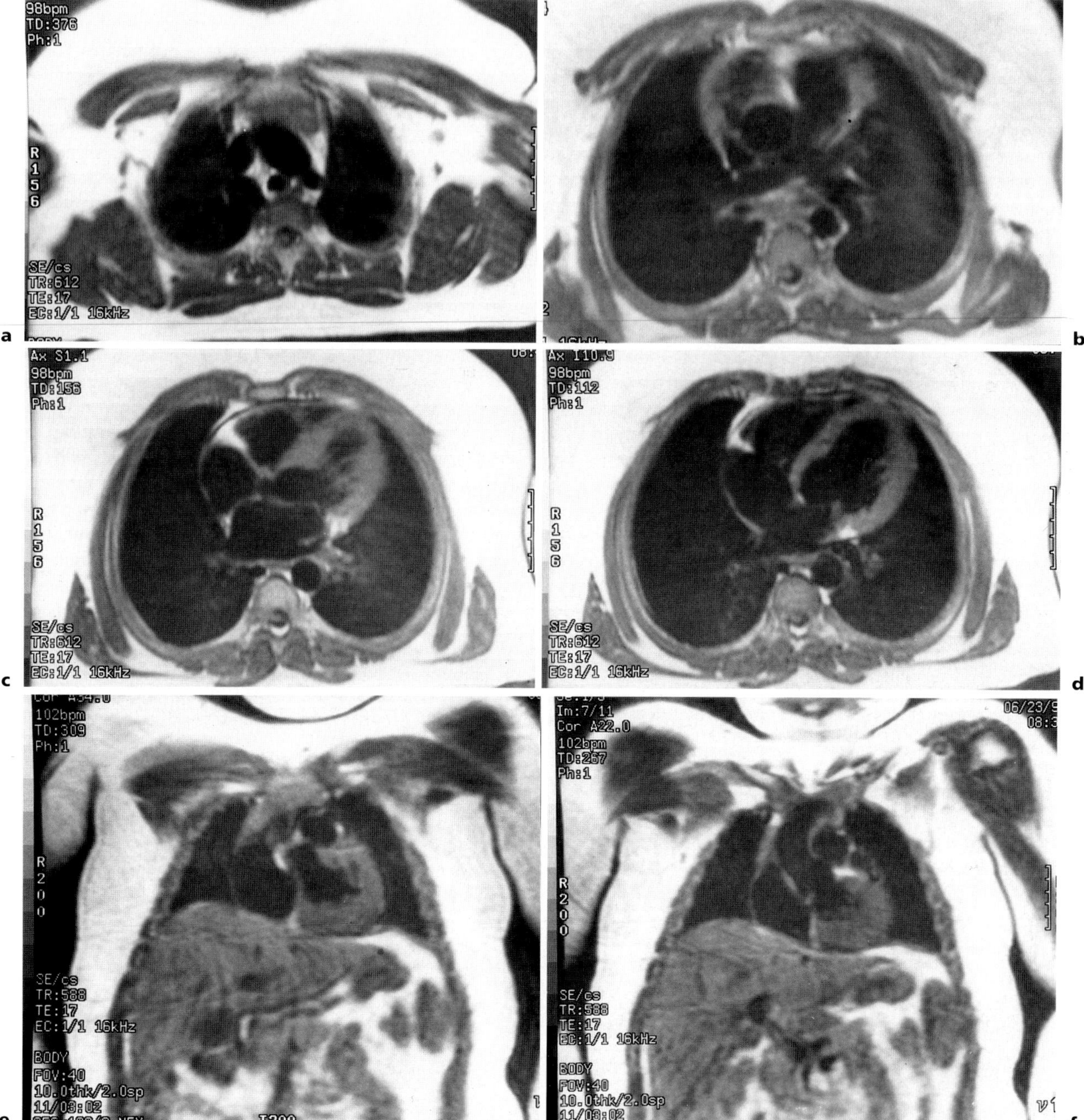

Fig. 2.29 a–k. Normal MR of the mediastinum (axial, coronal and sagittal sections). Remember: *black*, flowing blood. **a** The cephalic-most section reveals the rectangular, homogenous thymus anteriorly beneath the sternum and in front of vessels. The vertebral body and dural sac are seen posteriorly on all the sections. **b** The next section is at the level of the main pulmonary artery. The ascending and descending aorta, as well as the right and left pulmonary arteries are demonstrated. **c** The next caudad plane is at the level of the left atria. **d** Section through four chambers of the heart. **e** Most anterior coronal section showing thymus and right atrium. **f** Next posterior section through the ascending aorta defines cardiac anatomy. **g, h** Section through the superior vena cava and trachea. **i** Posterior section showing the vertebral bodies. **j** Oblique midline sagittal section showing the aortic arch. **k** Static sagittal scan of a cine MR imaging with the computer enhanced blood appearing white. Note the aorta

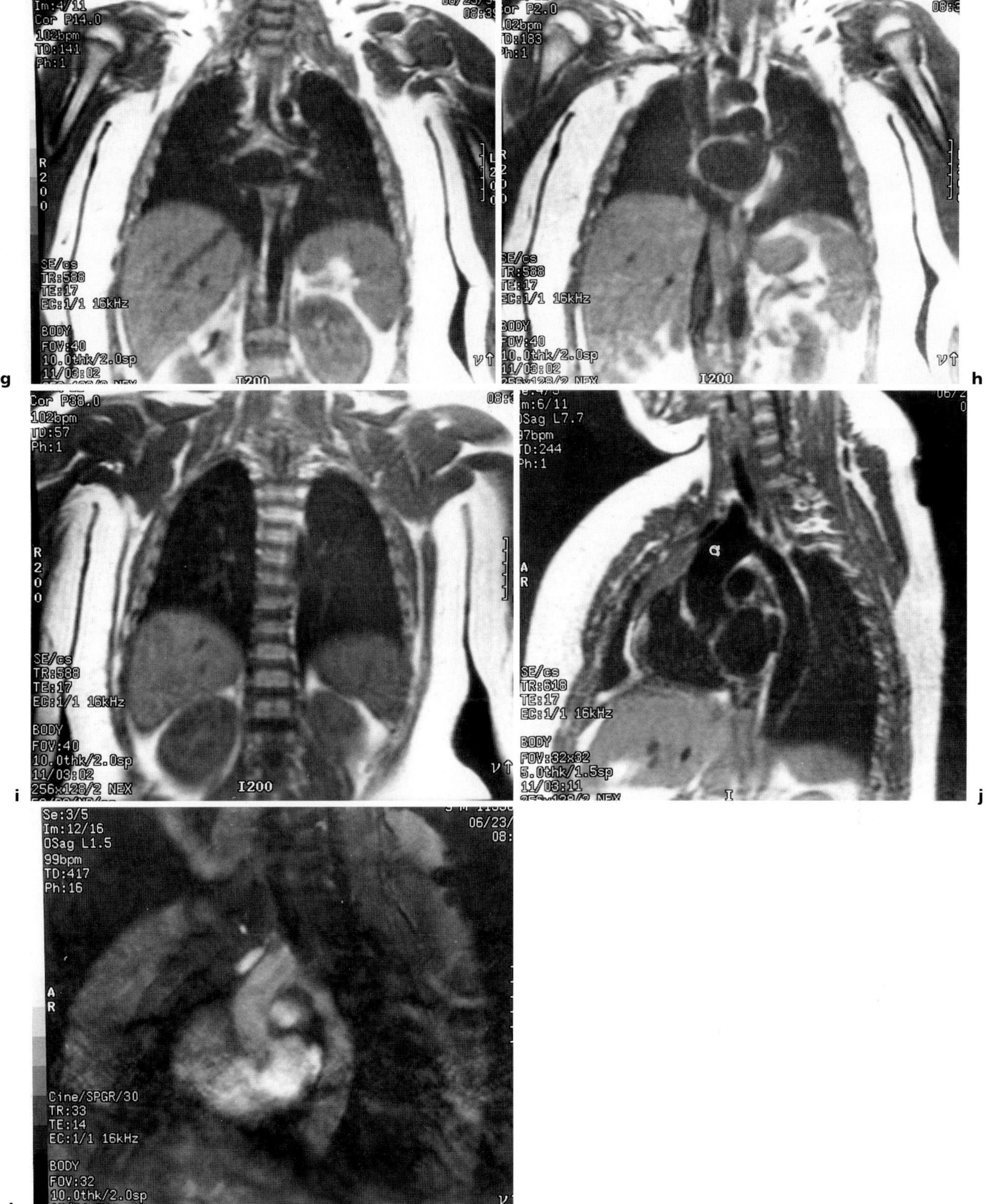
g
h
i
j
k

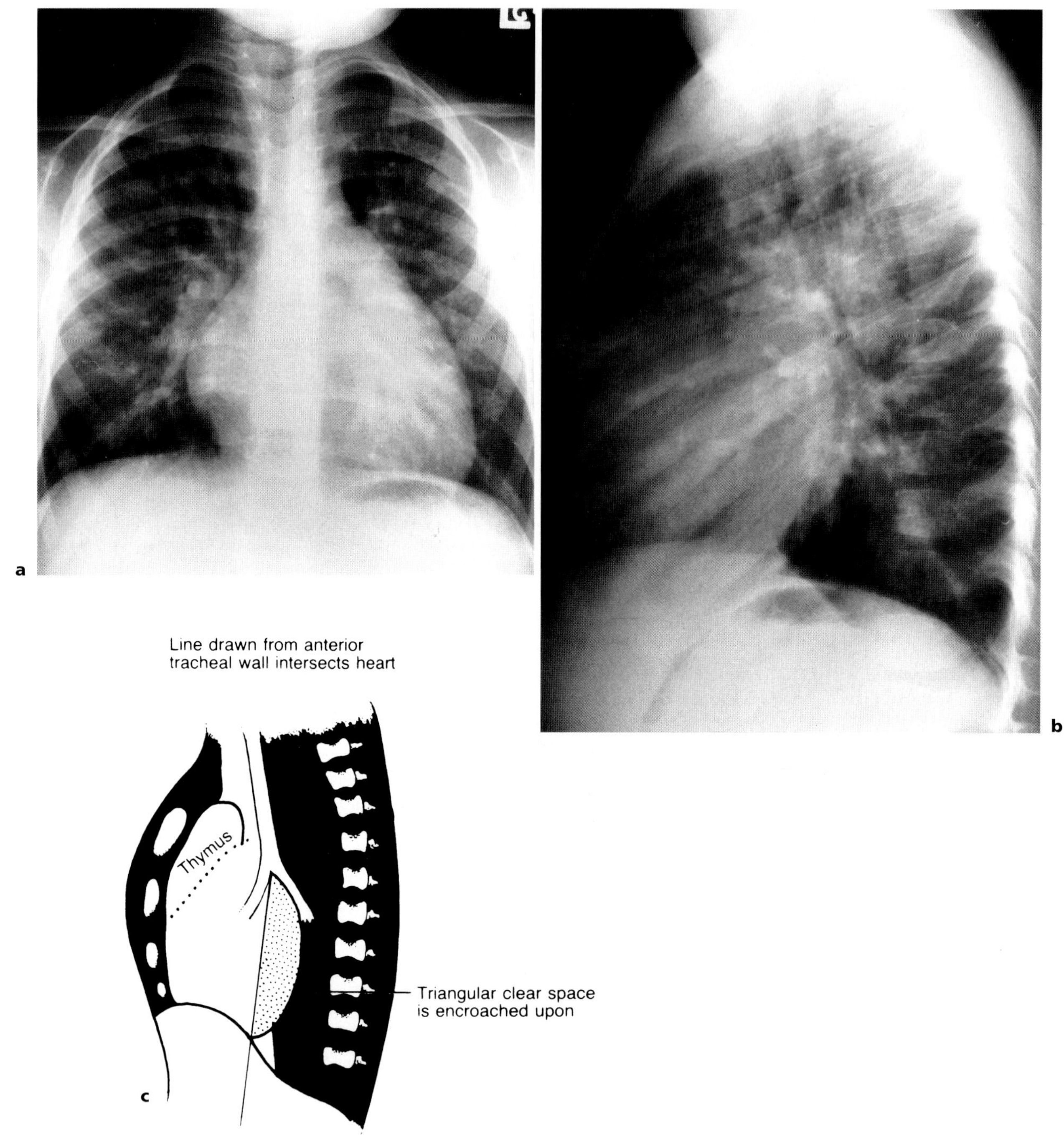

Fig. 2.30 a–c. Evaluation of cardiac enlargement on lateral film. **A,B** When the heart extends behind the line drawn from the carina vertically to the diaphragm, there is cardiomegaly. In addition, the trachea may be pushed back by a large heart. Frontal (**a**) and lateral (**b**) films of the chest show cardiomegaly with indistinct pulmonary vessels. The vessels in the upper half of the lung are more distinct than those in the lower due to pulmonary venous congestion causing the fluid to leak into the interstitium of the lung obscuring the pulmonary vessels. A large heart with fuzzy vessels suggests congestive heart failure. **c** Diagram of cardiac enlargement on the lateral film

Heart

The heart must also be evaluated for *position, size,* and *contour.* Its position is normally in the left hemithorax with a small right thoracic border. The appearance of the heart on the frontal film depends greatly on the degree of inspiration and on the size of the thymus. For these reasons, on the lateral roentgenogram, the air space behind the heart and the position of the anterior margin of the trachea play a major diagnostic role. A line dropped from the carina (where the trachea ends on the lateral film) inferiorly to the diaphragm, it should not intersect the heart (Fig. 2.30). This rule works only on a nonrotated lateral film. Additionally, the trachea should not be pushed back against the spine (see Fig. 2.1). An enlarged heart pushes the trachea back, as do other mediastinal abnormalities. Therefore if a frontal film shows questionable cardiac enlargement, look at the lateral! If the lateral film is normal, the heart size is normal, as defined by Reed's Rule No. 4:

▶ *Reed's Rule No. 4:* A mass must be seen in two planes, i.e., if the heart is really large, it must appear large in two planes.

The *contour* of the heart on plain films, in our experience, is not helpful in determining the *specific* nature of congenital anomalies. Echocardiography, MR, and cardiac catheterization are more accurate methods of diagnosing congenital defects. Nonetheless, evaluating the contour of the heart in an older child where the thymus is smaller can be valuable. In children the left atrial appendage is not a prominent bulge on the left side because it is usually obscured by even a small thymus. The pulmonary artery, however, may be prominent normally in adolescents (especially girls) (Fig. 2.31).

Pulmonary vascular changes, on the other hand, may give a clue to the exact nature of the cardiac disease. Normally one sees pulmonary vessels in the hila and the middle third of the lungs but not in the more peripheral portion. Signs of increased arterial flow include: (a) enlarged central vessels, (b) enlarged vessels in the medial third of the lung, and (c) on the erect film, equalization of vessel size between upper and lower lobes. Venous congestion associated with clinical findings of congestive heart failure can be indicated by: (a) loss of distinct vessels at the bases (interstitial edema), (b) alveolar filling (pulmonary edema), or (c) right-sided pleural effusion (see Fig. 2.30). Remember: language here is important! Overcirculation, increased arterial flow, and increased vascularity all suggest left to right shunt. Congestion and pulmonary venous distention suggest congestive heart failure.

It is much more difficult to detect *decreased* pulmonary vascularity. Correlating pulmonary vascularity with heart size and the clinical status of the patient (cyanotic vs. acyanotic) is frequently helpful in determining specifics of congenital heart disease. Note: Overcirculation is usually associated with cardiomegaly. If you suspect overcirculation but the heart appears normal, something is usually wrong with your observations.

Great Vessels

The great vessels that are easily identified are the inferior vena cava (on the lateral view) and the aorta (on the frontal film). The position of the trachea is the key to locating the aortic arch (see Fig. 2.25). A right aortic arch is often associated with congenital heart disease or vascular ring which presses on both the airway and the esophagus. For this reason, pay special attention to the tracheal air column and the bulges along either side. The right and left pulmonary arteries are easily identified, and the main pulmonary artery is one of the moguls (bumps) of the left heart border (Fig. 2.31).

Fig. 2.31. Moguls (bumps) along the heart border

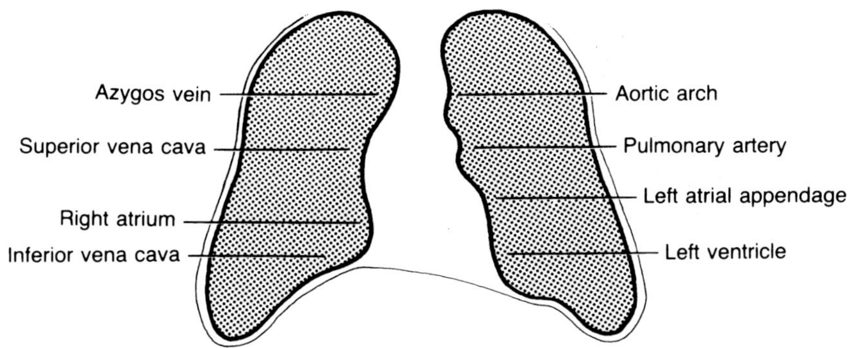

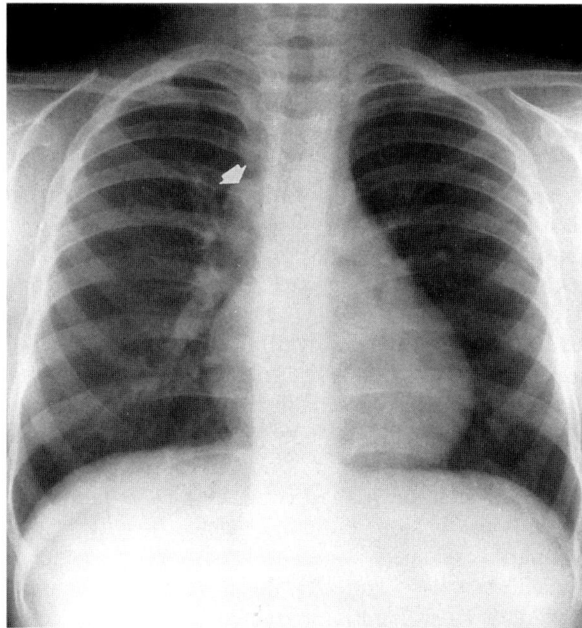

Fig. 2.32. What is the unusual dilatation (*arrow*) above the right main-stem bronchus? In this 4-year-old asymptomatic girl, a bulge was noted in the junction of the right main-stem bronchus and trachea. It did not pulsate, nor did it affect the esophagus. It was not seen on the lateral film. At ultrasonic examination, the abdominal vena cava was found to be atretic, leaving just an infrarenal vena cava. The mass is the azygos vein, which returns blood from the abdomen to the heart. This condition is called azygos continuation of the inferior vena cava

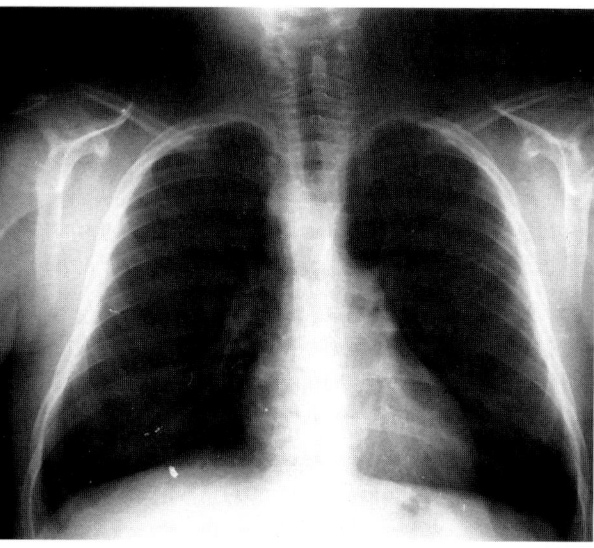

a

Fig. 2.33 a–c. MR of vascular ring. **a** Plain film examination shows the mass to the right of the airway with the carina to the left of midline. **b** Coronal section anteriorly shows a circular impression to the right and to the left of the trachea (*t*). **c** A more posterior coronal section shows the two arches joining and descending. This is a double aortic arch

What is the unusual dilatation above the right main-stem bronchus in Fig. 2.32? MR is superb for defining the side of the arch as well as abnormalities of the great vessels (Fig. 2.33).

Esophagus

The esophagus is another structure seen in the mediastinum. It lies in back of the trachea and may contain air in younger children. An air fluid level in the esophagus, however, is always abnormal. Since esophageal problems may manifest as cardiorespiratory symptoms, barium swallow is a valuable diagnostic examination in cases of unexplained respiratory disease (Fig. 2.34).

► *Reed's Rule No. 5:* An esophagram must be performed on any child with unexplained respiratory disease.

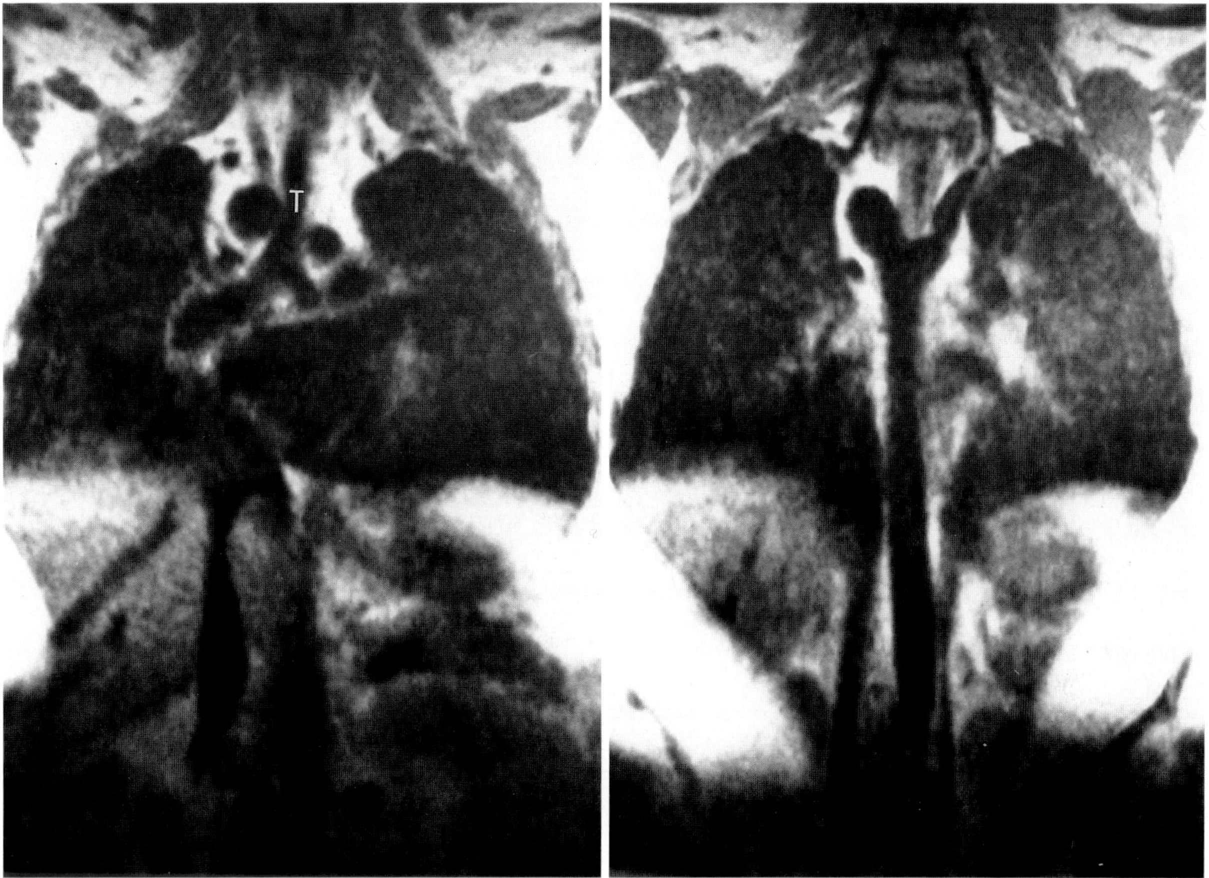

Lymph Nodes

Mediastinal lymph nodes are not visible on plain films unless they are enlarged. They are well seen on CT and MR.

Lungs

Let's review the anatomy of the lungs (Fig. 2.35). The upper and middle right lobes are separated by the minor fissure frequently seen in a normal chest radiograph. The major fissure separates the right lower lobe from the right middle lobe and upper lobe. On the lateral, the left major fissure is more vertical and posterior. These can often be seen on the lateral film. The pulmonary vessels are easily seen branching in the inner two-thirds of the lung. Most of the time the right hilum is lower than the left; it is never higher. The major bronchi are seen centrally because of the density of the mediastinum surrounding these air-filled bronchi; they cannot be seen peripherally. There are few visible lung markings in the peripheral third of the lung, especially in young children. Normally the pleura is not visible in the lower lobes. The hemidiaphragms change contour with respiration but are nicely dome-shaped on both frontal and lateral films.

Because the lungs are air filled, they offer sharp contrast to the soft tissue density of the heart and diaphragm, whose margins are quite sharp (see Fig. 2.1). If the margins are fuzzy or obliterated, the lung adjacent to these margins is abnormal (the silhouette sign).

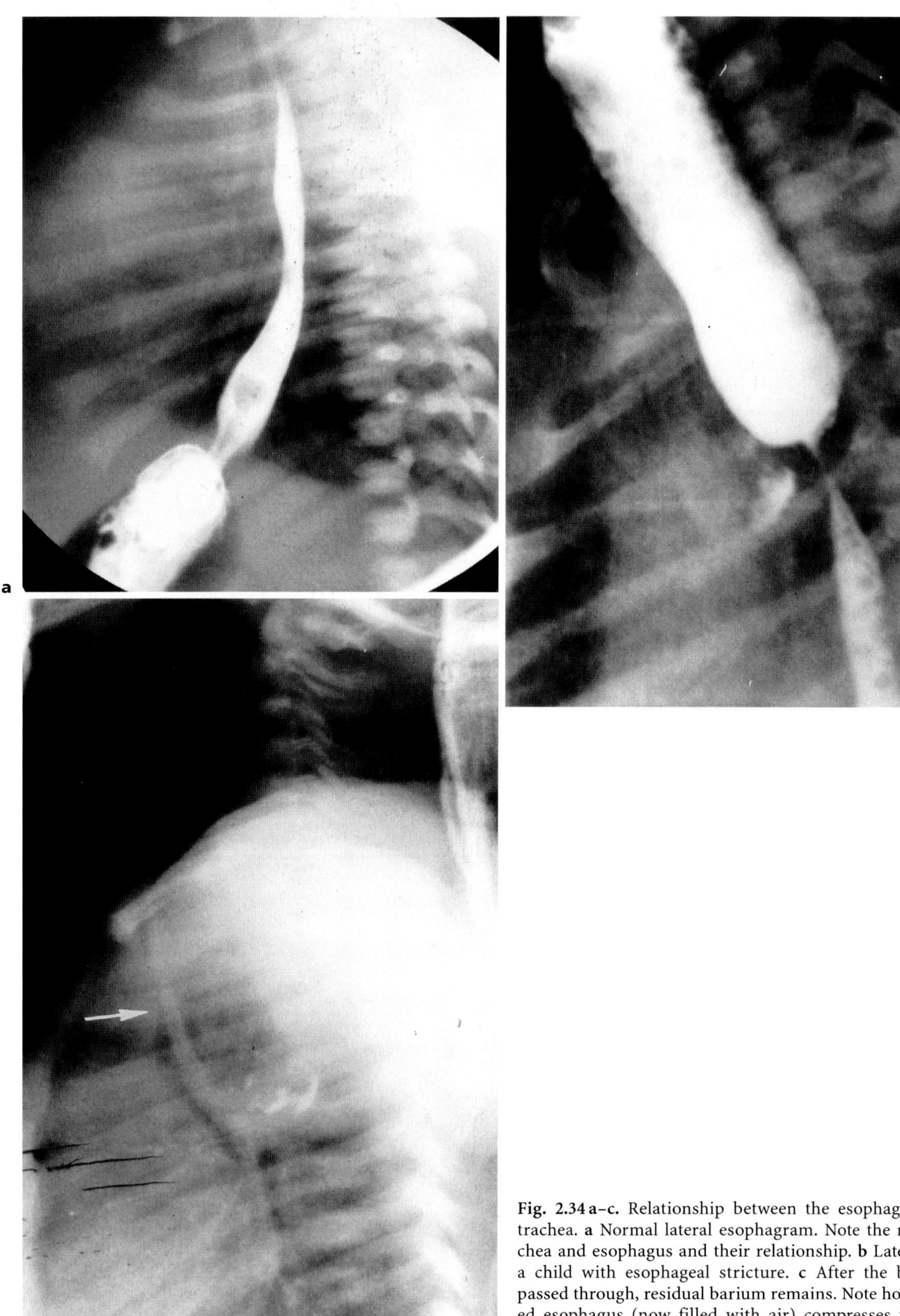

Fig. 2.34 a–c. Relationship between the esophagus and the trachea. **a** Normal lateral esophagram. Note the normal trachea and esophagus and their relationship. **b** Lateral view of a child with esophageal stricture. **c** After the barium has passed through, residual barium remains. Note how the dilated esophagus (now filled with air) compresses the trachea (*arrow*)

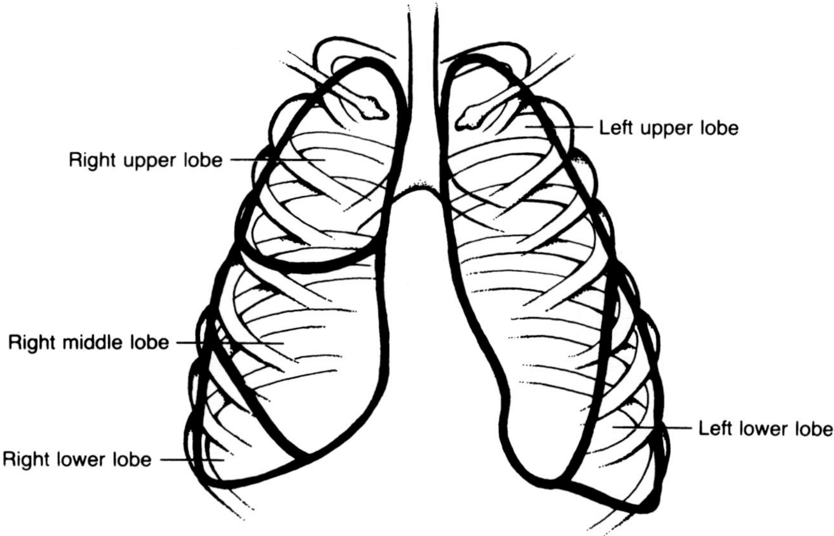

Fig. 2.35. Schematic drawing of lobar anatomy, including fissures

Common Pathological Conditions

Fine detail of lung anatomy is seen best with CT (Fig. 2.36). High-resolution CT demonstrates the lung detail of the secondary lobules with their concomitant vessels and bronchioles. The bronchioles and arteries are central with the interlobular septum composed of connective tissue and pulmonary veins peripherally placed (Fig. 2.37). High-resolution CT facilitates diagnosis of bronchiectasis, diffuse lung disease, defining the full extent of pulmonary disease, as well as explaining worrisome findings on the plain film. It is the most sensitive test for pulmonary metastatic disease.

Hyperexpansion

Hyperexpansion of the lungs results from "air trapping," i.e., the air cannot exit as rapidly as it enters. This may be caused by any functional or organic airway obstruction. Logically, hyperexpansion is manifested by flattening or inversion of the diaphragm, widening of the rib interspaces, and larger clear spaces in front and in back of the heart. The heart itself may be compressed and reduced in transverse diameter. The lungs may appear darker than normal, but check that the film was not overexposed (see Fig. 2.3). In general, it looks as if the child took a very deep breath when he clearly seems too young to have followed the technician's instructions. The air trapping must be seen on both frontal and lateral views to be sure this finding is real.

When hyperexpansion occurs chronically, cor pulmonale may result. Hyperexpansion may be unilateral or bilateral. Common causes of *bilateral* hyperexpansion are (a) asthma, (b) bronchiolitis, and (c) cystic fibrosis. Isolated hyperexpansion of one or two lobes *unilaterally* is commonly found in children who have a foreign body or hilar nodes compressing the bronchus. Because of unilateral hyperexpansion, the mediastinum may be shifted. In addition, unilateral hyperexpansion may result from atelectasis or collapse of the contralateral segment of lung (Fig. 2.38). Recognizing unilateral hyperexpansion of the lung is extremely important in pediatrics because children frequently aspirate foreign material (see Fig. 2.38).

▶ *Reed's Rule No. 6:* In unilateral hyperexpansion of the lungs, you must see how the air moves. Mediastinal position is critical to this determination.

The movement of air within a lung can be visualized by various procedures, such as (a) inspiratory and expiratory radiographs (mediastinal position), (b) fluoroscopy of the chest (mediastinal position and diaphragmatic motion), and (c) decubitus films (the down side is the "expiratory" side of the radiograph). With these maneuvers one should be able to see which side is abnormal, i.e., air in the abnormal side does not move appropriately (see Fig. 2.38).

If there is too much air in one hemithorax, be sure there are lung markings within the area; one may be overlooking a pneumothorax. It is mandatory to identify the visceral-pleural margin.

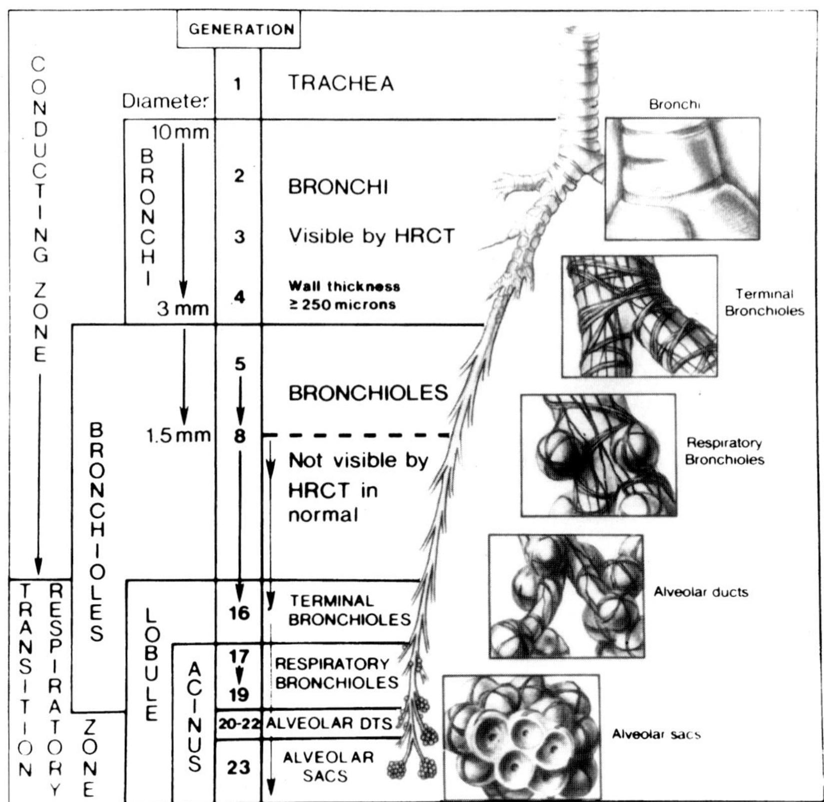
GENERATION
CONDUCTING ZONE
Diameter
10mm
BRONCHI
3 mm
1.5mm
BRONCHIOLES
1 TRACHEA
2 BRONCHI
3 Visible by HRCT
4 Wall thickness ≥ 250 microns
5
8 BRONCHIOLES
Not visible by HRCT in normal
16 TERMINAL BRONCHIOLES
17 19 RESPIRATORY BRONCHIOLES
20-22 ALVEOLAR DTS
23 ALVEOLAR SACS
TRANSITION
RESPIRATORY ZONE
LOBULE
ACINUS
Bronchi
Terminal Bronchioles
Respiratory Bronchioles
Alveolar ducts
Alveolar sacs
a

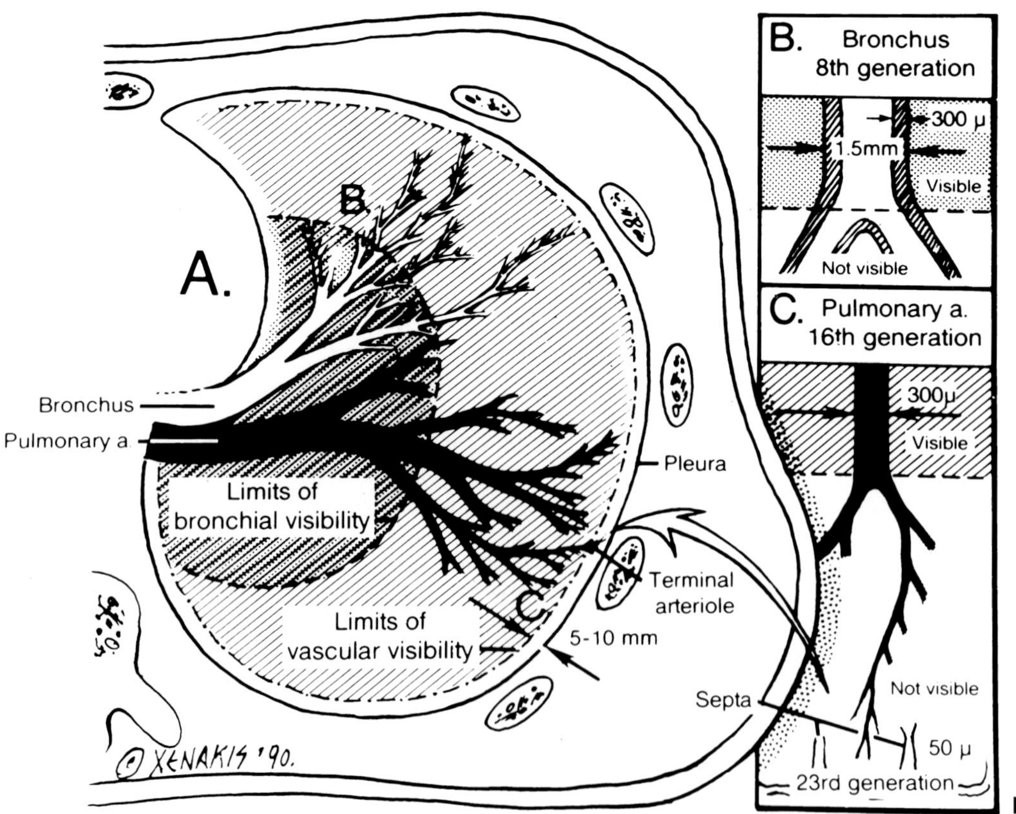
A.
B.
C.
Bronchus
Pulmonary a
Limits of bronchial visibility
Limits of vascular visibility
Pleura
Terminal arteriole
5-10 mm
Septa
B. Bronchus 8th generation
300 μ
1.5mm
Visible
Not visible
C. Pulmonary a. 16th generation
300μ
Visible
Not visible
50 μ
23rd generation
© XENAKIS '90.
b

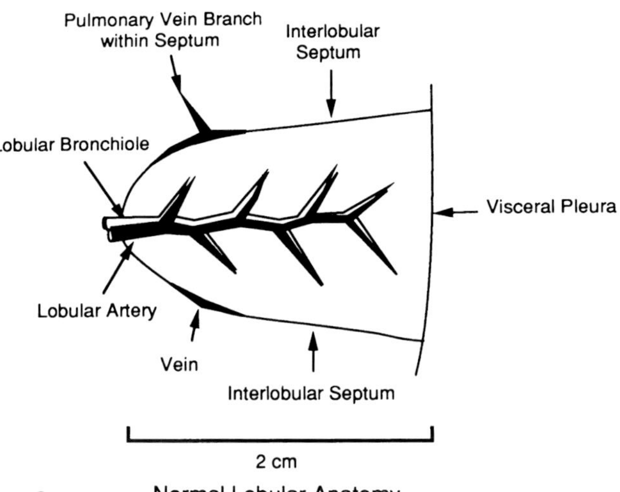

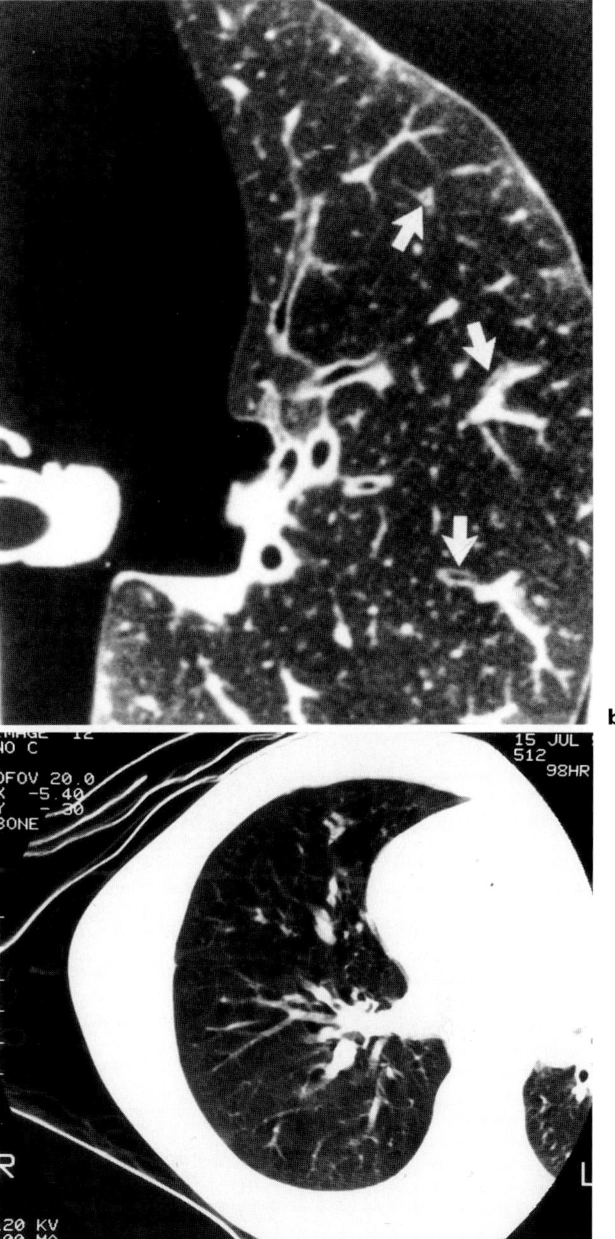

◀ **Fig. 2.36 a, b.** Anatomy as seen high resolution CT. This shows the ability of CT to visualize small structures within the lung. (From [7])

Fig. 2.37 a–c. High-resolution CT. This is the anatomy of the secondary pulmonary lobule. **a** Anatomy of the secondary pulmonary lobule. **b** Normal appearance in an isolated lung preparation (*arrows*, pointing to small bronchus). **c** Normal appearance in a 10-year-old child (From [8])

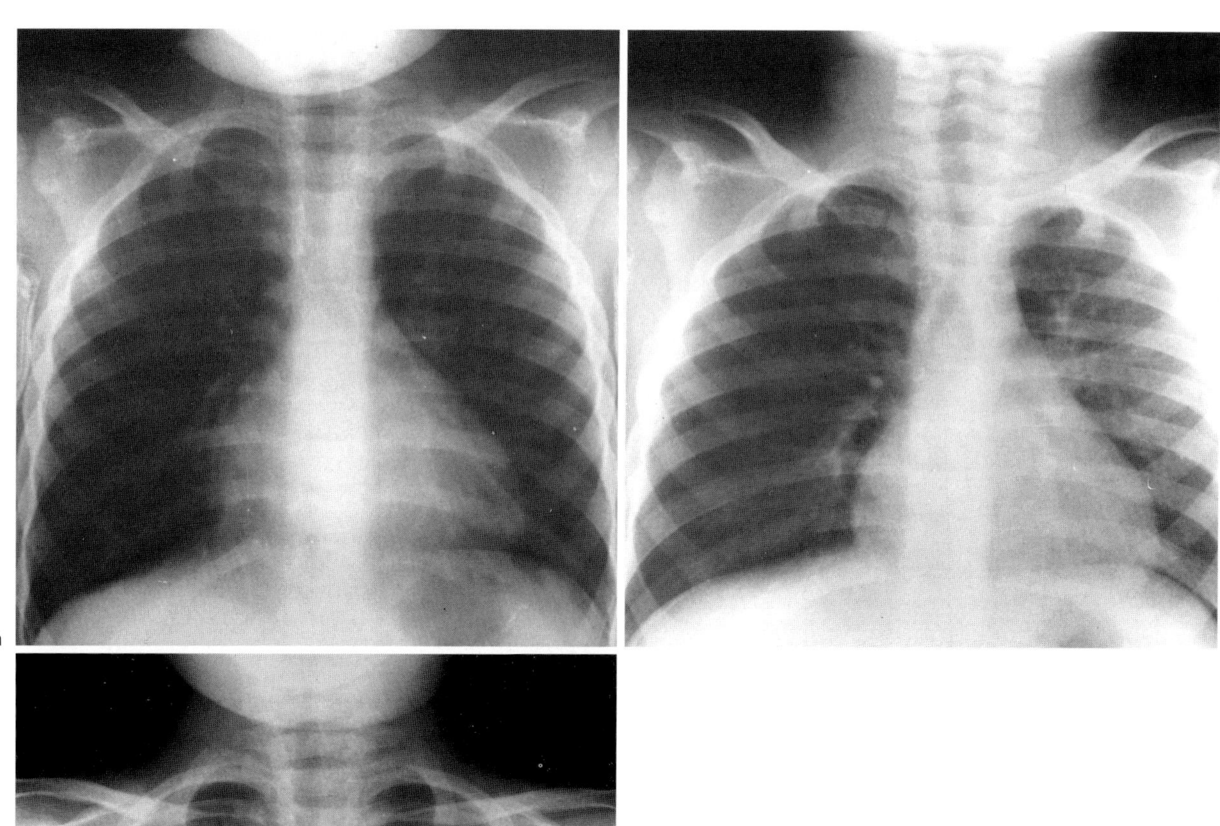

Fig. 2.38 a–c. A 3-year-old who started choking after eating peanuts. **a** Inspiratory frontal film has subtle changes: the right lung is hyperexpanded and blacker than the left, although there is no mediastinal shift. **b** Expiratory film reveals that air did not leave the right lung; it remains trapped during the expiratory phase of respiration. The mediastinum is shifted to the left (the left lung has gone through expiration properly). **c** Two days after a peanut was removed from the right main-stem bronchus the expiratory film shows no difference in aeration

Lobar Collapse

It is often helpful to think of the lobes of the lungs as being attached at the hila as if they were a fan. When these lobes collapse, they still retain their hilar attachment, and the other lobes often expand to compensate. The patterns of lobar collapse are identified in two ways: by seeing the collapsed lobe in a recognizable pattern and by noticing subtle shifts of intrathoracic structures and loss of normal roentgenological borders (silhouette sign) (Figs. 2.39, 2.40). Five questions should be asked when an opacity is seen that appears to be a lobar collapse:

- To which side is the mediastinum shifted?
- In what directions are the major and minor fissures deviated?
- What normal structures are silhouetted?
- Is the hilum shifted up or down?
- Is the diaphragm elevated (see Figs. 2.39, 2.40.)?

A common cause of lobar collapse in children is mucus plugging in postoperative and asthmatic patients. Always look for foreign bodies by carefully examining the right and left main-stem bronchi. Masses such as lymph nodes (due to tuberculosis, other infections, or lymphoma), or extrinsic masses such as bronchogenic cysts, can also cause lobar collapse.

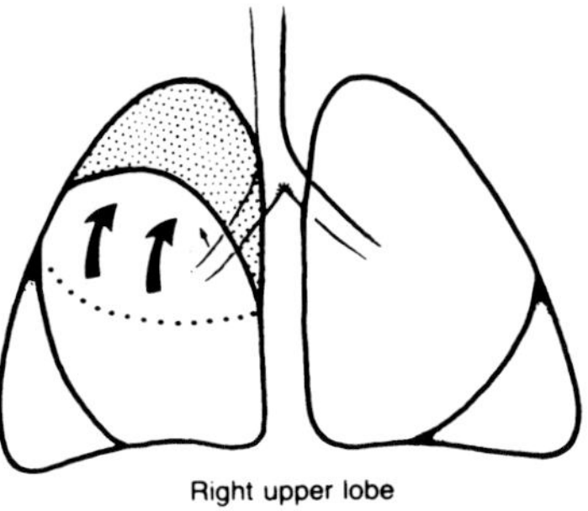

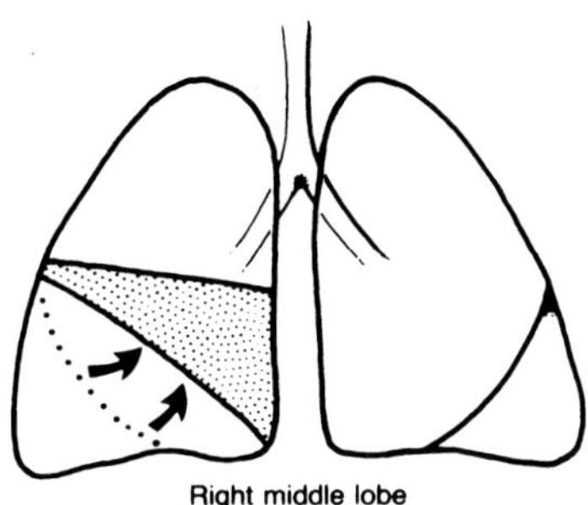

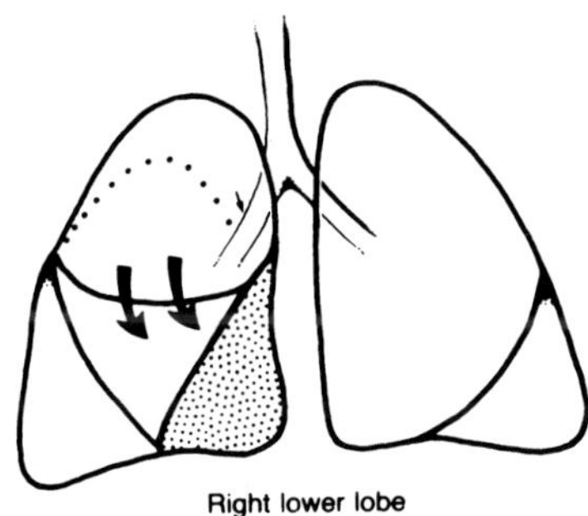

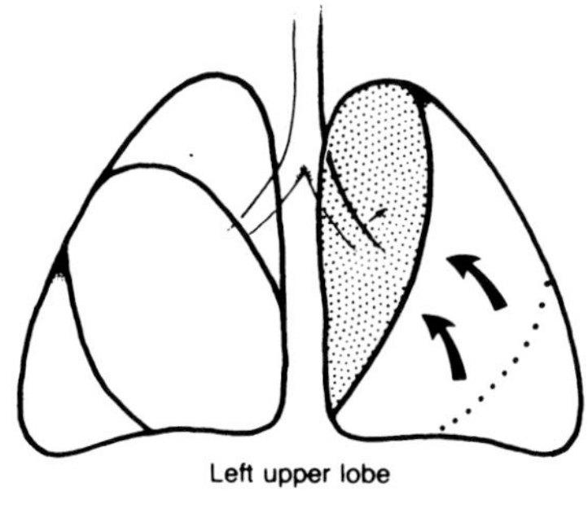

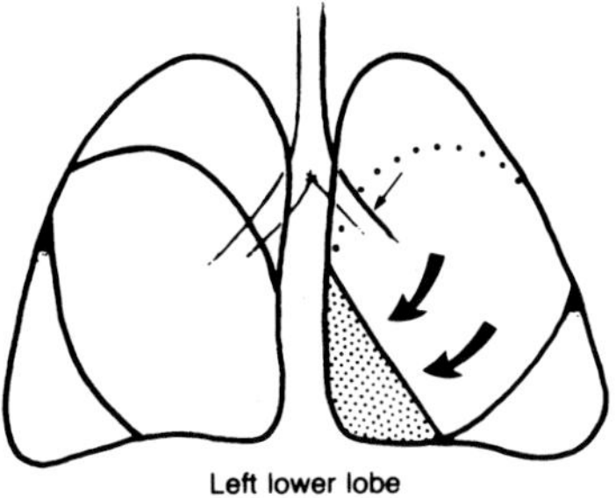

Fig. 2.39. Lobar collapse. Note bronchus (*small arrow*) and fissure (*large arrow*) shift

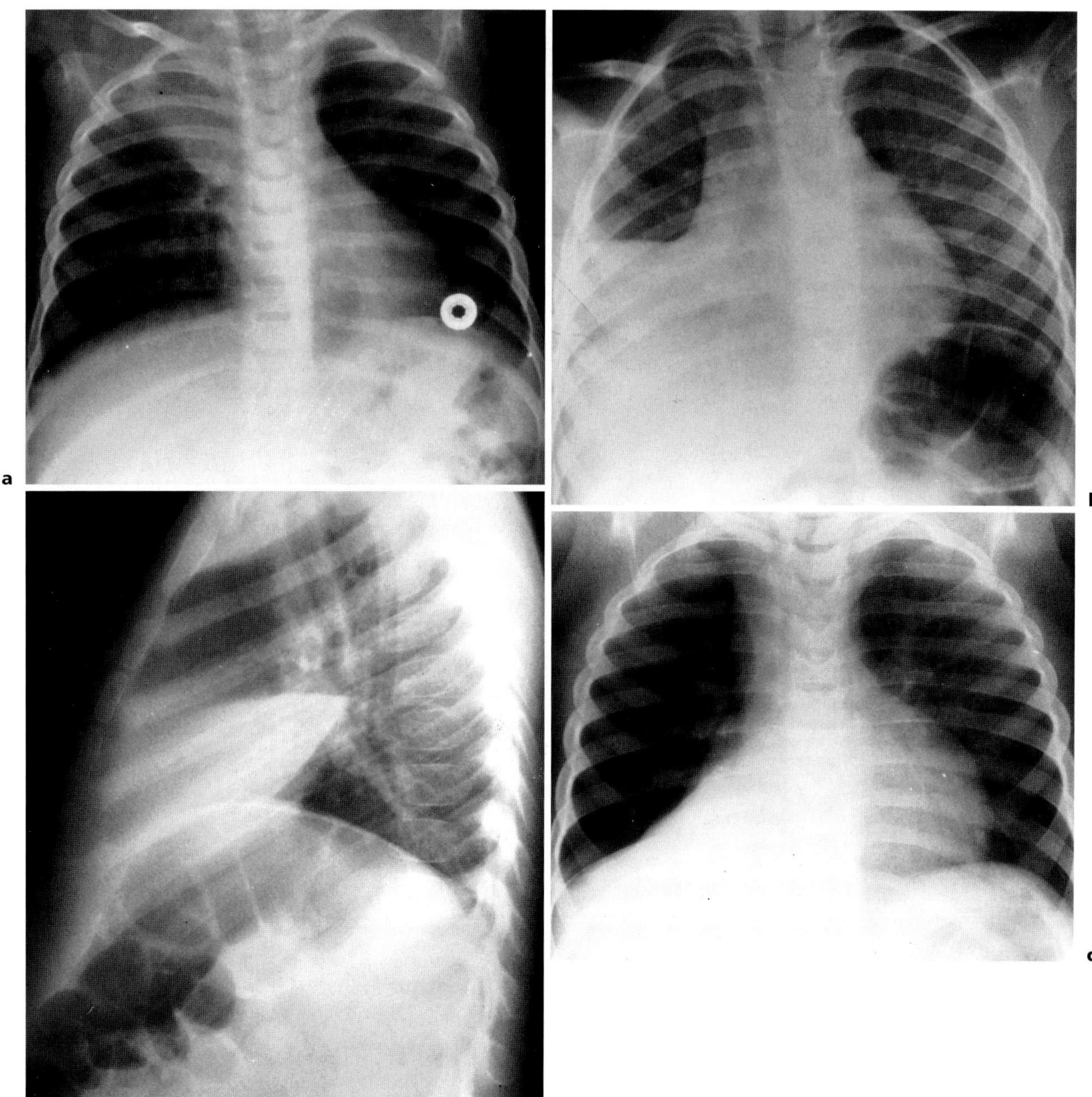
a
b
c
d

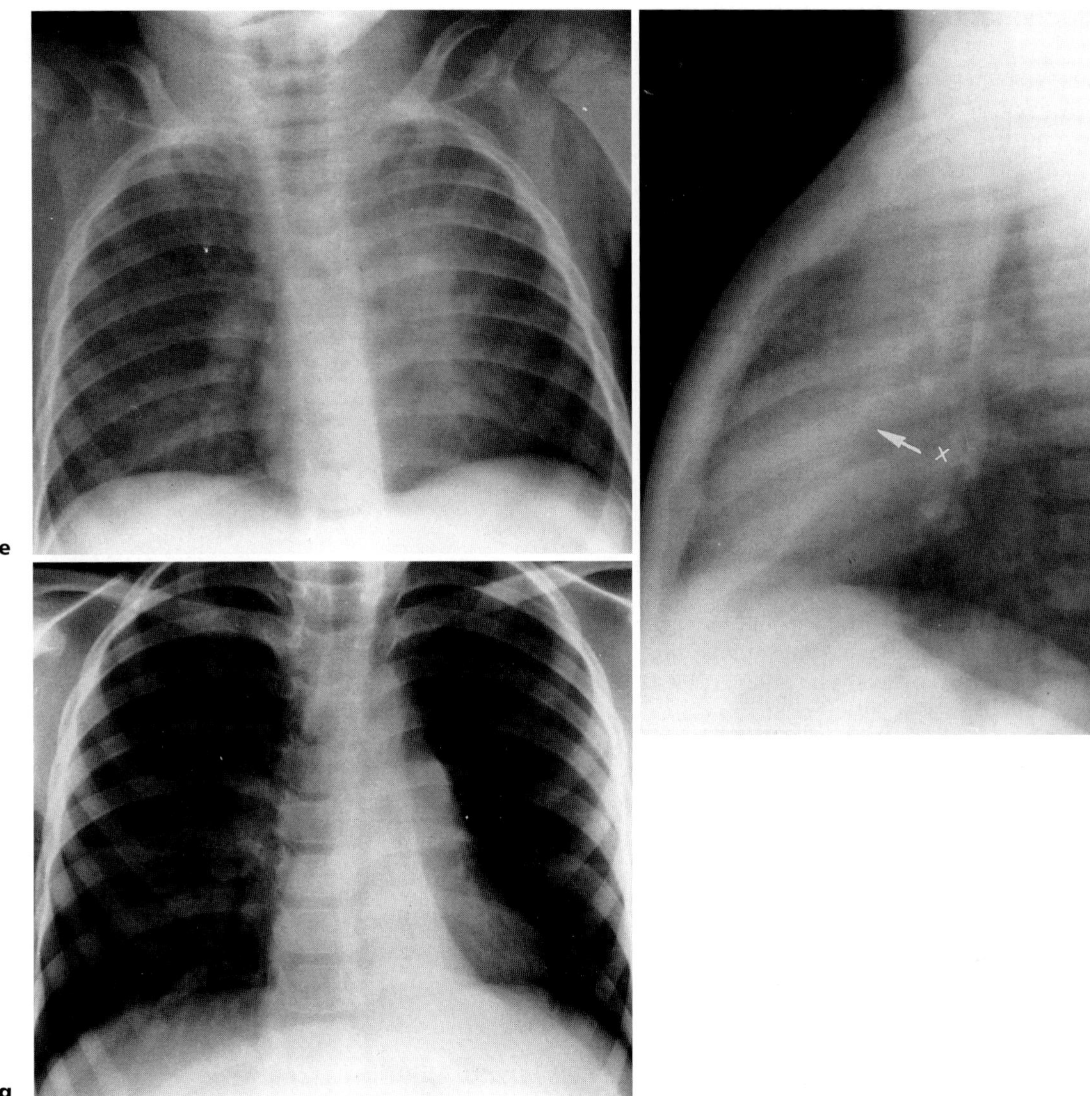

Fig. 2.40 a–g. Examples of lobar collapse. **a** Frontal film showing right upper-lobe collapse with elevation of the minor fissure (*arrows*). **b** Frontal film with right middle lobe collapse and loss of right heart border (the silhouette sign). **c** Lateral film of right middle-lobe collapse and wedge of opacity over the heart. **d** Frontal film with right lower-lobe collapse. The heart margin is not preserved as the medial portion of the right middle lobe is also collapsed. **e** Frontal film with left upper-lobe collapse and loss of the left heart border (the silhouette sign) and a hazy opacity over the left upper lung. **f** Lateral film of left upper-lobe collapse. Major fissure (*arrow*) is far anterior to its normal position (*x*). **g** Left lower-lobe collapse with opacity behind the heart. The left heart border is not obscured

Change in Pulmonary Densities

An opacity is represented by the image appearing too white, and a lucency by its appearing too black. An opacity in the lung may be caused by (a) pneumonic consolidation, (b) atelectasis, (c) neoplasm, or (d) a localized collection of fluid. Sometimes the causes of opacities are indistinguishable. In fact, two processes often are coexistent. When discussing this problem with colleagues, beware of the word "infiltrate." This has come to mean a pneumonic process, but some radiologists understand it to mean atelectasis or edema.

Opacities within the alveolar space frequently show air bronchograms, which occur when air within the bronchi is seen against a background of airless lung or fluid-filled alveoli. Most alveolar opacities are confluent and larger than individual vessels. Any material, such as pneumonic consolidation or fluid from congestive heart failure, may be manifest by alveolar air space opacity. In diseases such as viral pneumonia and tuberculosis, edema or pus in the interstitium of the lung creates discrete linear streaks. These "increased interstitial markings" represent peribronchial thickening, atelectasis, fibrosis, and what is commonly termed "the radiological dirty lung," a common finding in patients with asthma. Remember: "increased interstitial markings" are *a sign*, not a specific disease!

Lobar pneumonia can silhouette the mediastinum, mimicking lobar collapse (Fig. 2.41). However, there is no mediastinal shift of the same magnitude, nor is there a significant loss of lung volume associated with changes of position of the fissures.

The most overdiagnosed (nonexistent) pneumonias are: (a) "right lower lobe pneumonia" at the medial lung base, often caused by pulmonary arterial branches seen on a film taken with a poor inspiratory effort and (b) perihilar pneumonia, also caused by slight rotation of the chest and poor inspiration, making the hilar vessels stand out. Therefore be careful before diagnosing a perihilar infiltrate on a rotated film! Be leery of opacities in the perihilar regions and the right lower lobe. A clue is: if upon close inspection of the film it appears that the opacity in the right lower lobe is really a bunch of individual white lines, it probably is *not* pneumonia. The most *overlooked* pneumonia is that found in the left lower lobe (see Fig. 2.41). This is easily recognized when you remember that the heart should have the same density throughout. *Be aware of changes in density!* Loss of pulmonary artery visibility or a sudden change from gray to white in any portion of the heart should make you suspicious of retrocardiac pneumonia. When reading a chest film, train yourself to *look through things*, i.e., the heart and liver. Also, keep your eye on the left hemidiaphragm; it should be seen as clearly as the right. Any disruption may mean adjacent pneumonia or atelectasis (silhouette sign).

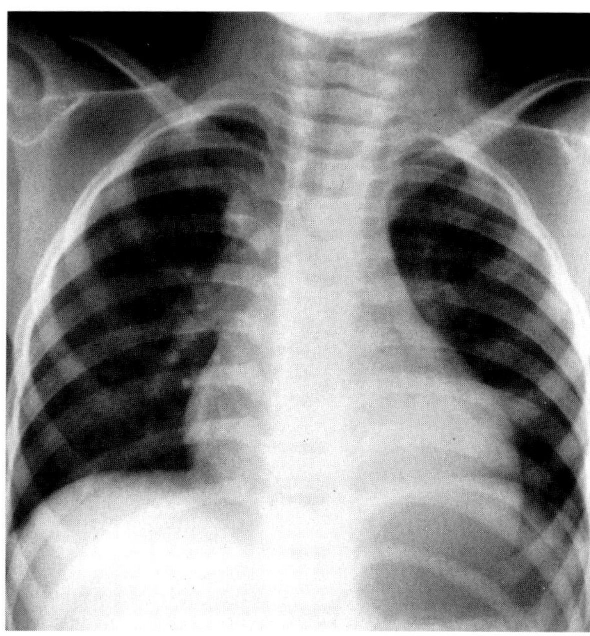

Fig. 2.41. Left lower infiltrate. This 3-year-old has fever and a cough. There is a great deal of opacity behind the left side of the heart. You can look through the right side of the heart and see the lung and its vascularity. This is not the case on the left – a finding consistent with left lower-lobe pneumonia

Masses and Pseudomasses

Commonly a "mass" in the lungs of children is in fact a pseudomass caused by the "round" pneumonia (Fig. 2.42). This type of opacity is sometimes so perfectly round that it simulates a neoplasm. Appropriate treatment is given, and follow-up films are obtained after 10 days to document whether the mass disappears. Another pseudomass is caused by loculated fluid in the fissure. Often this fluid has a teardrop shape and conforms to the anatomy of the fissure; the density is often sharply demarcated for one-half to three-quarters of its borders (see Fig. 2.42).

A common juxta-diaphragmatic pseudomass is due to partial eventration – thinning of the muscles of the diaphragm; it is most often seen on the right as a "bump" on the diaphragmatic surface. Such a phenomenon is *usually asymptomatic and does not require therapy*, but a large eventration can act as a diaphragmatic hernia, causing mediastinal shifts (Fig. 2.43).

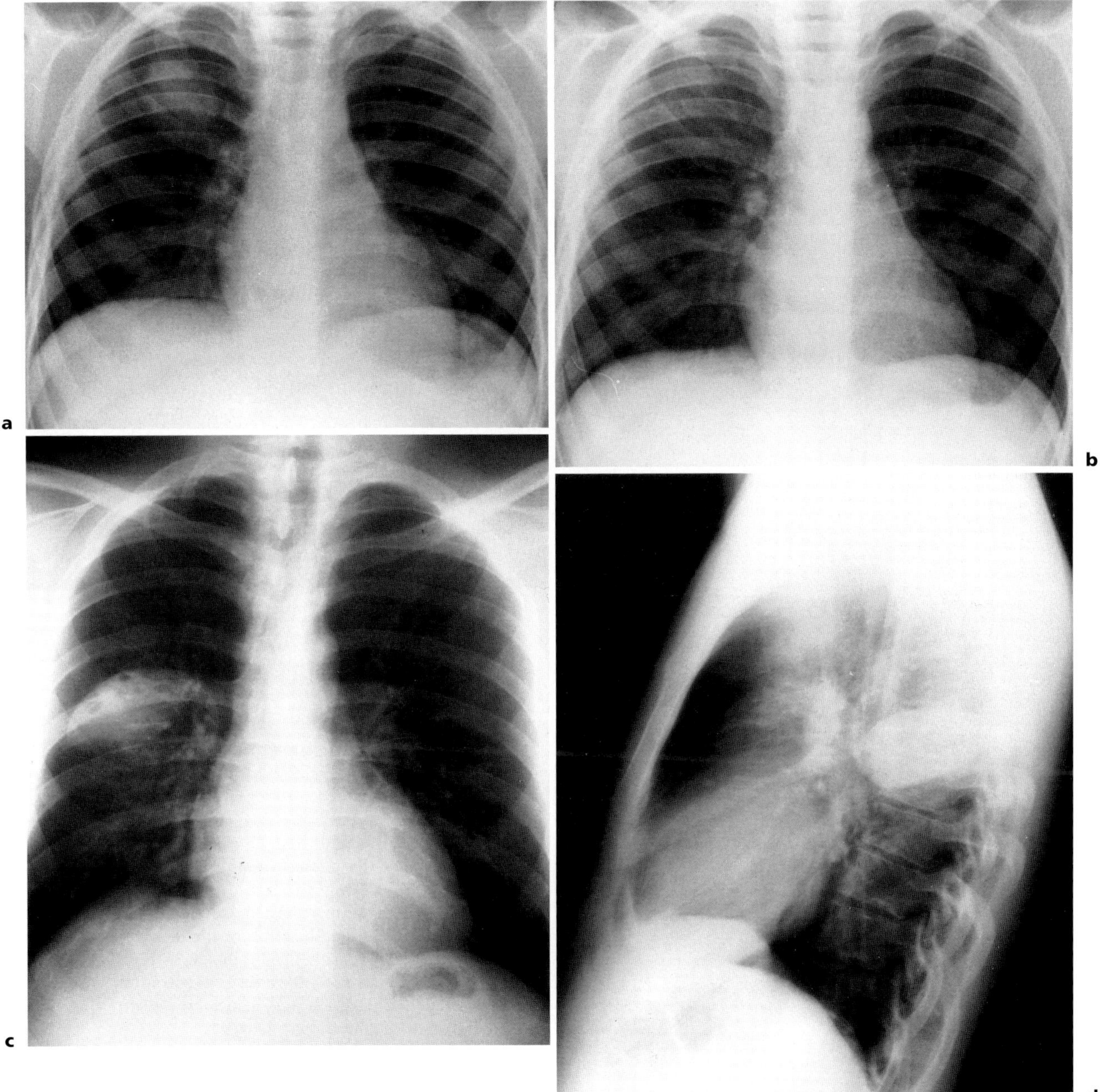

Fig. 2.42 a–d. Unusual pulmonary densities. **a** Round pneumonia. Frontal chest film shows a rounded density that might, at first glance, be mistaken for a tumor or metastasis. Antibiotic therapy resulted in a normal chest on subsequent films. **b** Frontal film eight days later. **c** Loculated pleural fluid. This child had unexplained fever and cough for 2 weeks after antibiotic therapy for pneumonia. Chest films show an elliptical density on the right. Note how it conforms to the position of the minor fissure. This is characteristic of a loculated effusion (in this case, infected fluid) in the fissure. **d** Lateral film of another child with loculated pleural fluid in the posterior portion of the major fissure

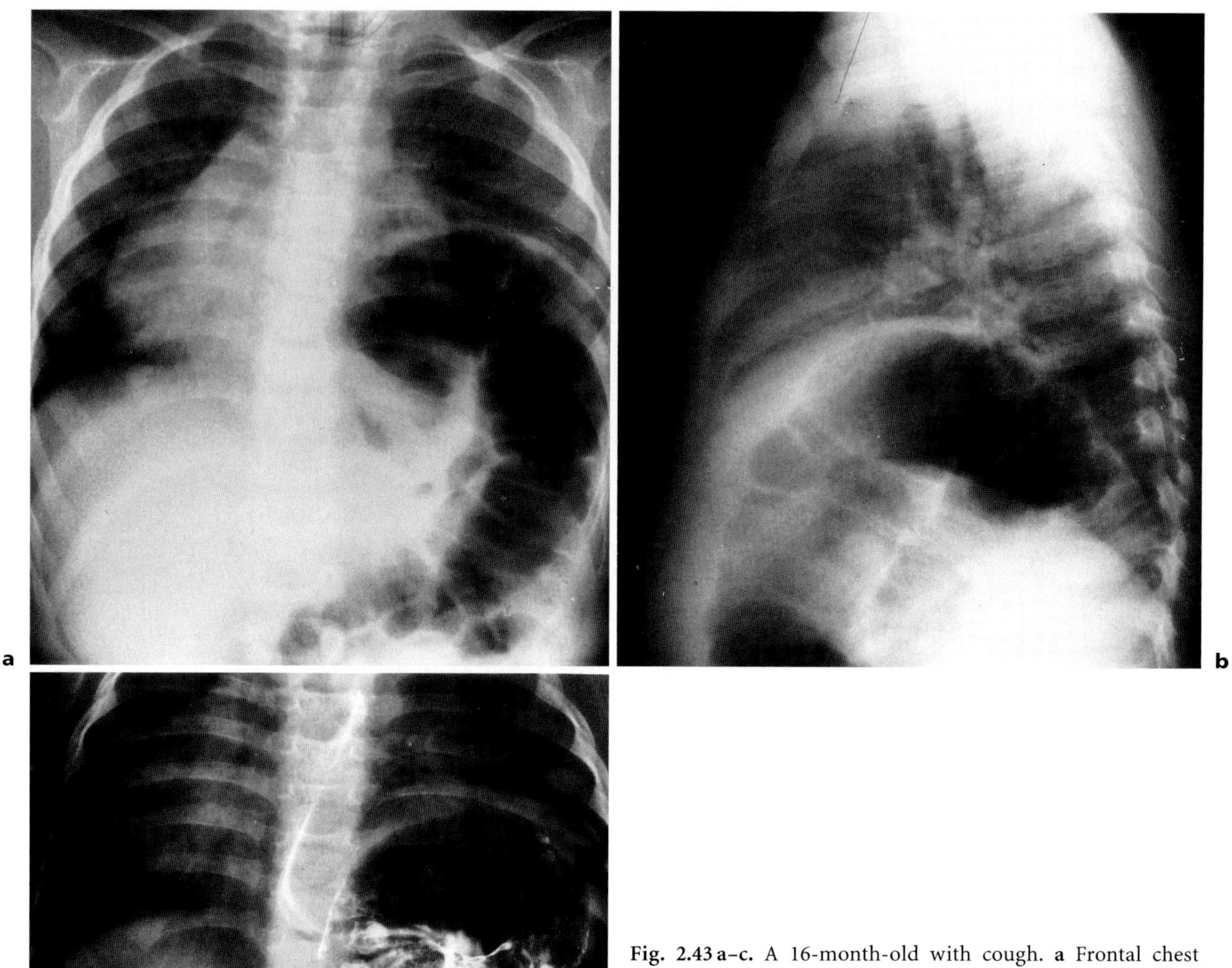

Fig. 2.43 a–c. A 16-month-old with cough. **a** Frontal chest radiograph shows the mediastinum shifted to the right and bowel loops compressing the left lower lung. **b** Lateral film shows bowel high in the chest. **c** Barium was given, confirming the intrathoracic location of the stomach and small bowel. At surgery there was an intact diaphragm, but it was very thin, consistent with a large eventration. When the eventration is this large, it acts as a mass causing the same symptoms as a diaphragmatic hernia

True primary pulmonary neoplasms are uncommon in children. The most common ones are extensions of mediastinal structures or are caused by defects of the diaphragm and are in fact extrapulmonary (Fig. 2.44). It is appropriate, then, to discuss mediastinal masses in this category. These masses arise in any of the three components of the mediastinum. The most common posterior mediastinal mass is a neurogenic tumor such as a neuroblastoma, ganglioneuroma, or neurofibroma. The hemidiaphragm inserts posteriorly at the L1-2 level; therefore, a posterior basilar intrathoracic mediastinal mass may masquerade as an abdominal mass. Remember the normal inferior extent of the thoracic cavity! Middle mediastinal masses are most commonly of lymphoid origin (e.g., lymphoma), but lesions of any of the other structures of the middle mediastinum – such as esophageal duplication – may occur. The most common anterior mediastinal masses are "terrible" lymphomas, teratomas, thymomas (in children aged over 10 years), and cystic hygromas (with extension down from the neck). True parenchymal masses are frequently due to metastasis such as that from Wilms' tumor (Fig. 2.45). Congenital primary masses are discussed in the next Chap 3.

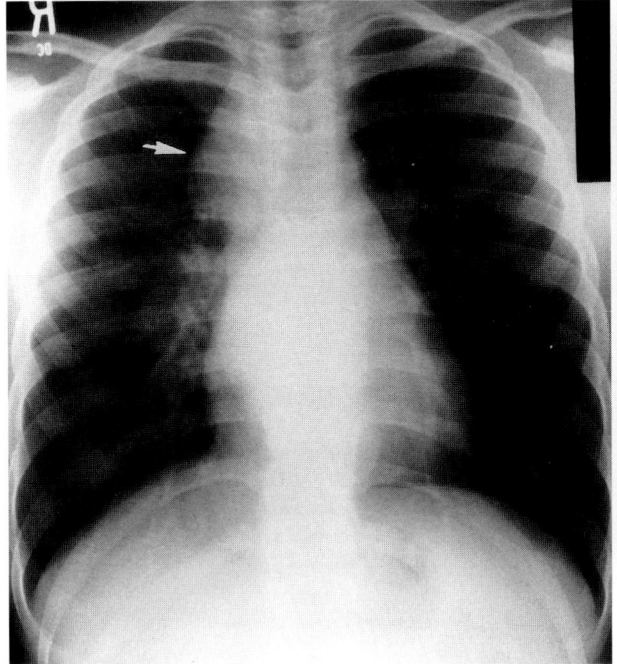

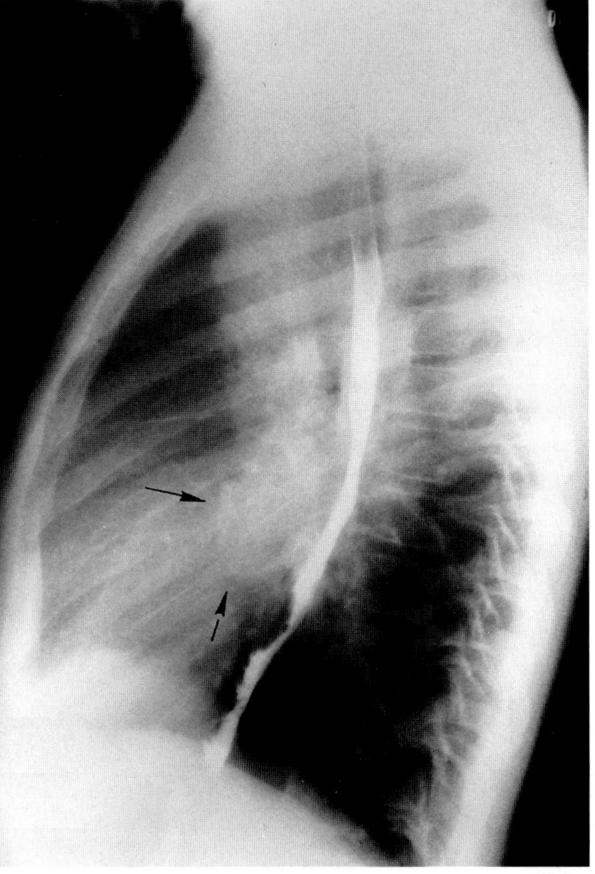

Fig. 2.44 a, b. Mediastinal mass. **a** This 10-year old has a widened mediastinum. He is too old to have a large thymus and, in fact, has an enlarged right hilum with paratracheal adenopathy (*arrow*). The subcarinal region is also "too white" when compared to the rest of the heart. **b** Lateral roentgenograph shows the density in the middle mediastinum – a common presentation for a lymphoma (*arrows*)

The outline below is a useful summary of the etiology of mediastinal masses:

- Anterior mediastinum (the four T's and a C)
  - Teratoma
  - Thymoma
  - Thyroid (often mentioned, never seen!)
  - "Terrible" lymph node enlargement by either infection or malignancy
  - Cystic hygroma
- Middle mediastinum (an abnormality for each organ)
  - Esophagus: duplication cysts
  - Great vessels: aneurysmal dilatation
  - Hila: enlarged lymph nodes (leukemia, lymphoma, tuberculosis, etc.)
  - Trachea: bronchogenic cysts
  - Pericardium: cyst
- Posterior mediastinum (T, E, N)
  - Tuberculosis (Pott's disease) or any spinal infection
  - Extramedullary hematopoiesis (almost always in adults)
  - Neural tumors: neuroblastoma, ganglioneuroma, neurofibroma, neurenteric cyst
- Tips when viewing mediastinal masses
  - Middle mediastinal masses silhouette the heart border and aorta.
  - Posterior mediastinal masses may spread ribs.

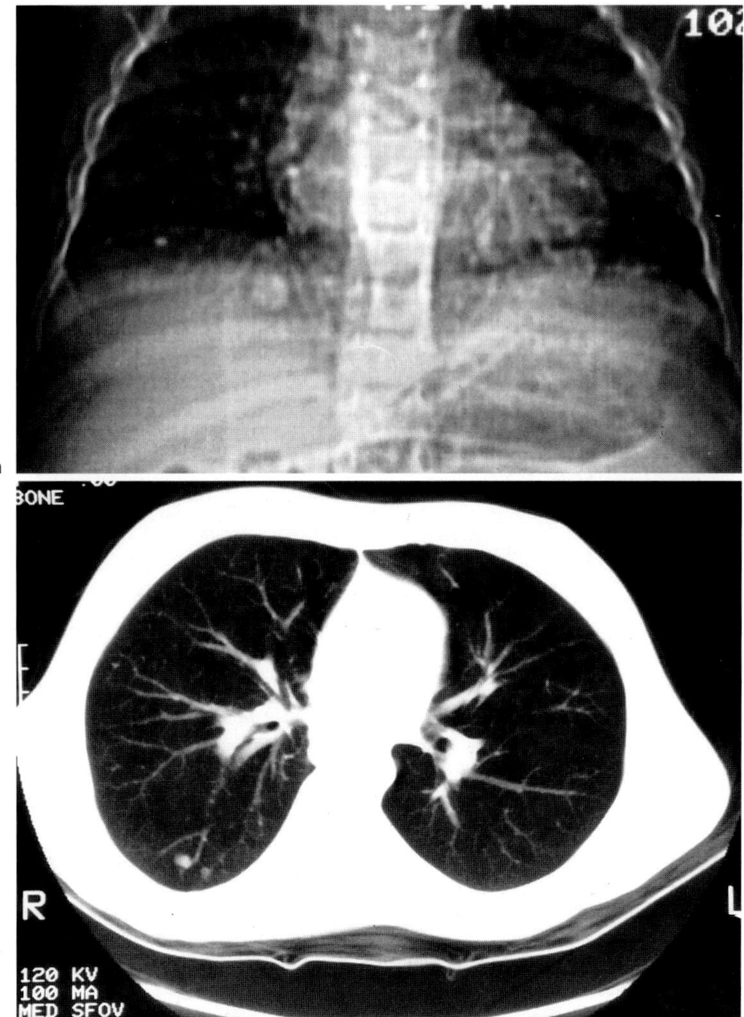

Fig. 2.45 a, b. Metastatic lung disease. **a** Scout film prior to CT in this 3-year-old who had a Wilms' tumor removed 7 months previously. There are multiple rounded densities in the chest. **b** CT reveals multiple lung metastases

Pleura

Pleural reaction (effusion or thickening) is best indicated by a density between the aerated lung and rib border (Fig. 2.46 b). Thickened pleura, loculated pleural fluid, or empyema appear similar radiographically and cannot always be differentiated by normal radiographic techniques. Decubitus films demonstrate free-flowing fluid but may not show loculated pleural fluid, viscous empyema, or thickened pleura. An excellent way to detect small amounts of fluid or limited pleural thickening not visible on the frontal film is to look carefully at the posterior lung sulci on the lateral film. Then check the thickness of the pleural line in relationship to each rib; it should be snug against the rib. Fluid can also accumulate beneath the inferior surface of the lung and can simulate an elevated hemidiaphragm. Such collections are called subpul-

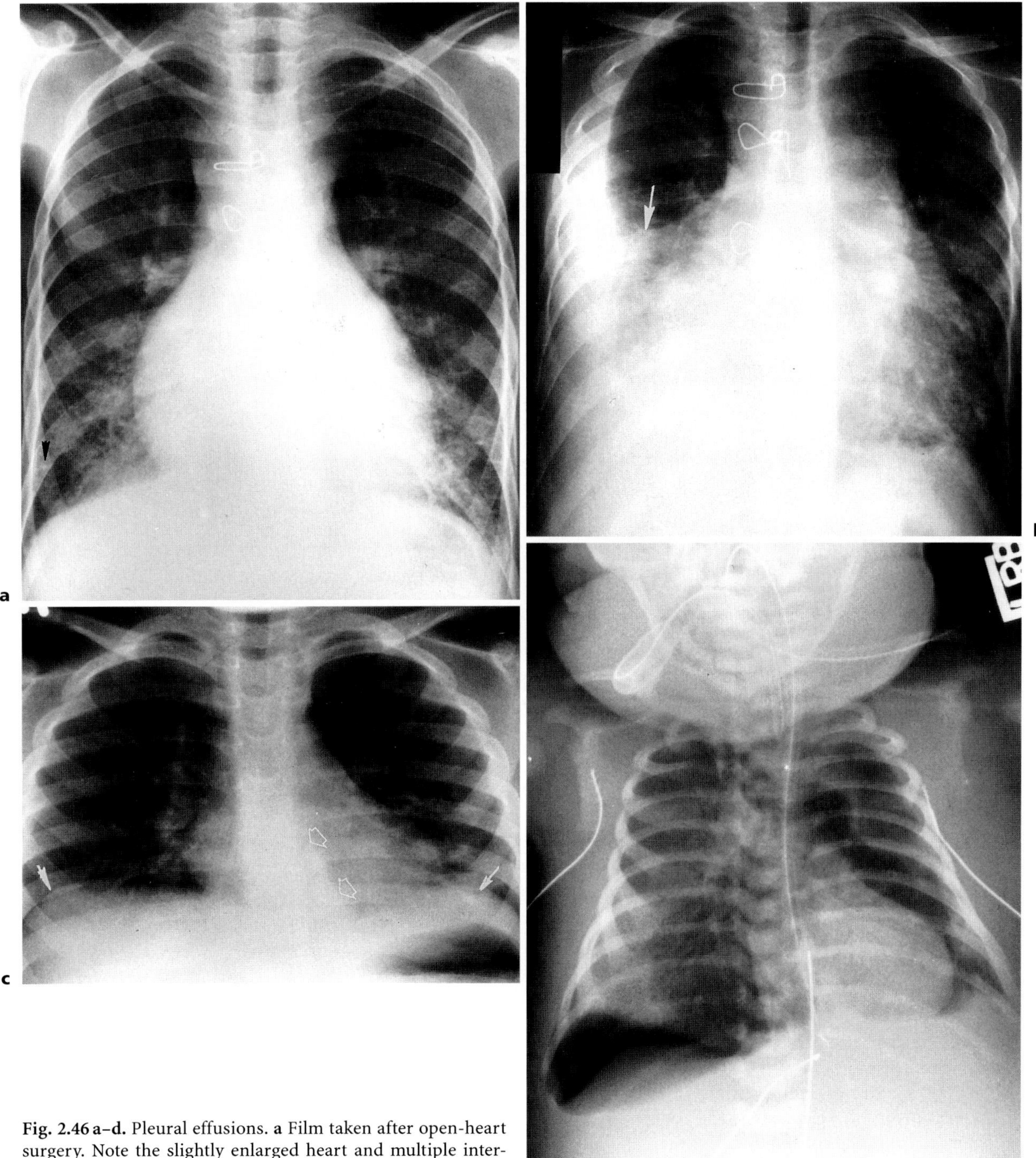

Fig. 2.46 a–d. Pleural effusions. **a** Film taken after open-heart surgery. Note the slightly enlarged heart and multiple interstitial lines in both lower lungs. The lines, which are horizontal and extend to the pleura (*arrowhead*), are called Kerley's B lines. **b** Postpericardiotomy syndrome. A few days after the first film, this child developed an extensive right-sided pleural effusion. The fluid dissected into the region of the minor fissure (*arrow*). **c** Subpulmonic effusion. Careful attention to the apex of the "dome of the diaphragm" shows that it is somewhat laterally situated on both sides of the chest (*arrows*). Note also that the stomach bubble is separated from the "dome of the diaphragm" by a space. There is also a paramediastinal density (*open arrows*). This child had nephritis resulting in a pleural effusion that filled the space below the lung and above the diaphragm. This fluid simulates a diaphragmatic border, but, in fact, the diaphragm is not visible. **d** This premature infant has a right pneumothorax. It is situated beneath the lung (subpulmonic) but above the diaphragm. Note the similar shape of the air and the fluid in **c**

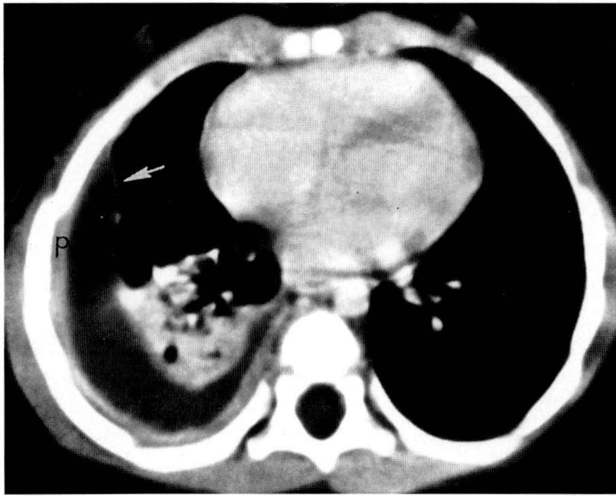

Fig. 2.47. Empyema with split pleural sign on CT. Axial CT shows right enhancing parietal pleura (*p*), the lower density fluid (empyema), and the enhancing visceral pleura (*arrow*). Anterior to the visceral pleural is atelectatic lung

monic effusions and are recognized by the laterally shifted "diaphragmatic dome" (see Fig. 2.46 c).

The most common cause of pleural effusion in children is infection, and almost any infection can cause a small pleural effusion. Pleural effusions are also frequently seen in patients with congestive heart failure (if unilateral, always on the right) and chronic renal disease. In difficult cases enhanced CT can differentiate pleural disease from effusion from parenchymal disease (Fig. 2.47). Ultrasound can often be used as well to find fluid for diagnostic taps.

Summary

A thorough radiographic work-up should include the following, in order of priority:

- Good erect, nonrotated inspiratory frontal and lateral chest films
- Inspiratory and expiratory films (if persistent hyperexpansion of atelectasis is the problem) and/or fluoroscopy of the chest to observe mediastinal shift and diaphragmatic excursion (decubitus films may help)
- Specialized study of the airway, if the air passage itself needs evaluation (see Chap. 9)
- An esophagram in any unsuspected airway disease
- MR or CT for mediastinal masses
- High-resolution CT for complete work-up of unusual or questionable pulmonary parenchymal abnormalities

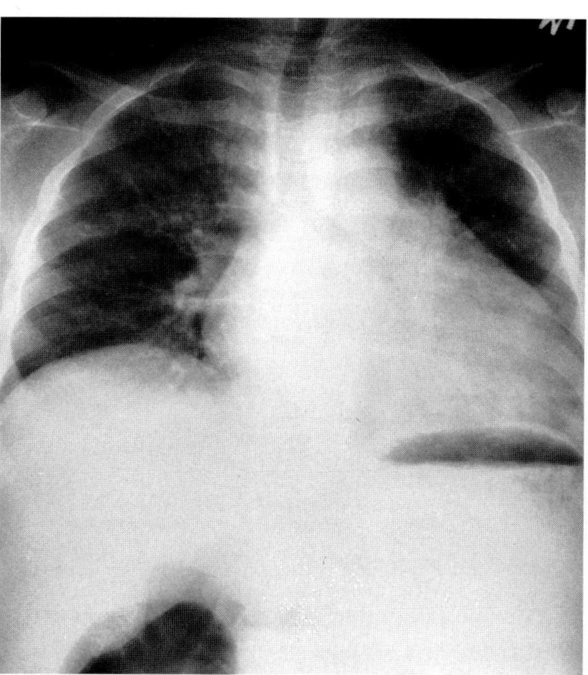

Fig. 2.48. Unusual densities. (see "Appendix 2")

Remember: the chest radiograph can be a very tricky thing. It is easy to get "seduced" by obvious pathology such as a mass opacity, a large heart, or a large pleural effusion. You must resist the temptation to describe the obvious abnormality and force yourself to do a routine, orderly scan of the entire chest film and not be "seduced" by the obvious lesion. This method will help train you to spot more subtle findings, such as a rib fracture. A convenient way to read systematically is to evaluate the technical factors of lung volume, patient position, and the way the film was exposed. Use the radiologist's circle and ABC's: A = abdomen, B = bones and soft tissues, C = chest (airway, mediastinum, lungs, and diaphragm). Now evaluate Figs. 2.48–2.52. Approach each one systemically and describe the abnormalities you see. The answers are in the "Appendix."

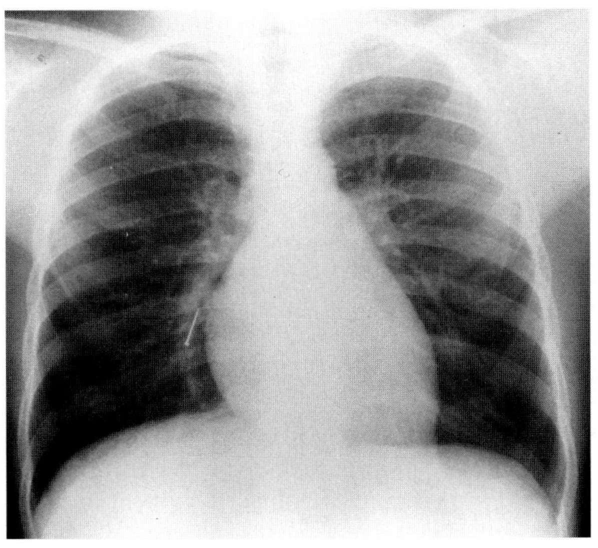

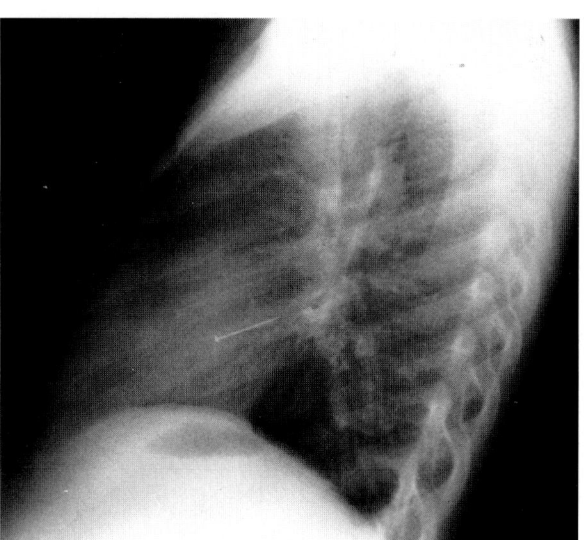

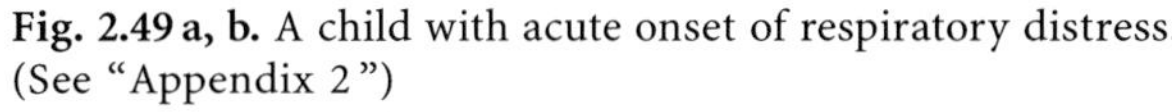

Fig. 2.49 a, b. A child with acute onset of respiratory distress. (See "Appendix 2")

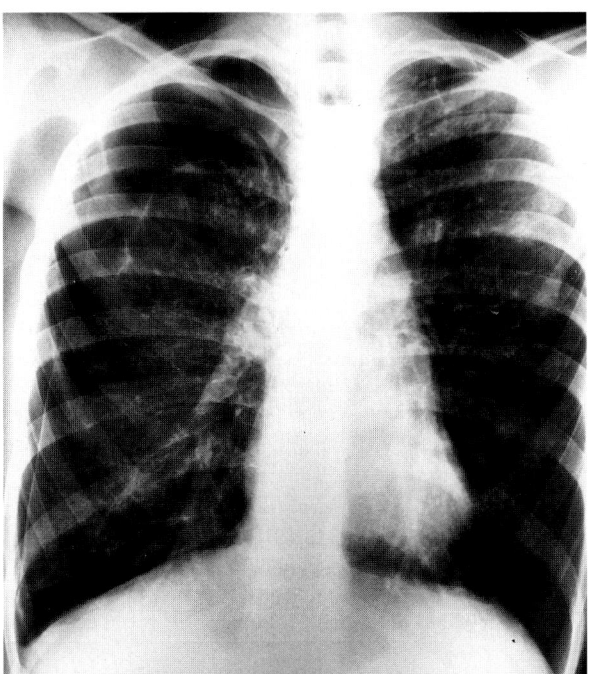

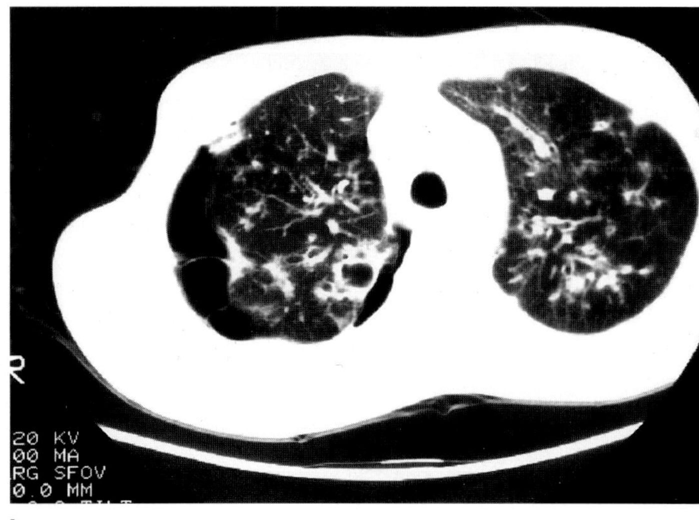

Fig. 2.50 a, b. Chronic lung disease. (See "Appendix 2")

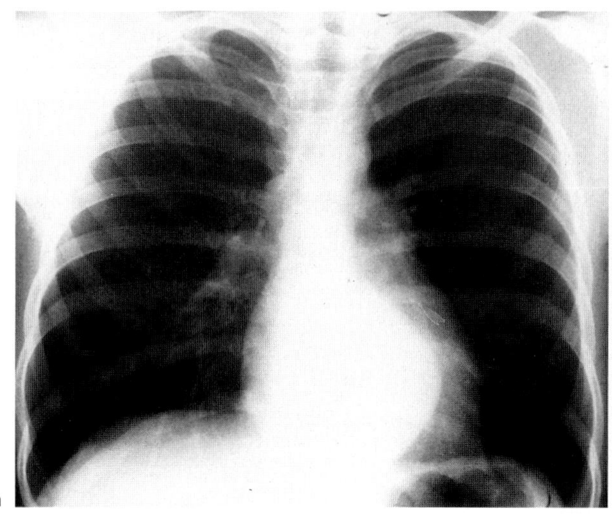

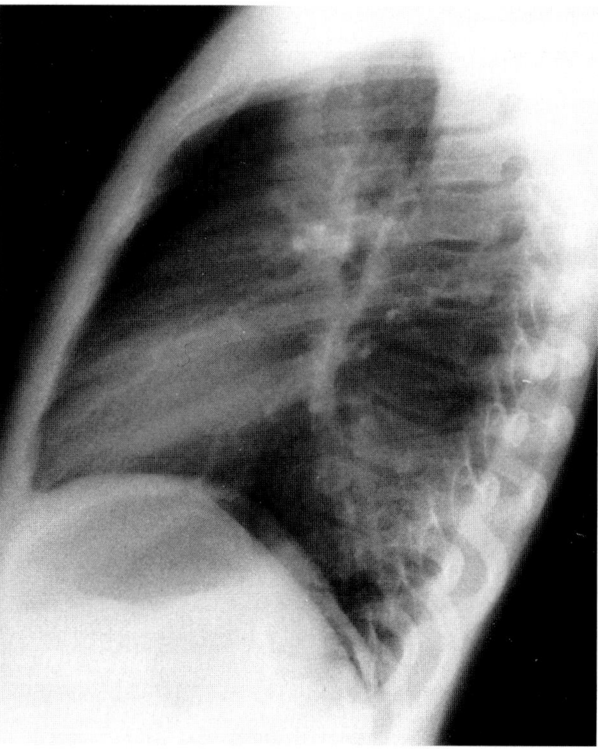

Fig. 2.51 a, b. A child with a cough. (See "Appendix 2")

References

1. Riggs W Jr. (1979) Pediatric chest roentgenology: recognizing the abnormal. Green, St. Louis
2. Felson B, Weinstein AS, Spita HB (1965) Principles of chest roentgenology – a program text. Saunders, Philadelphia
3. Squire LF (1988) Fundamentals of radiology, 4th edn. Harvard University Press, Cambridge
4. Silverman FN, Kuhn JP (1993) Caffey's pediatric X-ray diagnosis, 9th edn. Mosby, St. Louis
5. Slovis TL, Haller JO Berdon WE, Baker DH, Joseph PM(1979) Noninvasive visualization of the pediatric airway. Curr Probl Radiol 8:17
6. Slovis TL (1977) Nonivaseive evaluation of the pediatric airway. a recent advance. Pediatrics 59:872
7. Naidich DP, Zerhouni EA, Siegelman SS (1991) Computed tomography and magnetic resonance of the thorax, 2nd edn. Raven, New York
8. Webb WR, Müller NL, Naidich DP (1992) High-resolution CT of the lung. Raven, New York

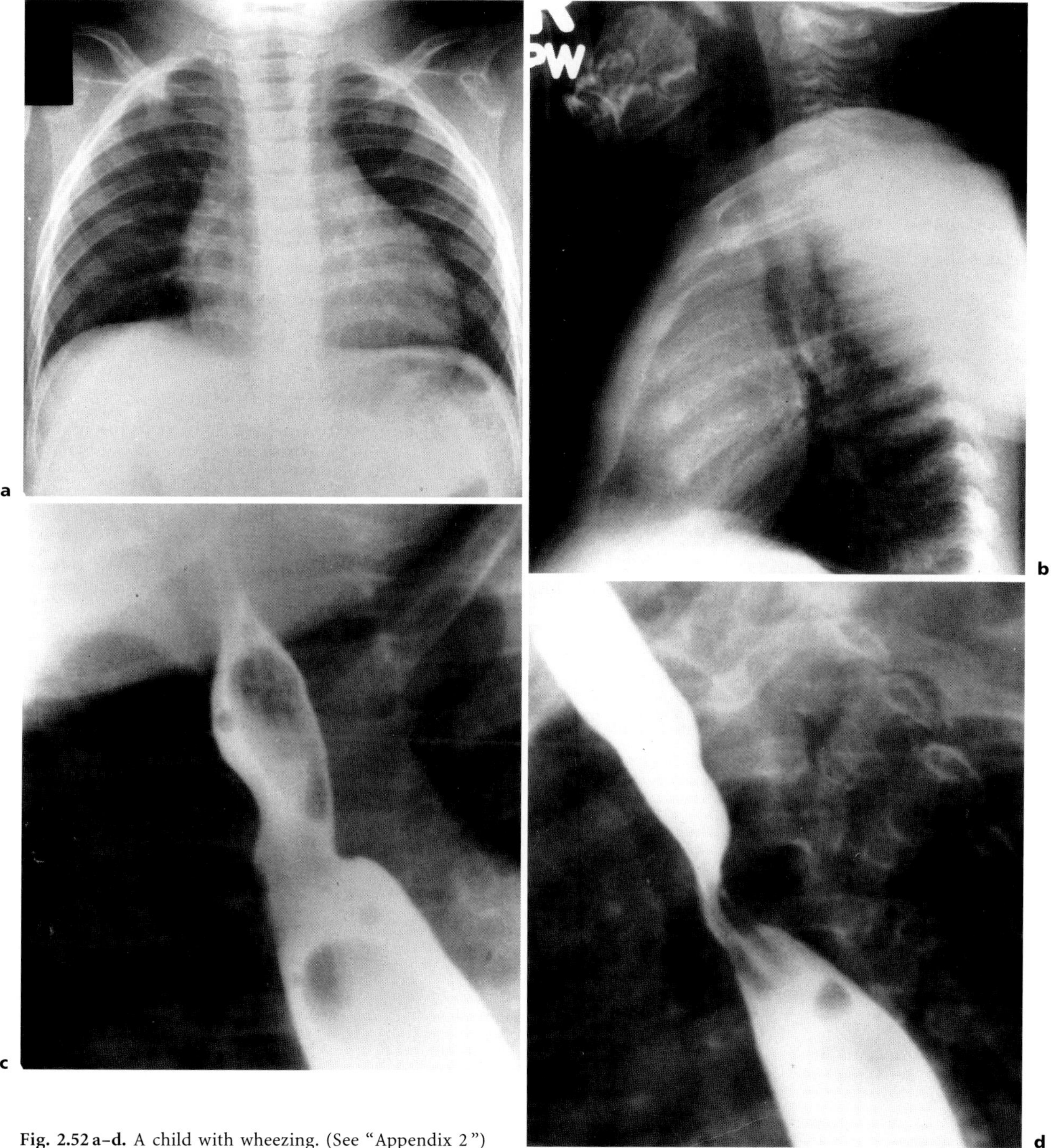

Fig. 2.52 a–d. A child with wheezing. (See "Appendix 2")

3 The Chest in the Neonate and Young Infant

Rapid physiological changes occur in the first minutes and hours of a newborn's life. The fluid-filled lungs empty of surfactant-rich fluid and fill with air. The circulatory system is dramatically changed when the ductus arteriosus closes. The lungs now receive a major influx of blood, and gaseous exchange occurs. During subsequent days to weeks, the pulmonary artery pressures fall from near systemic values. This drop in pulmonary vascular resistance permits clinical recognition of left-to-right shunts, such as ventricular septal defects and atrial septal defects.

The newborn infant breathes and cries. Both of these processes fill the lungs and the gastrointestinal tract with air. The lungs fill with air during the first breath. The gastrointestinal tract fills more slowly, and it may take up to 24 h for gas to reach the rectum (although it occurs by 12 h in most healthy infants).

The sequence and timing of these expected physiological and anatomical changes allow the radiologist to detect the infant making an abnormal transition to extrauterine life.

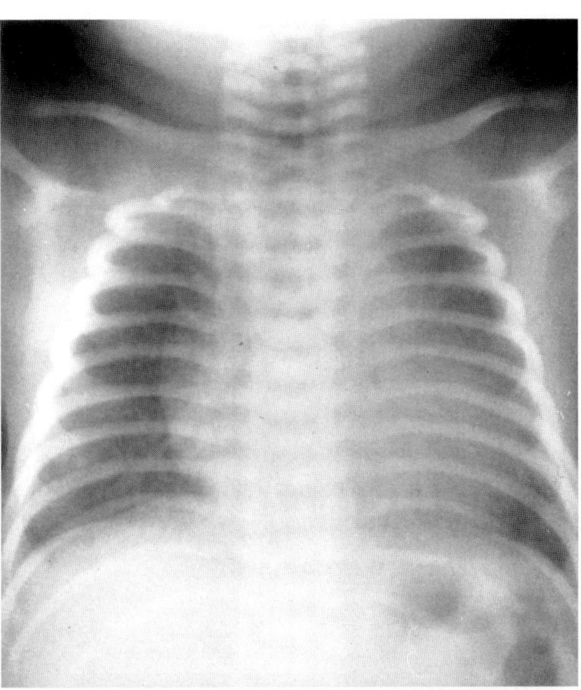

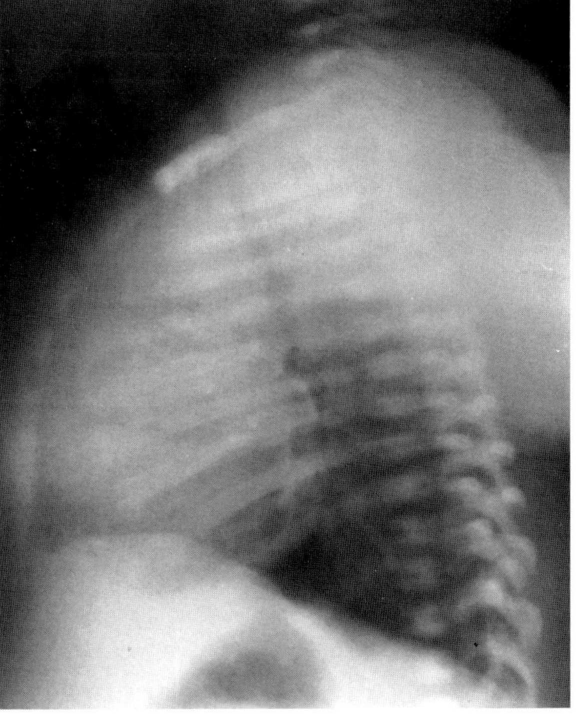

Fig. 3.1 a, b. Normal chest. a On this frontal supine film the mediastinum is wide, and the lateral margins of the heart are obscured by the thymus. The thymic border is rather indistinct, blending into the lung on the left. b On the lateral view, however, the thymus clearly occupies the anterior mediastinum. There is a triangular air space behind the heart

Technical Factors

The method for taking chest films in a neonate differs from that in older children (Chap. 2). The baby remains supine, the film (which is under the baby) is exposed with the X-ray tube above for the anterior-posterior projection. The tube-film distance is 36–40 in. because the equipment must be fixed within the restraints of the isolette and life-support systems (Fig. 3.1). A lateral film may be taken by turning the baby onto its side. It may also be taken as a "cross-table lateral," i.e., with the baby supine and the beam directed through the baby's side. The cross-table lateral technique is particularly important when there is a

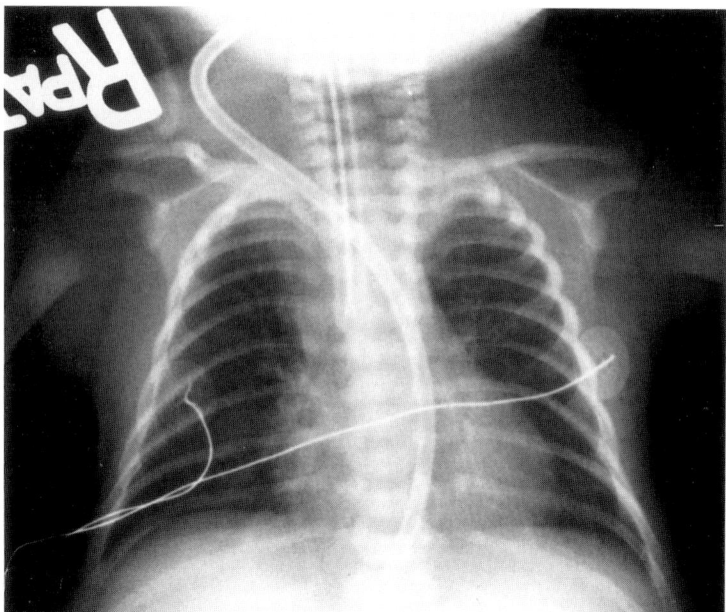

Fig. 3.2. Digital radiograph in a newborn with respiratory distress. The patient has a ventricular peritoneal catheter and an endotracheal tube. What is wrong with the endotracheal tube? The tip is in the right main-stem bronchus

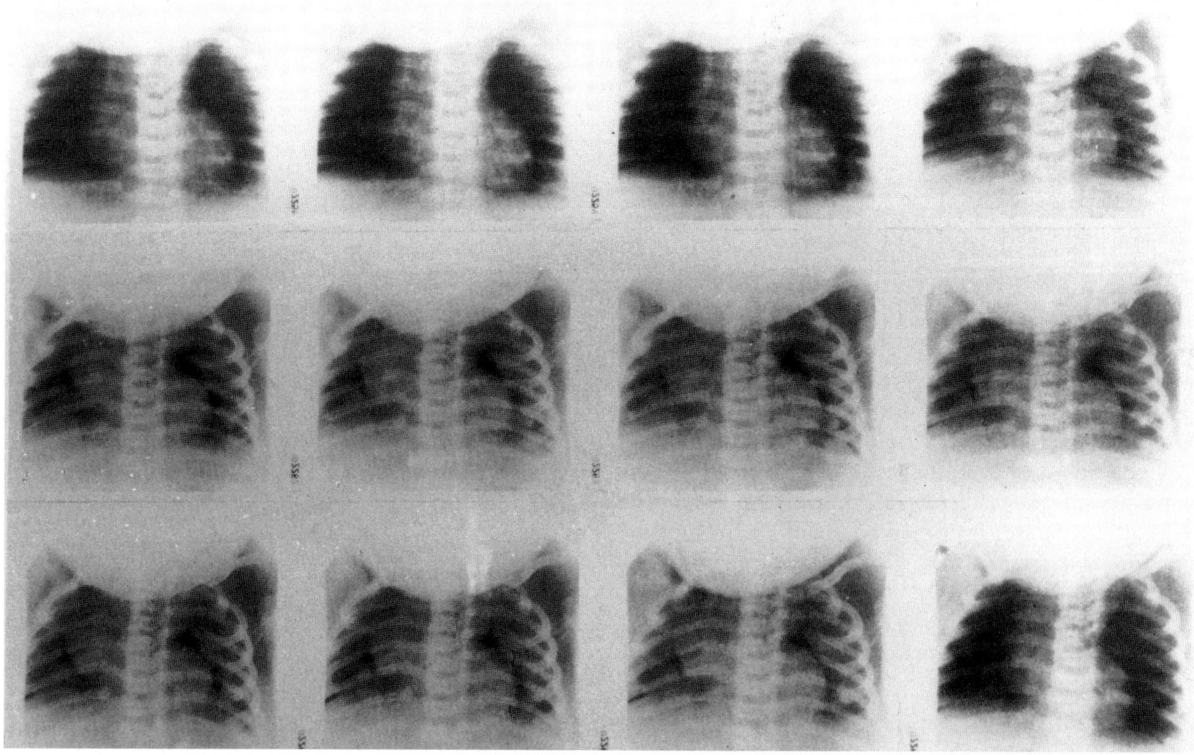

Fig. 3.3. Phases of respiration. Multiple films obtained during a 12-s interval while this infant with a pneumomediastinum was crying. *Top row,* the heart size is normal, and the lungs are well aerated. *Middle row,* during expiration, the lungs are becoming opaque and filling with blood. The hemidiaphragms are elevated, and a pneumomediastinum outlines the heart. *Bottom row,* by the last film the patient is again in the inspiratory phase of respiration cleaning the lungs. (Courtesy of Walter E. Berdon, M.D., and David H. Baker, M.D., Babies and Children's Hospital, New York)

possibility of free air (pneumothorax or pneumomediastinum). Since the child is supine, and air rises, air can be seen under the sternum.

We are now able to perform digital radiography for neonates, a technique which uses a computer to help create the image. This technique diminishes the radiation dose by 50%. The single view neonatal chest film exposes the patient to only 3.4 mr (Fig. 3.2).

On all supine portable films there is inherent magnification of mediastinal structures and absence of the effect of gravity on both the pulmonary vascularity and on fluid within the bowel. Why is this important? (Answers in "Appendix 2".)

Newborns are unique in other ways: (a) a normal neonate breathes at a rate of 30–50 times per minute, and it is therefore more difficult to get a "good inspiratory film"; (b) the trachea in the neonate and young infant is "too long" for the contracted chest in expiration and therefore buckles; and (c) normal neonates have a large anterior mediastinal mass – the thymus, which is accentuated by the anterior-posterior projection (Fig. 3.3).

How then does one determine the normal film? What criteria should be used? The approach is the same as that outlined in Chap. 2; lung volume and patient position, i.e., rotation, must be evaluated first (review "Technical Factors" in Chap. 2). The radiologist's circle must be followed, and since there are multiple films on the sick neonate, strict attention must be paid to the name, date, and time of examination. The ABC approach is important in evaluating the neonatal chest as well.

► *Reed's Rule No. 1:* On every chest film, read the abdominal portion as you would read an abdominal film.

Interpreting the Film

Abdomen

The neonate frequently has an orogastric or nasogastric tube for decompression of a distended stomach or

Fig. 3.4 a, b. Perforation by nasogastric tube. **a** Frontal film shows the tip of the nasogastric tube (*arrow*) in the right side of the chest and/or abdomen. **b** Contrast injected into the nasogastric tube spills into both the pleural and peritoneal spaces

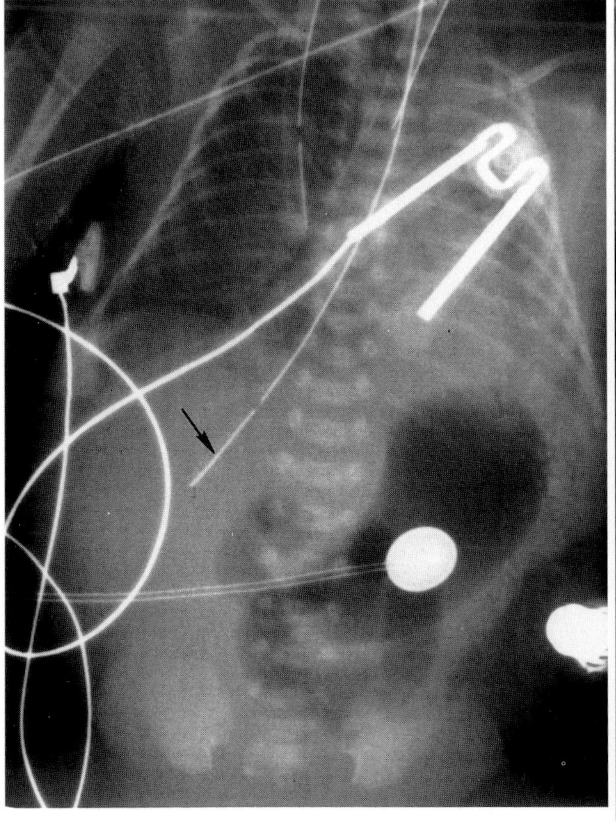
a

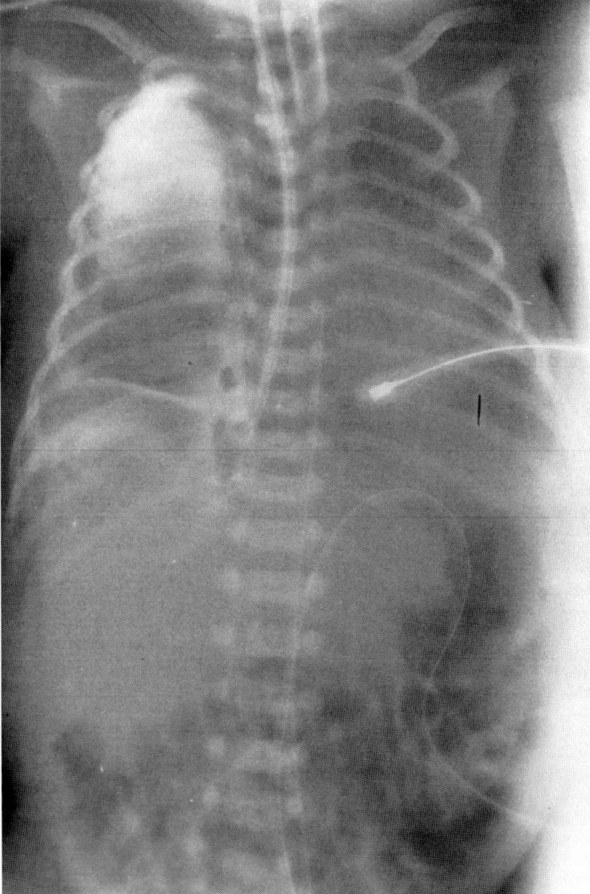
b

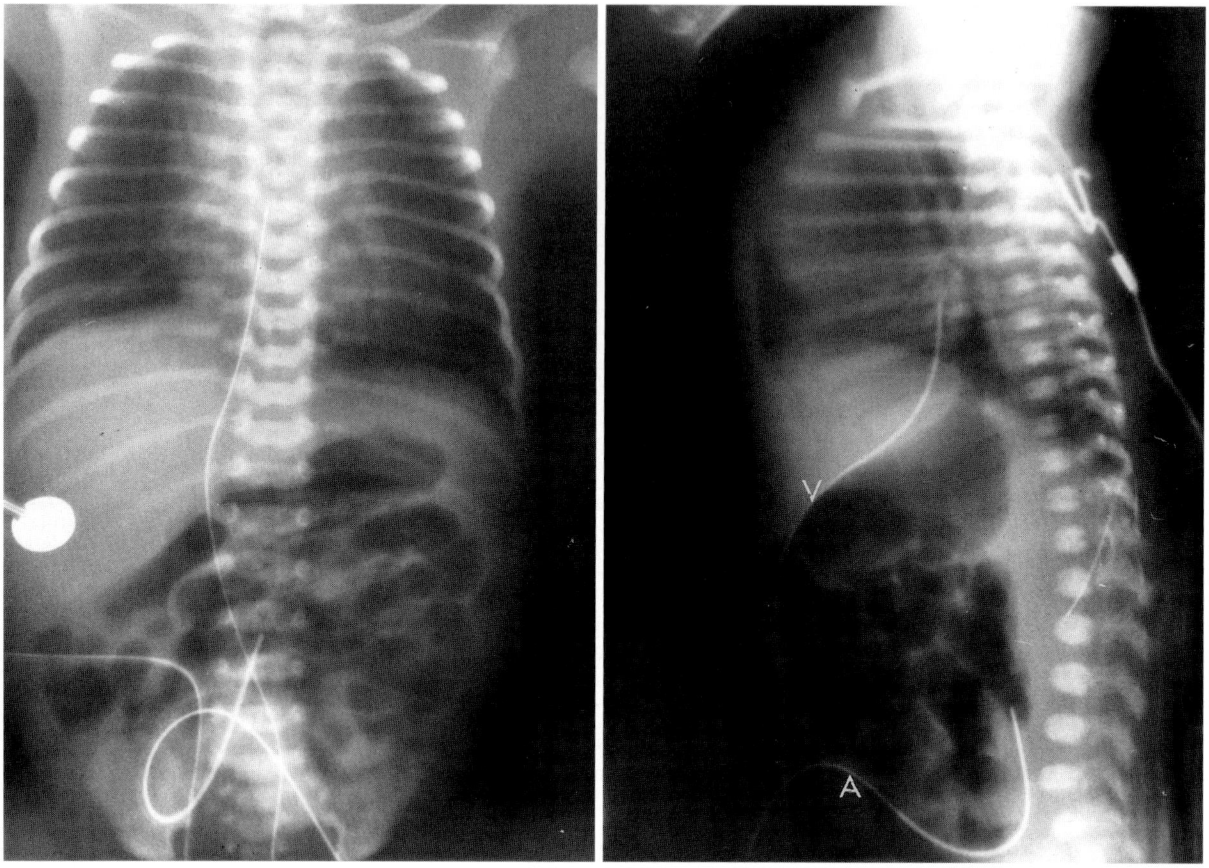

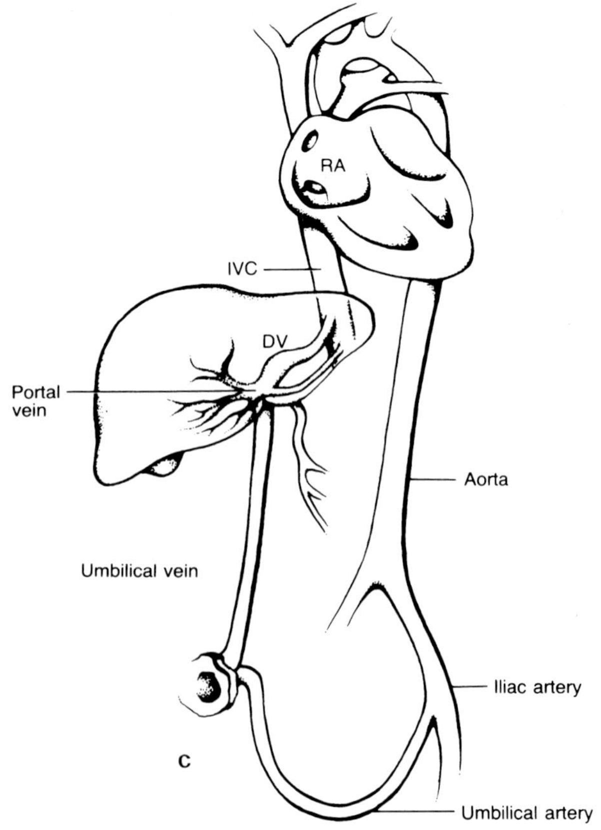

Fig. 3.5 a–c. Catheters and tubes. **a** Frontal radiographs of the chest and abdomen. Two tubes can be seen: one whose tip ends in a vessel within the abdomen, and one in a vessel within the chest. **b**, the lateral film confirms which tube is arterial (*A*) and which is venous (*V*). The anterior catheter starts in the umbilical vein and extends to the liver into the inferior vena cava, via the ductus venosus and into the right atrium. The arterial line dips inferiorly in the iliac artery and then rises posteriorly in the abdominal aorta. **c** Anatomy of the umbilical vessels. A catheter in the umbilical vein crosses the portal vein and enters the ductus venosus on its way to the right atrium. The umbilical artery dips down to join the internal iliac artery then the main aorta. *IVC*, Inferior vena cava; *DV*, ductus venosus; *RA*, right atrium

for feeding. Its position must be noted, as it may be in the esophagus (a good situation for aspiration), deep within the small bowel or, worse, extraluminal (Fig. 3.4). Venous catheters may be either in an umbilical vein, within the portal venous system, in the inferior vena cava, or in the heart. These venous catheters are seen anteriorly as they pass into the left portal vein, through the ductus venosus and into the inferior vena cava, while the umbilical artery catheters are placed posteriorly (Fig. 3.5). The arterial catheter enters through the umbilical artery, proceeds caudad in the iliac vessels, and then ascends through the abdominal aorta. The catheter course is to the left of the midline.

Bones and Soft Tissues

As one continues in the imaginary circle around the periphery of the film, the bones and soft tissues should be considered as important clues to the well-being of a baby. There is little subcutaneous fat in normal neonates but abundance of fat in infants of diabetic mothers. Usually the soft tissues are quite inconspicuous. However, clinical evidence of hydrops fetalis or hypoproteinemia indicates edema (anasarca). A rather common soft tissue density is an umbilical clamp and the residual umbilical cord. It may project as a "mass" in the midabdomen.

Because the neonatal radiograph is the first opportunity for detecting congenital abnormalities, be sure to check the bones for such abnormalities as hemivertebrae, absence of the clavicles, and fractures secondary to trauma of the birth process. The bones also provide a clue to a possible congenital infection (TORCHS infections: *to*xoplasmosis, *r*ubella, *cytomegalic* inclusion disease, *h*erpes, and *s*yphilis).

Chest

Airway

Again, the parameters used to evaluate the extrathoracic and intrathoracic airway are patency, position and size (Fig. 3.6).

▶ *Reed's Rule No. 3:* The airway should be visible on all chest films. To examine the airway in detail, it is frequently useful to use your finger as a pointer so that each structure receives your undivided attention.

In assessing *patency* one should see the airway from the oropharynx and nasopharynges to the right and left main-stem bronchi. The baby with an obstructed nasopharynx presents with severe respiratory distress because it breathes primarily through the nose. The only part of the airway not seen with plain film is the nasal airway. This is best seen with CT. The CT demonstrates not only the various sites of nasal obstruction but also the kind of obstruction – bony or membranous (see Chap. 2).

Regarding *position*, remember that the trachea is *not* a midline structure (the carina projects adjacent to the right pedicles). Buckling of the trachea is normal (see Fig. 3.6).

Airway *size* is difficult to ascertain, as it is a dynamic structure that changes in caliber. However, if on all views of the airway it is persistently small, further investigation is necessary. It is *normal* for neonates and young infants to occasionally have some air in the esophagus (not so in older children).

Sick neonates often require an endotracheal tube. It is crucial to tell the clinician about the relationship of the tube to the carina because these tubes can move. If they slip into the main-stem bronchus on either side (more frequently on the right, as it is a straighter drop), obstructive emphysema on one side with atelectasis on the other may occur (Fig. 3.7). The ideal position of the endotracheal tube is at the level of the inferior margins of the clavicles.

The Mediastinum

The heart and mediastinal structures demand attention as to *position, size,* and *contour.*

The *position* is easily determined on a nonrotated film. The aortic arch frequently cannot be seen in a neonate, and its position must be inferred by the position of the carina. On a normal study the carina overlies the right pedicles, and the aortic arch is therefore positioned on the left. Similarly, a right-sided aortic arch may be inferred if the position of the carina is midline or to the left. A right aortic arch should alert the physician to the possibility of congenital heart disease and/or a vascular ring. The thymus constitutes the major portion of the mediastinal silhouette in a normal newborn (see Fig. 3.1). It may extend from the lung apex to the diaphragmatic surfaces, be insinuated into the minor fissure on the right (giving a "sail sign"), be bilaterally symmetrical or predominantly one-sided. The normal thymus is situated in the anterior mediastinum and never "pushes" on the airway or any other intrathoracic structure. Because the thymus is so ubiquitous and large, evaluating cardiac size becomes more difficult in the neonate and young in-

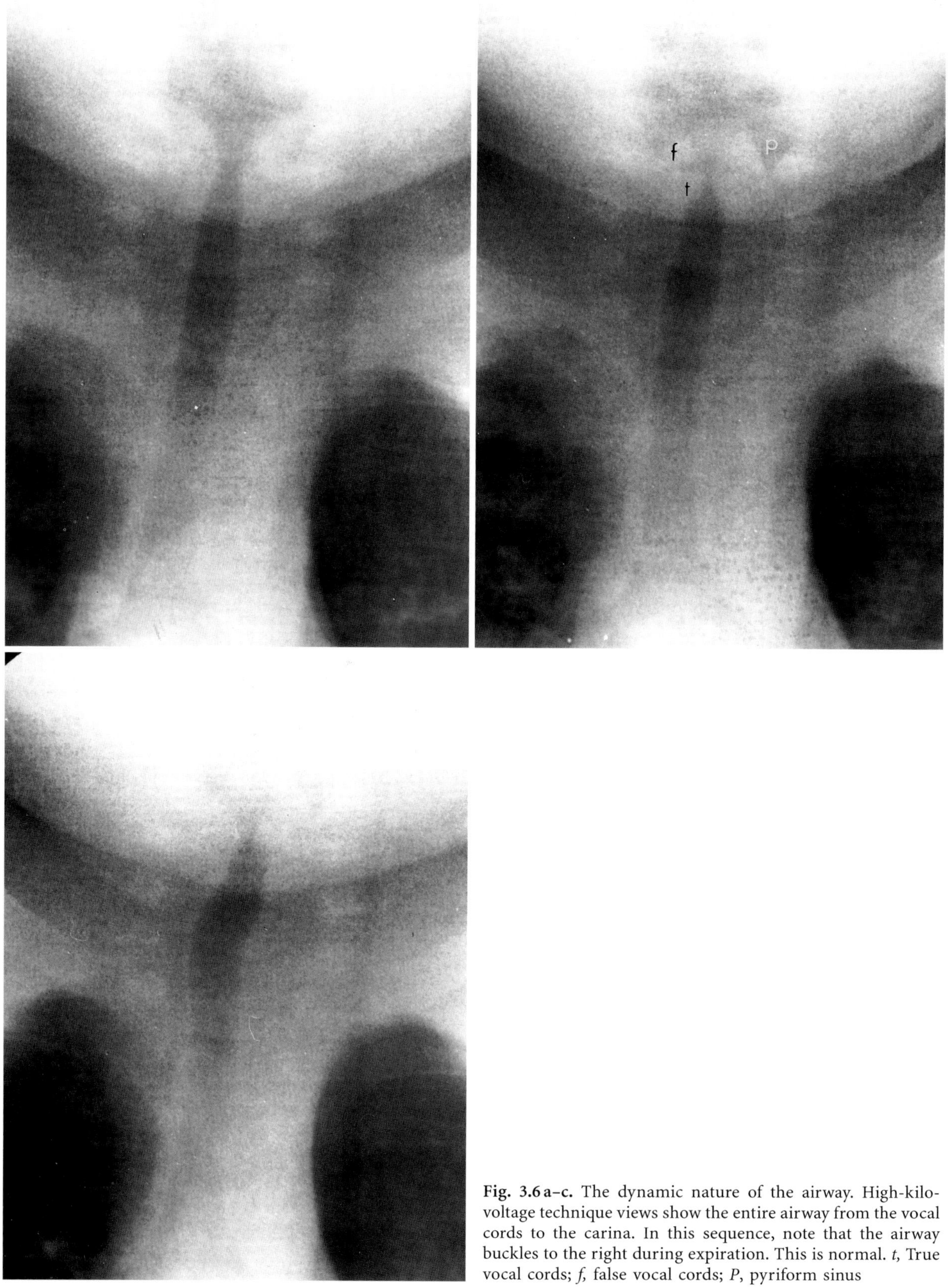

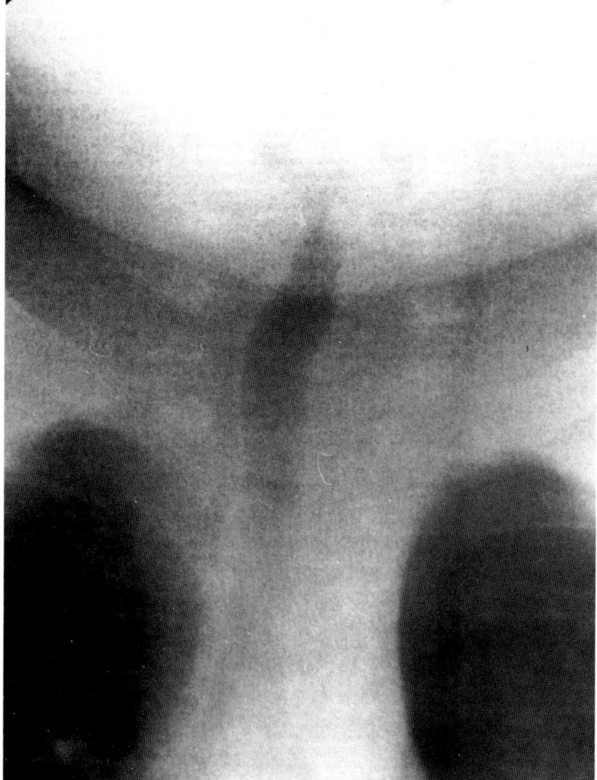

Fig. 3.6 a–c. The dynamic nature of the airway. High-kilovoltage technique views show the entire airway from the vocal cords to the carina. In this sequence, note that the airway buckles to the right during expiration. This is normal. *t*, True vocal cords; *f*, false vocal cords; *P*, pyriform sinus

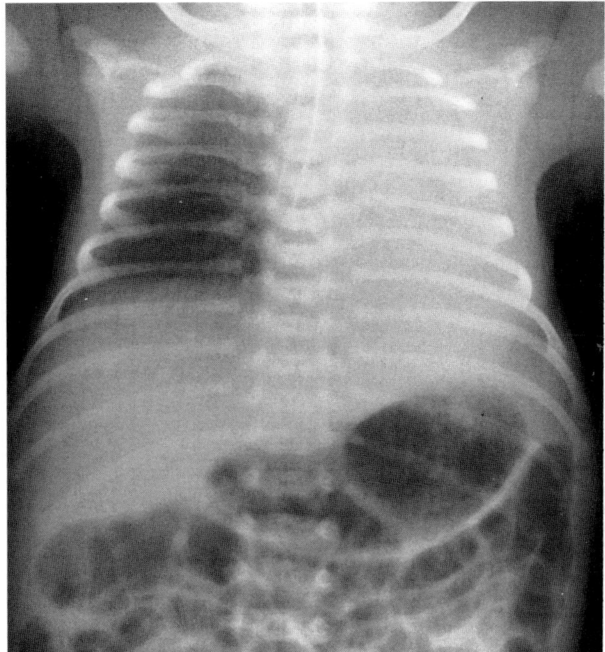

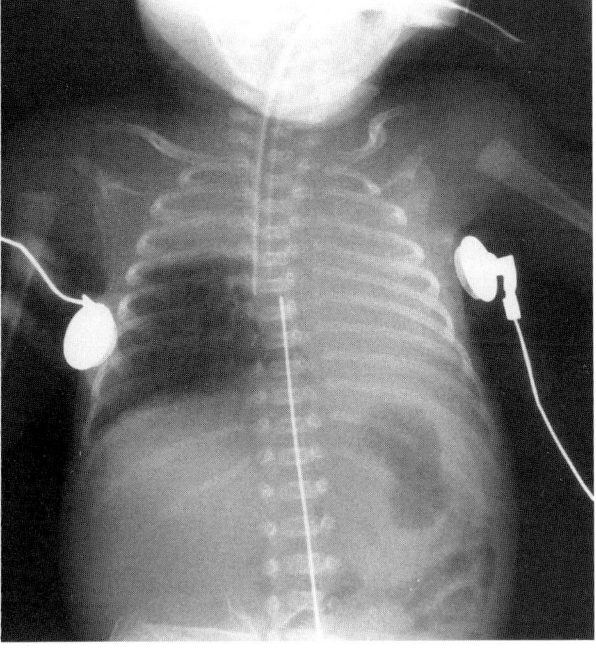

Fig. 3.7 a, b. Endotracheal tube. **a** This is an infant with a tube in the right main-stem bronchus. The left lung is atelectatic. **b** The endotracheal tube in this child is in the same position as in **a**. He has both right upper lobe atelectasis and left lung collapse. The airway is so small that a tube plus normal secretions can cause obstruction or ball valve effect in any lobe

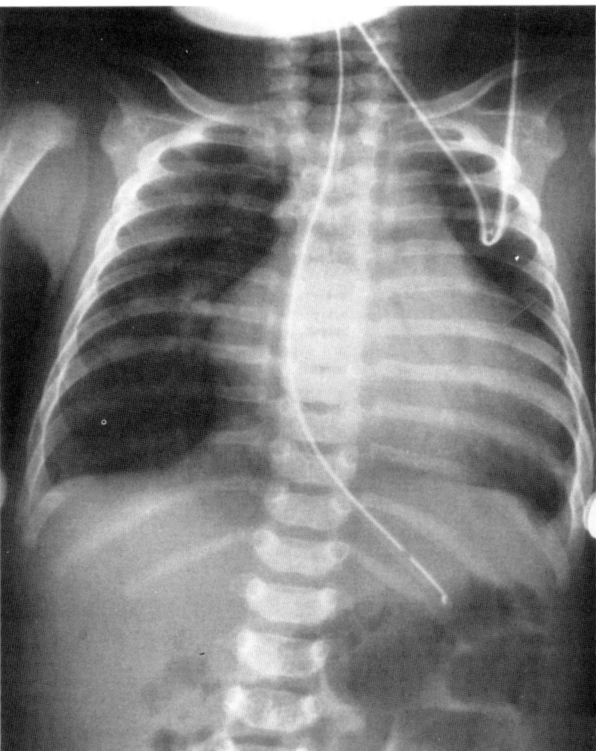

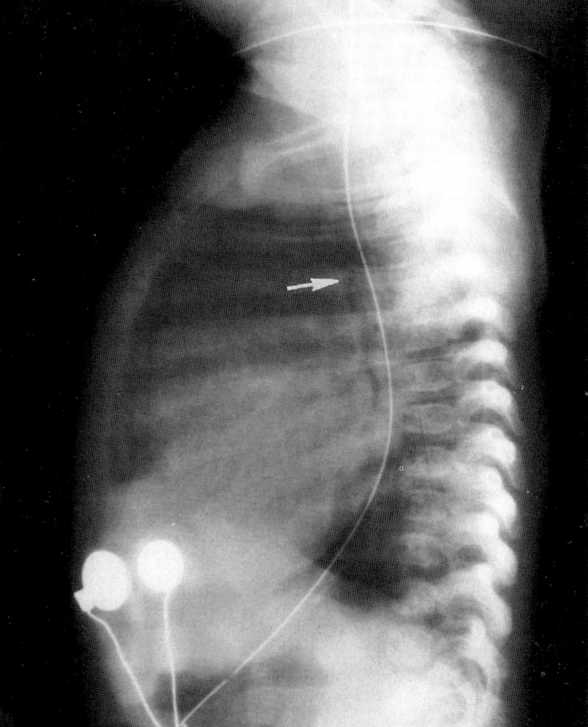

Fig. 3.8 a, b. Cardiac enlargement. **a** Frontal radiograph reveals a nasogastric tube in the stomach. The heart occupies some of the right hemithorax and extends to the left lateral chest wall. The density behind the heart is atelectasis secondary to impingement on the left main-stem bronchus by the large heart. **b** On the lateral film, see how the heart extends posterior behind the airway, almost reaching the spine. The airway is pulled backward (*arrow*) ▼

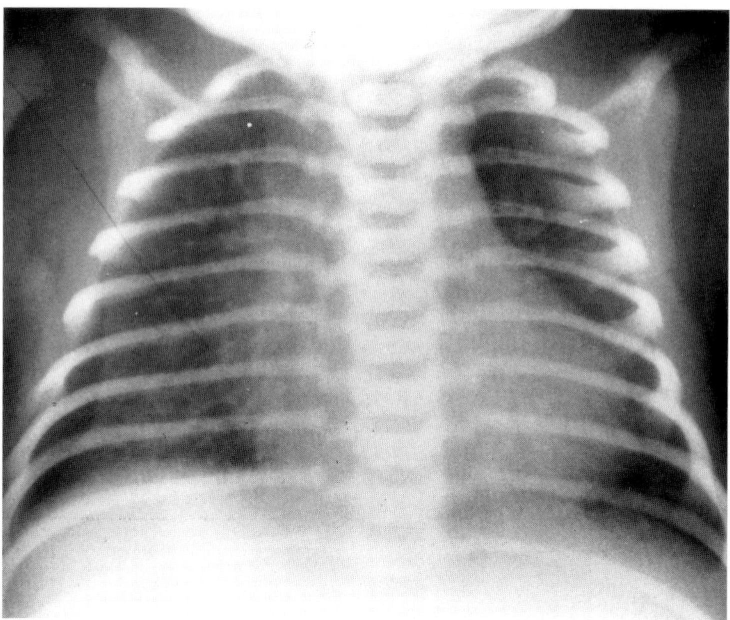

Fig. 3.9. Skin fold. The apparent pneumothorax on the right is actually a skin fold, easily determined when one sees that the margin does not conform to that of a collapsed lobe or lung. If uncertain, repeat the film after moving the baby to a different position, for example, decubitus view

fant (the thymus may be seen in some children up to the age of 4–5 years).

Size is the second parameter used in evaluating the mediastinal silhouette.

► *Reed's Rule No. 4:* A mass must be seen in two planes, i.e., if the heart is really large, it must appear large in two planes.

If the heart is large, it should appear so in both *frontal* and *lateral views.* Since the thymus is in the anterior mediastinum, it is difficult to evaluate heart size on the frontal film. The lateral roentgenograph is most valuable in this regard (Fig. 3.8). The retrocardiac air space should be seen, and a line drawn from the carina straight down to the diaphragm should not intersect the heart (see Chap. 2).

The *contour* of the heart, the third parameter, is widely considered to be helpful in determining the specific nature of congenital heart defects. A narrow cardiac base is described in transposition of the great vessels and a "boot-shaped" heart in tetralogy of Fallot. Clinically these signs may not be very important as echocardiography most often can give a specific diagnosis. However, in infants as in older children, pulmonary vascular changes may give the clue to the general category of the cardiac disease, for example, a left-to-right shunt. In contrast to the older child, the pulmonary vessels of a newborn can be seen at the hila and only in the medial third of the lungs. Vessels should be hard to find in the lateral two-thirds of the normal lung. When there is vascular congestion secondary to congestive heart failure or overcirculation from a left-to-right shunt, the vascularity becomes much easier to see in the lateral two-thirds of the lung. It is much more difficult, however, to detect decreased pulmonary vascularity (as found in severe pulmonic stenosis or atresia).

Deceptive Shadows

One of the most common mistakes is diagnosing a pneumothorax which in reality is only a skin fold (Fig. 3.9). This error can be avoided by realizing that the border of the fold does not conform to the position that a collapsed lobe or lung would assume. In addition, the skin fold is frequently seen extending off into the axilla. If you are uncertain, a repeat film with the baby in another position is helpful, or perform a cross-table lateral.

Another important finding on a neonatal chest film is the "ductus bump" seen best on the frontal view at the level of the pulmonary artery (Fig. 3.10). This is formed by the superimposition of the main and left pulmonary artery on the patent ductus arteriosus, and it usually is not visible by day 3. It cannot be seen on

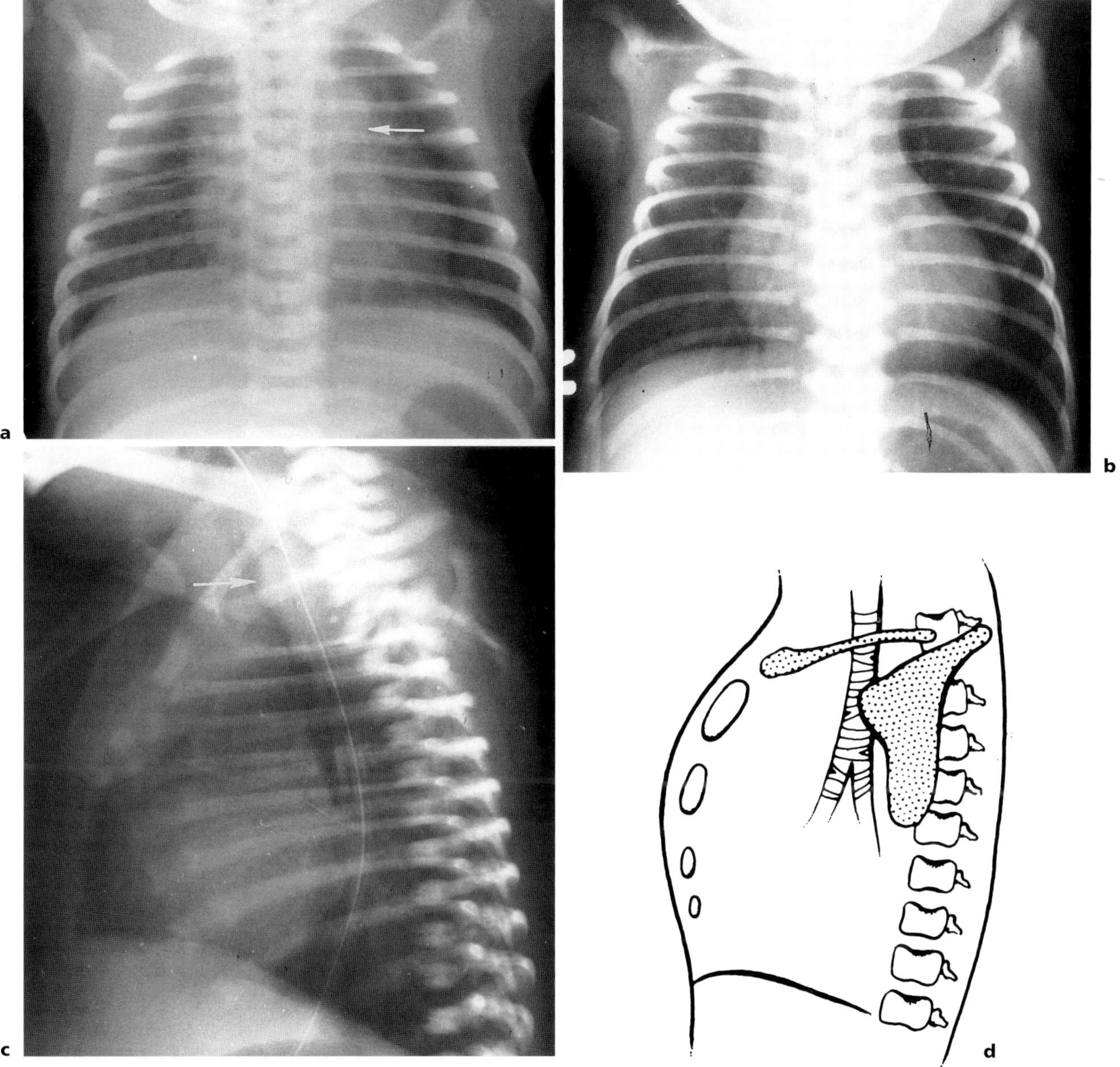

Fig. 3.10 a–d. Pseudomasses. **a, b** "Ductal bump." Frontal views of the chest in an infant 1 day old (**a**) and 3 days old (**b**). The "bump" (*arrow*) in the upper mediastinum is no longer visible. It was caused by the superimposition of the main pulmonary artery, left pulmonary artery, and ductus arteriosus. The latter gradually retracts, and the mass disappears. **c** This lateral film shows another pseudomass. The trachea looks as if it is being compressed posteriorly by a mass (*arrow*). **d** In fact, the "mass" is caused by superimposition of the scapula over the airway

the lateral film. The scapula, however, may create a pseudomass in this region.

The following summarizes the assessment of the neonatal chest and also lists questions to ask oneself about each film and specific parameters for evaluating the airway, mediastinal silhouette, and lungs. Remember the ABC's and Reed's Rule No. 1. General considerations are:

- Lung volume: Are the lungs hyperinflated?
- Position of patient: Is the patient rotated? Why?
- Exposure: Is the film properly exposed? How do you know?

Specific factors include:

- Airway
  - Patency
  - Position
  - Size
- Mediastinal silhouette
  - Position
  - Size
  - Contour
- Lungs (see Table 3.1)
  - Volume
  - Pulmonary density
  - Vascularity

An Approach to Common Neonatal Abnormalities

Correlation of the generalized lung volume (increased, decreased, normal) with type of pulmonary opacity leads to the differential diagnoses of neonatal lung disease (Table 3.1). Since the lung volume has already been assessed, differentiating the various forms of pulmonary opacity is the next task. You should ask yourself the following questions:

- Are the opacities uniform and homogeneous (Fig. 3.11)?
- Do the opacities correspond to the distribution of blood vessels or bronchi (Fig. 3.12)?
- Do they involve the whole lung or a portion of the lung (Fig. 3.13)?

Diseases with Generalized Increase in Lung Volume

Increased lung volume may be the first and only clue to significant parenchymal or cardiovascular abnormalities in the neonate. From a teleological point of view, the lungs are hyperexpanded as the infant tries desperately to adapt to its new environment and cannot oxygenate optimally. Any of the aspiration syndromes (discussed below), pneumonias, or congenital heart diseases may present with relatively clear lungs and hyperexpansion. However, there are frequently opacities within the lung parenchyma or other clues, such as pulmonary vascularity and cardiac size (see above), that point to the correct diagnosis.

Two conditions can be readily anticipated from the changes the fetus undergoes from intrauterine to extrauterine life. First, the neonate may not be able to clear all the fetal fluid from its lungs (see Fig. 3.12). Since one-third of the fluid exits through the tracheobronchial tree and is expelled when the thorax is compressed in the birth canal, tracheobronchial tree obstruction or a cesarean section (in which the baby's chest is not compressed) may lead to retained fetal fluid – the wet lung syndrome, radiographically. These babies have increased lung volume and strandy opacities emanating from the hila that follow the course of the tracheobronchial tree (with the vessels and lymphatics). Pleural fluid may also be present; it outlines the lung fissures. Retained fetal fluid usually clears within 24–48 h (transient tachypnea of the newborn is another name for this entity).

The second abnormality that can result from the birth sequence is aspiration (see Fig. 3.13). The most serious kind is meconium aspiration. A fetus passes meconium in utero because of some perinatal or parturitional stress. At the first breath this viscous material may be inhaled. The radiograph shows increased lung volume, but this time there are *patchy* opacities throughout both lungs. Meconium in the tracheobronchial tree and lung parenchyma presents a striking picture (see Fig. 3.13).

Early hyperexpansion of the neonatal lung may herald a localized infiltrate, such as a pneumonic consolidation that does not become visible for a few days (Fig. 3.14). In a neonate with congenital heart disease, the first radiographic sign may well be increased lung volume only. As pulmonary resistance decreases, signs of a left-to-right shunt or cardiac enlargement become evident. It is important to note that a large heart does not necessarily mean primary congenital heart disease; anemia, asphyxia, and other high-output states may cause cardiomegaly as well.

Table 3.1. Differential diagnosis of lung pathology based on lung volume and type of density

Lung volume	Type of density	Disease considerations
Increased (generalized) (first days)	None	Aspiration syndromes Congenital heart disease
	Multiple course areas (strandy densities following bronchovascular pattern)	Meconium aspiration Retained fetal fluid (TTN)
	Localized	Pneumonia
	Increased pulmonary vascularity	Congenital heart disease
Increased (generalized) >1st week–months	Fine, lacelike, strandy lines or cysts	Pulmonary interstitial emphysema (PIE) Bronchopulmonary dysplasia (BPD)
	None	Chronic aspiration, cystic fibrosis, congenital heart disease
Normal or decreased	Homogeneous fine granular (ground-glass) density with air bronchograms	Hyaline membrane disease (RDS and HMD) Group B β-hemolytic streptococcal pneumonia
Variable	Variable	Persistent fetal circulation Group B β-hemolytic streptococcal infection
Localized increase in volume	Air-filled	Lobar emphysema
	Fluid-filled	Bronchial obstruction (lobar emphysema initially, congenital cyst, bronchogenic cyst)
	Air and/or fluid filled	Cystic adenomatoid malformation

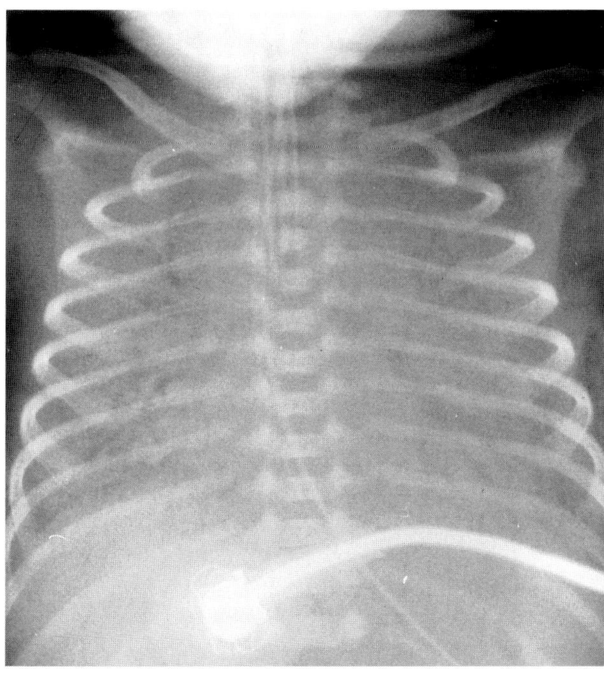

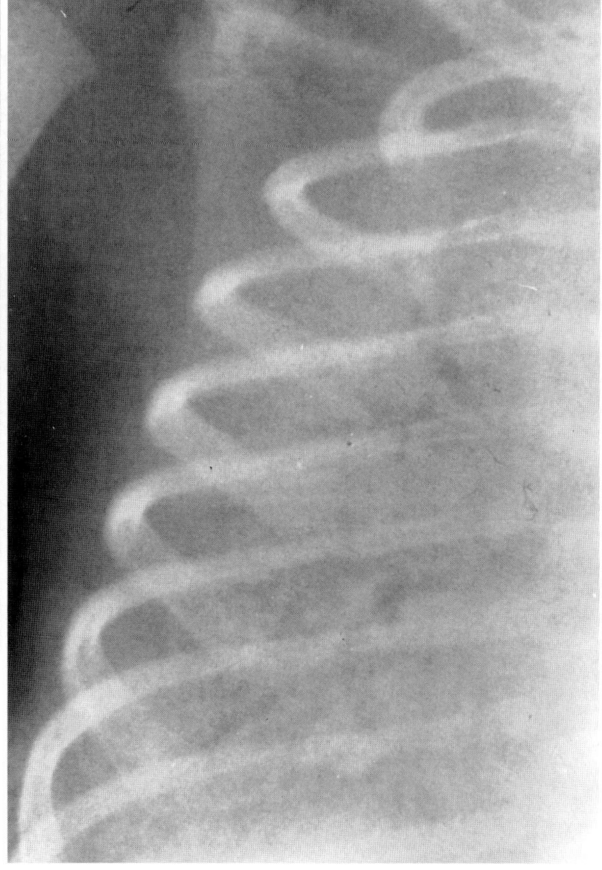

Fig. 3.11 a, b. Hyaline membrane disease. **a** Frontal radiograph of a premature infant demonstrates ground-glass appearance of both lungs with a normal volume. The endotracheal tube is at the carina. **b** Frontal magnified view of the granular appearance caused by the atelectatic surfactant-deficient alveoli (terminal air sacs)

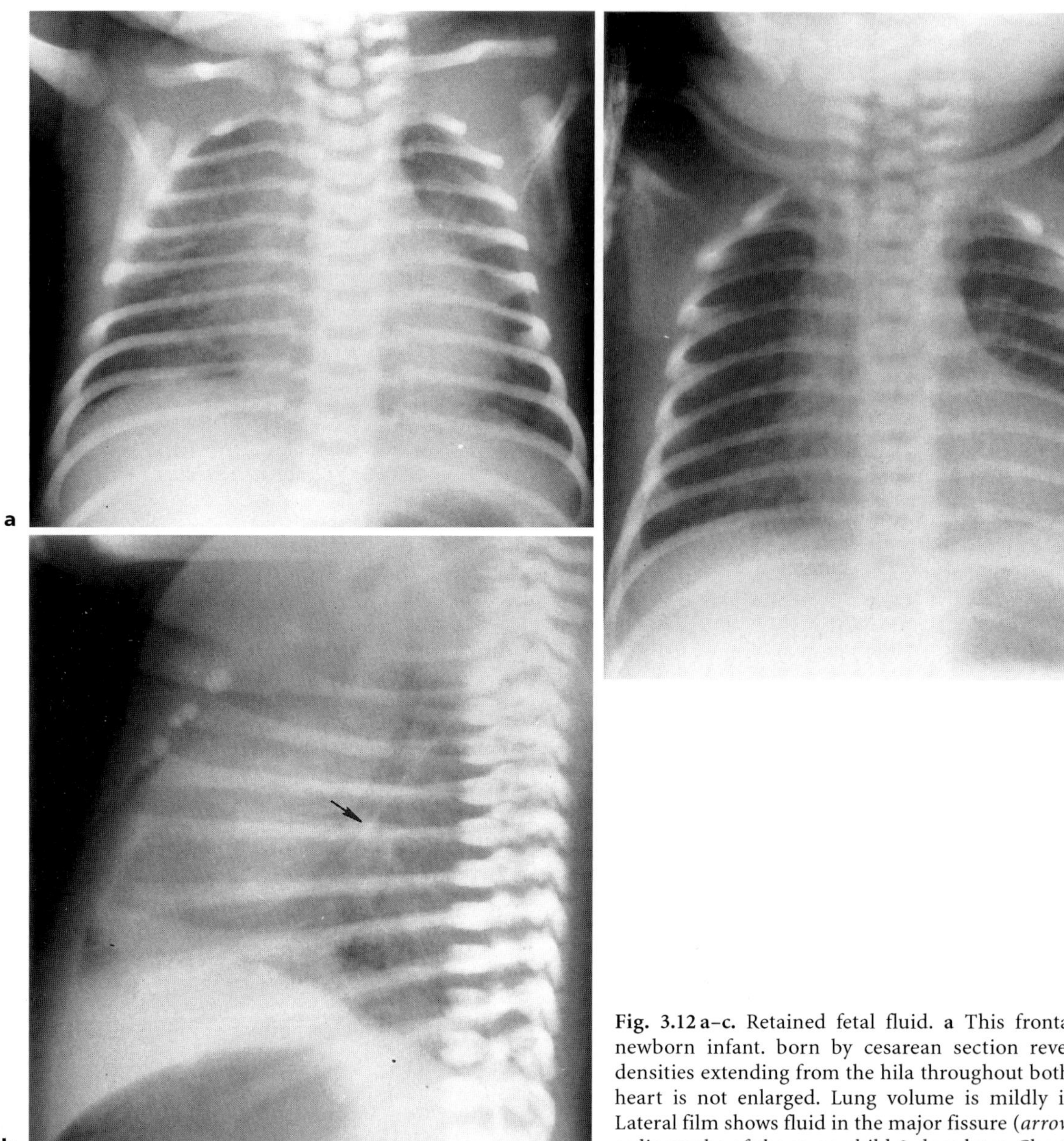

Fig. 3.12 a–c. Retained fetal fluid. **a** This frontal film of a newborn infant. born by cesarean section reveals strandy densities extending from the hila throughout both lungs. The heart is not enlarged. Lung volume is mildly increased. **b** Lateral film shows fluid in the major fissure (*arrow*). **c** Frontal radiographs of the same child 2 days later. Chest is normal

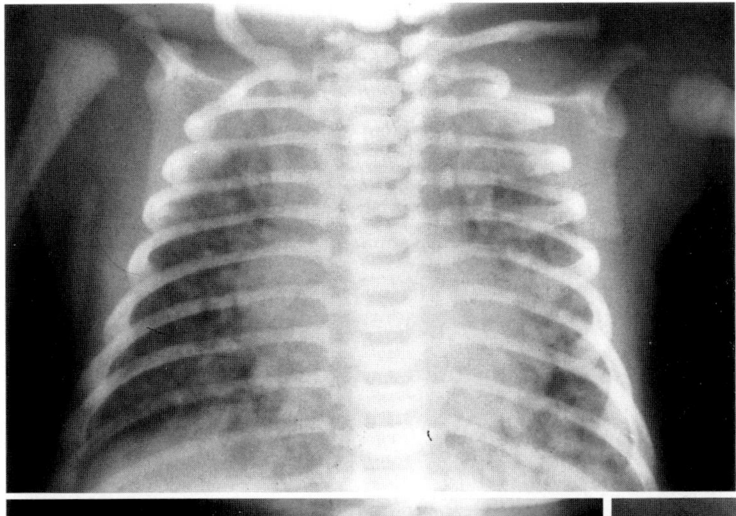
a

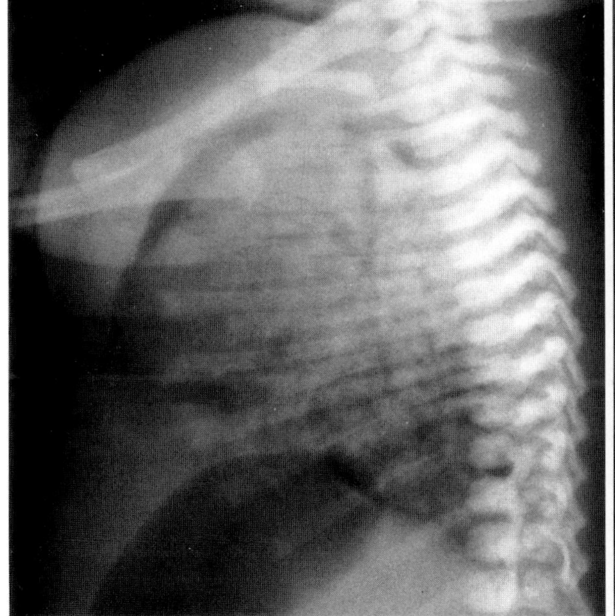
b

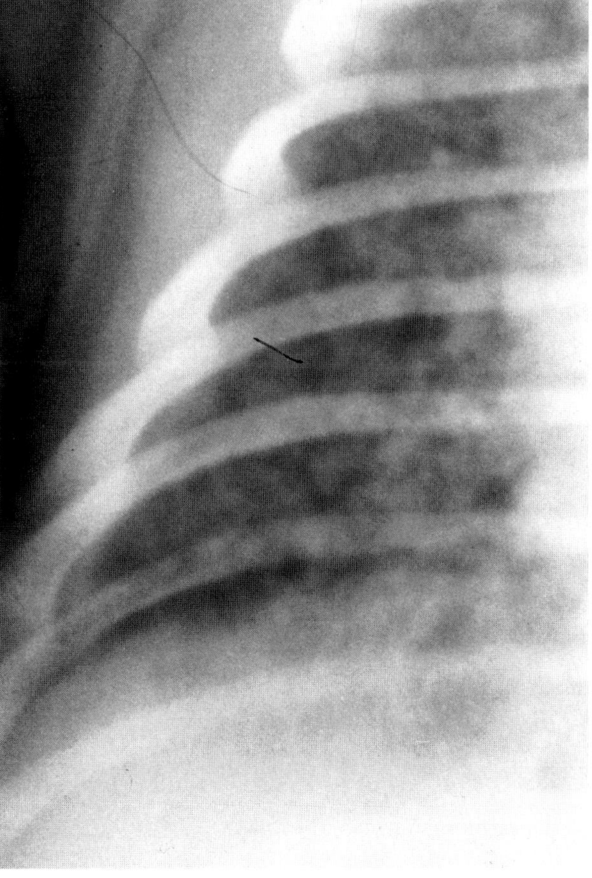
c

Fig. 3.13 a–c. Meconium aspiration. a Frontal radiograph shows coarse, globular, rounded densities dispersed throughout the lungs. Lung volume is increased. b Lateral view showing hyperexpansion and coarseness throughout the lungs. The heart may be enlarged (although not in this case) in meconium aspiration secondary to hypoxia. c Magnified view of a portion of lung shows the course of globular infiltrate

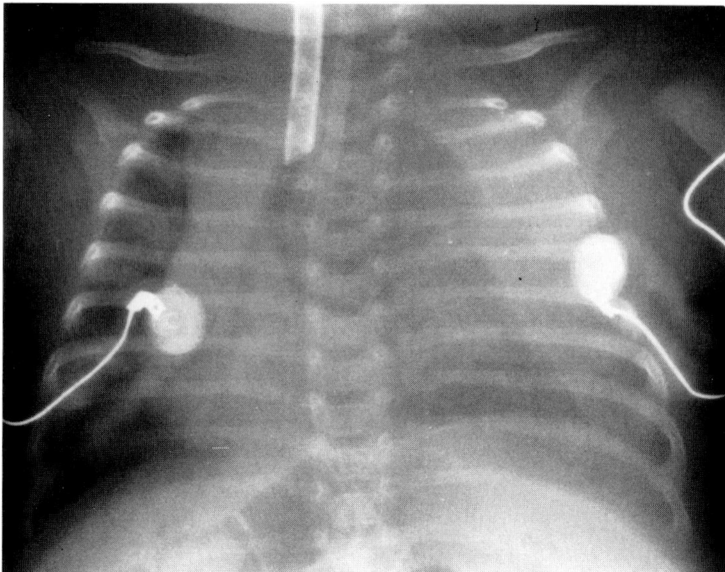

Fig. 3.14. Pneumonia. This frontal view of a 2-day-old shows extensive opacity in the left side of the chest due to both an infiltrate and a large pleural effusion. The mediastinum is shifted to the right. Group B β-hemolytic *Streptococcus* was the offending organism

Diseases with Normal or Decreased Lung Volume

The most common disease in this group is hyaline membrane disease. Unfortunately, group B β-hemolytic streptococcal pneumonia may appear indistinguishable from it. In both diseases homogeneous, fine opacities appear throughout the lungs with accompanying air bronchograms. This sign has been described as a "ground-glass appearance" (see Fig. 3.11). In hyaline membrane disease these changes are related to surfactant deficiency; therefore the terminal air spaces tend to collapse, resulting in a low normal to decreased lung volume. The collapse of the terminal air spaces accounts for the fine, homogeneous granularity. Remember to look for air bronchograms. You must see the granularity or white dots all the way out the edge of the lungs to make a diagnosis of hyaline membrane

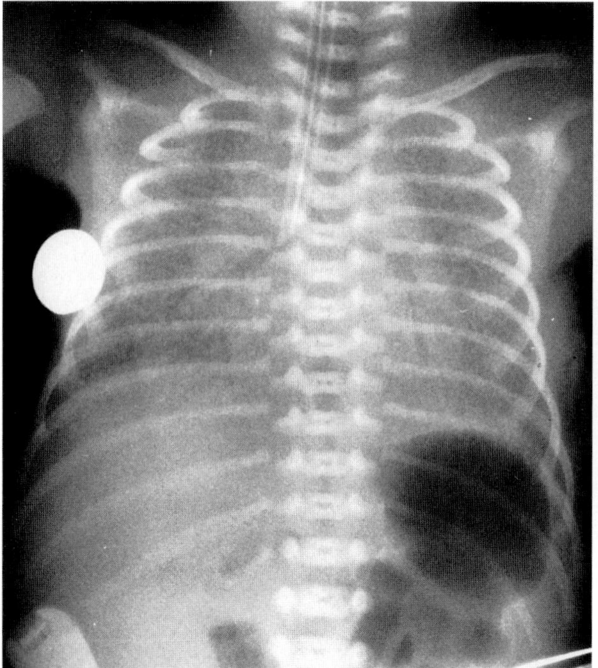

a

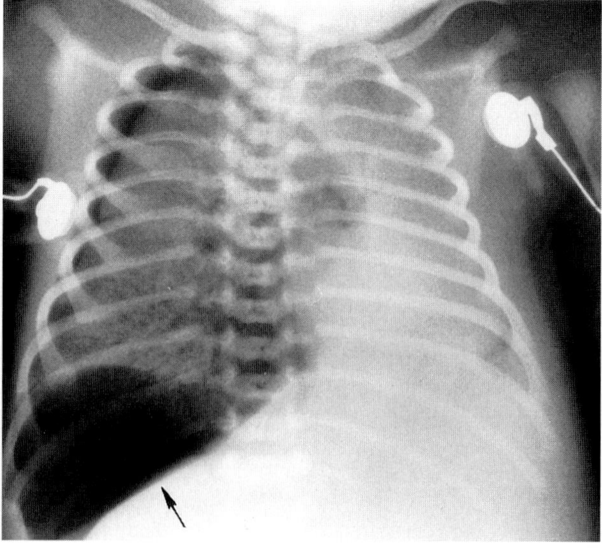

b

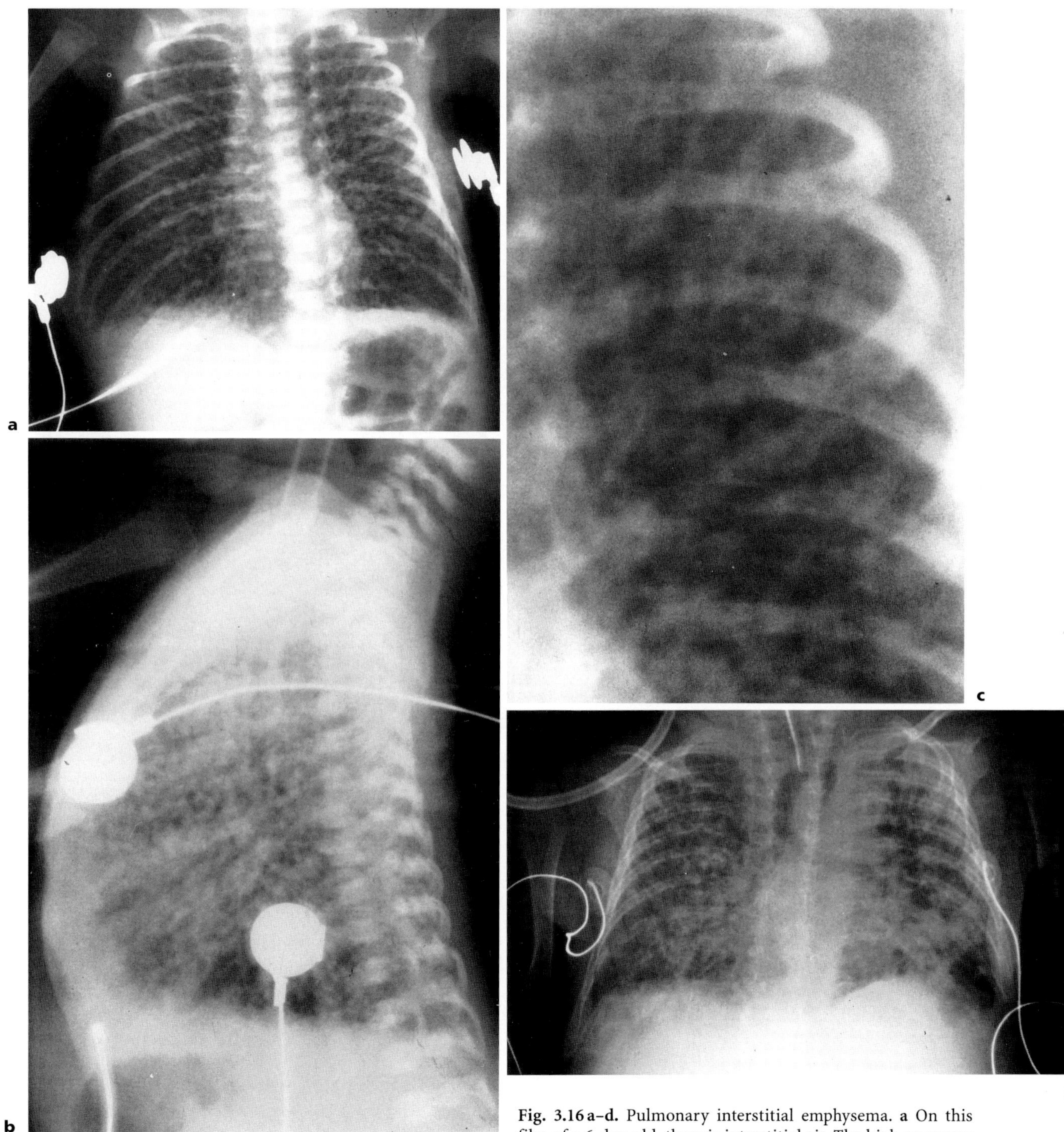

◀ **Fig. 3.15 a, b.** Complications of hyaline membrane disease and ventilation. This 1-day-old infant, with hyaline membrane (**a**) disease suddenly became very ill (**b**). The right lung has collapsed, and the mediastinum has shifted to the left, indicating a tension pneumothorax on the right. The large air space filling the right thoracic cavity is inverting the right hemidiaphragm (*arrows*)

Fig. 3.16 a–d. Pulmonary interstitial emphysema. **a** On this film of a 6-day-old, there is interstitial air. The high pressures necessary to ventilate the child caused air to leak into the interstitium. This may compress the bronchus and, in fact, hinder aeration. **b** The lateral view showing interstitial air as small black dots. This complication of mechanical ventilation occurs when high pressures are used and ventilation is prolonged. **c** Magnified image of "black dots." **d** A digital image of another patient with similar disease demonstrates the pulmonary interstitial emphysema at a lower radiation dose

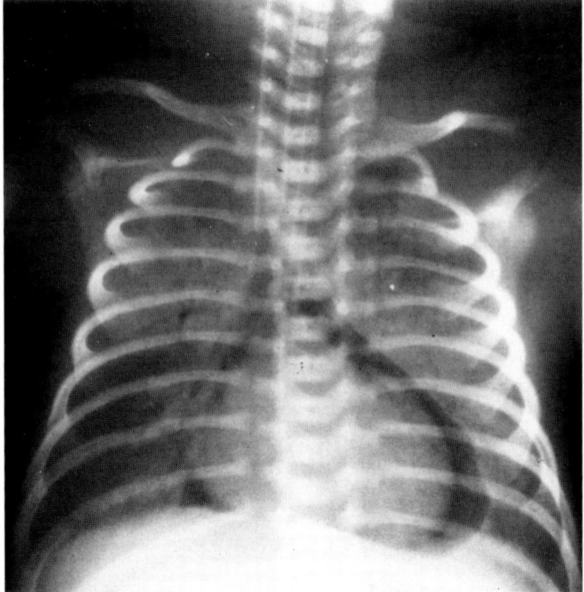

Fig. 3.17. Pneumopericardium. A frontal radiograph shows air around the heart. The air stops at the left aortic-pulmonary window where the pericardium attaches (*arrow*)

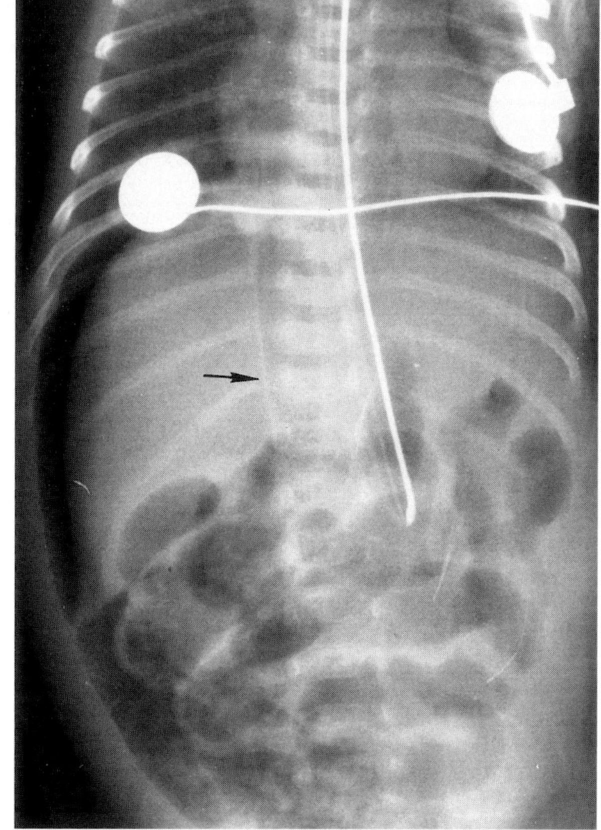

Fig. 3.18. Pneumoperitoneum dissect down the mediastinum ▶ into the peritoneal cavity. On this decubitus roentgenograph with the baby's right side up, air is noted above the liver. The falciform ligament is seen (*arrow*)

disease. Prematurity and maternal diabetes are two of the more common underlying etiological factors predisposing to this disease.

Mechanical ventilation often causes air to leak into the interstitium of the lungs (pulmonary interstitial emphysema), into the mediastinum (pneumomediastinum), into the pleural space (pneumothorax), and occasionally into the pericardium (pneumopericardium; Figs. 3.15–3.17). Rarely, air dissects into the peritoneal cavity (Fig. 3.18).

One of the most difficult conditions for the novice to recognize is the pneumomediastinum. Graphically, three different densities or shades of gray are visible on the frontal film (Fig. 3.19). The first is the white opacity of the heart. The second – the pneumomediastinum – is a radiolucent black area lateral to the heart and medial to the lungs that may elevate the thymus laterally and upward. The third is a gray opacity representing lung compressed laterally by trapped air.

A pneumomediastinum may be very small and may be difficult to differentiate from a pneumopericardium (see Fig. 3.17). When a pneumopericardium is present, separation of the aorta from the pulmonary vein is clearly seen on both frontal and lateral views, since the pericardium attaches at the base of the great vessels. In addition, the pericardial membrane may be visible when there is air on both sides of it.

Air dissects upward into the subcutaneous tissues of the neck (unusual in a neonate) and downward through the same diaphragmatic hiatus as the aorta and esophagus, resulting in a pneumoperitoneum (see Fig. 3.18).

The most important air leak, however, is that of a pneumothorax. Pneumothoraces are formed by rupture of air through the overlying pleura or by rupture of a subpleural bleb (see Fig. 3.15). Once there is a rupture of air by whatever mechanism into the pleural space, the lung begins to collapse. Since the infant is recumbent, an anterior and medial air space may ap-

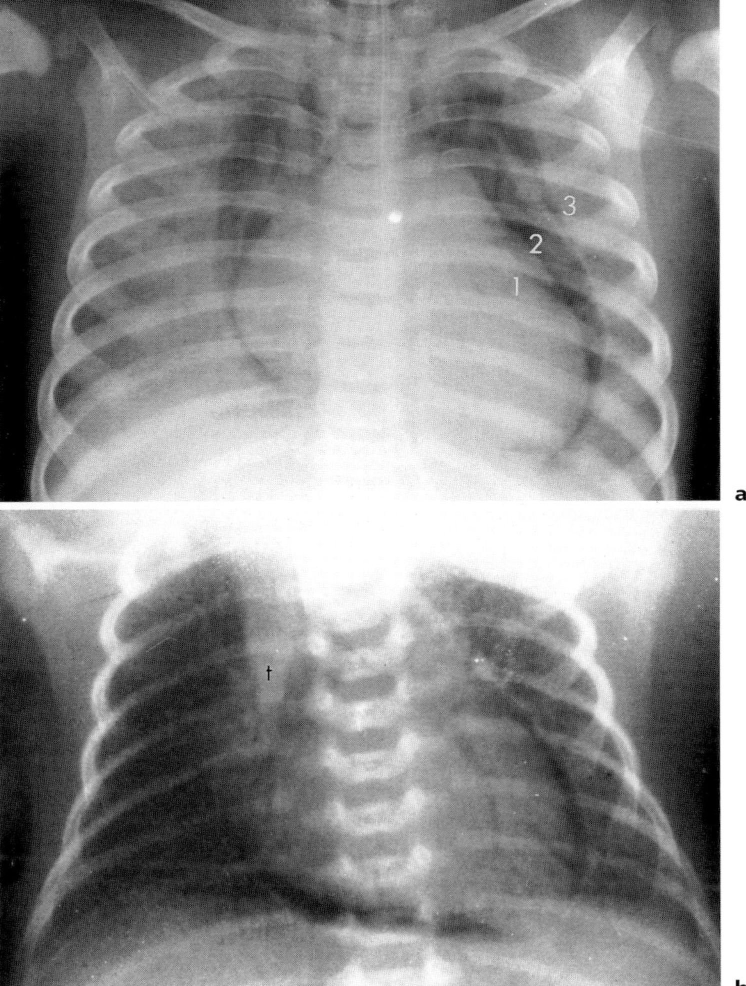

Fig. 3.19 a, b. Pneumomediastinum. a This frontal view of the chest reveals three densities: *1*, heart; *2*, pneumomediastinum; and *3*, compressed lung. b Pneumomediastinum in another child reveals the thymus (*T*) is elevated and outlined with air

pear first or may outline the inferior lung margins. *Look* for the pleural margins of the lobes. Beware of skin folds that may simulate pleura (see Fig. 3.9). As the quantity of air increases and the lung collapses to its fullest, i.e., the elastic limit is reached, the pressure builds up and a *tension pneumothorax* develops. This results in: (a) shift of the mediastinum away from the midline and (b) flattening or even eversion of the diaphragm on the affected side. (If by chance the pneumothorax is bilateral, there may be no or less mediastinal shift, but then the heart is compressed and appears smaller.) At first, these changes may be so subtle that the pneumothorax becomes apparent only in comparison with previous films.

▶ *Reed's Rule No. 7:* Always review all old films to properly assess the new one. Subtle findings can easily be missed when a single previous examination is reviewed.

A common problem in infants with hyaline membrane disease (HMD) is the patent ductus arteriosus (PDA), causing a left-to-right shunt. The classic roentgenographic signs of a PDA are an enlarging heart, enlarging liver, and increasing pulmonary vascularity. These, however, are late signs and may be masked by the parenchymal changes of HMD. In infants with HMD the only clues to a coexistent PDA may be (a) lack of improvement after 3 days of adequate therapy for HMD and (b) increasing perihilar haze. These roentgenographic findings are frequently noted before the clinical signs of a bounding pulse or a murmur.

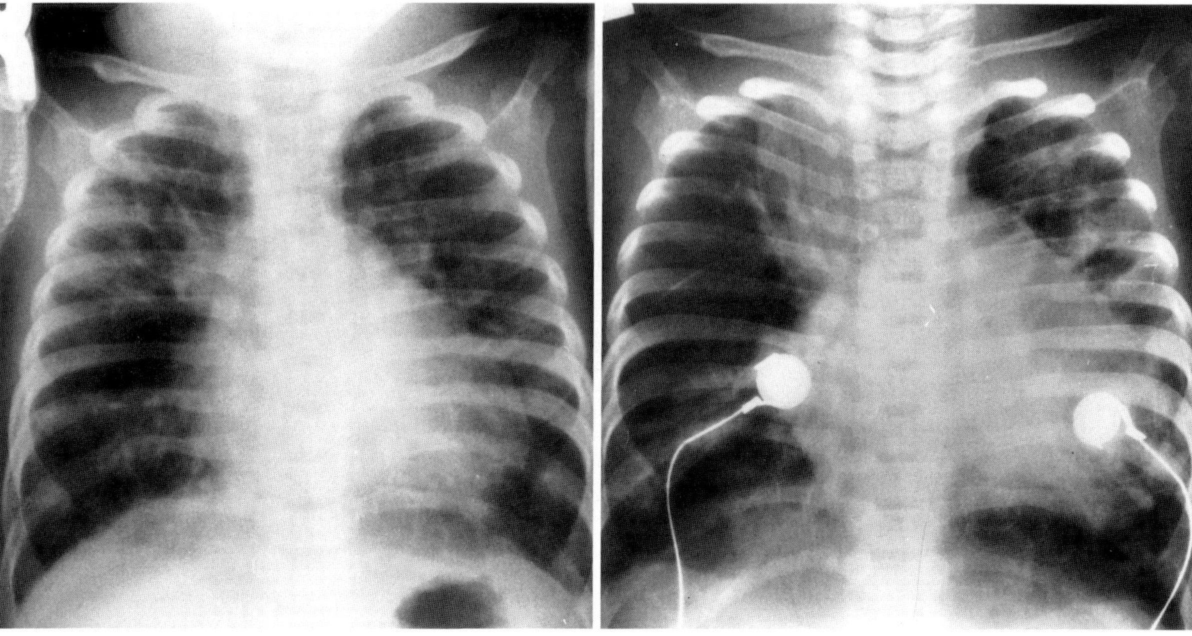

Fig. 3.20 a, b. Sequelae of hyaline membrane disease and mechanical ventilation. **a** This 6-month-old had severe hyaline membrane disease requiring assisted ventilation for over 1 month; he was still on supplemental oxygen. The heart is enlarged, and there are fibrous changes throughout both lungs with uneven expansion. The lungs are very hyperexpanded. **b** At 1 year of age further enlargement of the heart has occurred, and there is increasing emphysema. The areas of fibrosis have now coalesced. There is some cyst formation in the left midlung and left base. This child died at 18 months of age of chronic respiratory insufficiency

While most infants recover from HMD, 15% go on to develop bronchopulmonary dysplasia (Fig. 3.20). This disease is most likely the result of a combination of pulmonary insults due to severe hyaline membrane disease, high oxygen concentration, prematurity of the lungs, and prolonged high-pressure mechanical ventilation (barotrauma). Graphically, "cystic" areas appear in the lung parenchyma, intermixed with areas of fibrosis and atelectasis and generalized emphysema. The lungs become congested secondary to "leaking" capillaries.

Diseases with Variable Lung Volume

Persistent fetal circulation is not a radiographic diagnosis, and the neonate may present with variable lung volume.

Localized Changes in Lung Volume

Localized increase in lung volume can be either air filled or fluid filled (Fig. 3.21). Since in utero the lung is filled with fluid, an obstruction of a bronchus traps the fluid, delays resorption, and causes a localized increase in lung volume or a "*mass*" lesion. This mass compresses adjacent lobes and frequently shifts the mediastinum contralaterally. As the fluid is absorbed, it is replaced by air, but lung markings are not seen.

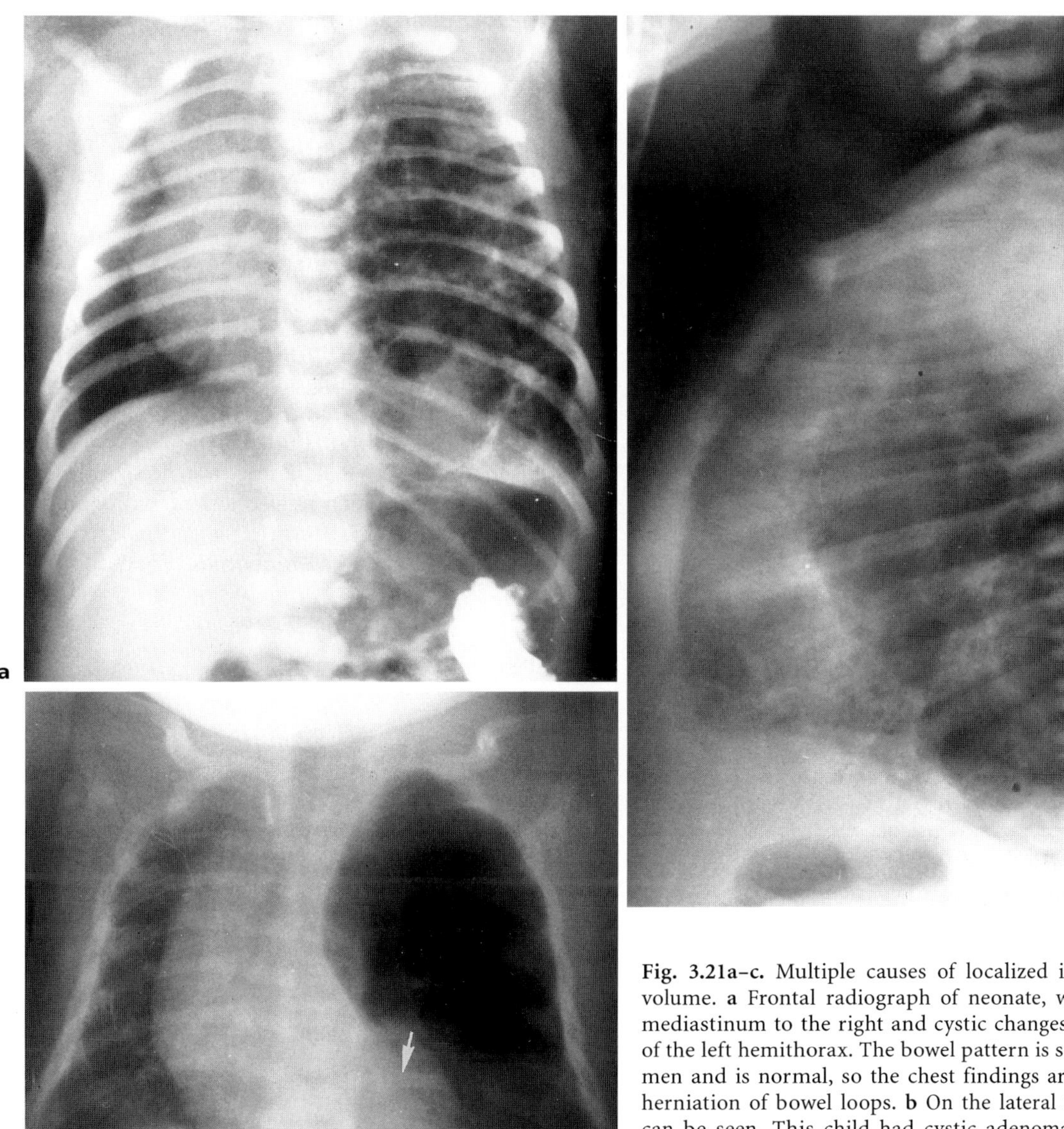

Fig. 3.21a–c. Multiple causes of localized increase in lung volume. **a** Frontal radiograph of neonate, with shift of the mediastinum to the right and cystic changes involving most of the left hemithorax. The bowel pattern is seen in the abdomen and is normal, so the chest findings are not caused by herniation of bowel loops. **b** On the lateral film, large cysts can be seen. This child had cystic adenomatoid malformation, a type of hamartoma of the lung. **c** Lobar emphysema. Note the localized increase in lung volume in the left upper lobe. The left lower lobe is compressed (*arrow*)

Classically this is associated with lobar emphysema or any condition obstructing a main-stem bronchus (e.g., intrinsic stenosis, bronchogenic cyst, pulmonary artery sling). Fine strands of tissue seen within the lucency indicate the presence of cysts. The commonest cyst lesion is congenital adenomatoid malformation. The lack of a defined *pleural* marking excludes pneumothorax.

► *Reed's Rule No. 5:* An esophagram must be performed in any child with unexplained respiratory disease. It is simple, inexpensive, and informative.

In the neonate as in the older child, unexplained airway disease should prompt an esophagram, which may be carried out initially with a tube in the esophagus so that the "H-type" fistula between the trachea and the esophagus can be excluded (Fig. 3.22). If this fistula is not found, the infant is given a bottle, and the swallowing mechanism is evaluated. Look at the position, course, contour, and motility of the esophagus. A vascular ring, i.e., an anomaly of the great vessels, masses, or nodes, often makes an impression on the esophagus. Check for gastroesophageal reflux – chalasia – during this examination (see Chap. 5). In addi-

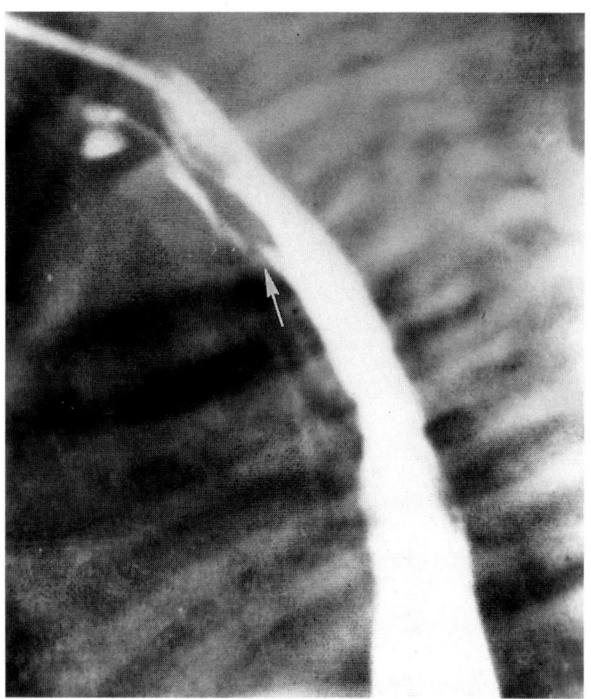

Fig. 3.22. "H-type" tracheoesophageal fistula in a child with chronic pneumonia. This lateral view of an esophagram demonstrates an unusual finding. A small barium-filled tract (*arrow*) can be seen from the esophagus running upward toward the trachea. Ingested formula could similarly be aspirated into the lungs

tion, under fluoroscopy, the diaphragm and mediastinum can be examined for diaphragmatic paralysis and unilateral air trapping.

If, after this study, further airway evaluation is necessary, or if the child continues to be a "noisy neonate," the airway can be studied fluoroscopically with the use of videotape and high-kilovoltage technique (see Chap. 9).

Remember: the most important question is: "Why am I ordering this set of films?" Once the diagnosis of hyaline membrane disease or severe bronchopulmonary dysplasia is established, radiographs should be used to show correctable conditions, such as airway obstruction, pneumonia, pneumothoraces, and vascular rings. Since the premature infant may be more acutely sensitive to the deleterious effects of radiation (Chap. 1), the timing and selection of radiographic examinations should be tempered with this consideration. Remember the ALARA concept (Chap. 1).

References

1. Swischuk LE (1989) Imaging of the newborn, infant and young child, 3rd edn., Williams and Wilkins, Baltimore
2. Silverman FN, Kuhn JP (1993) Caffey's pediatric X-ray diagnosis, 9th edn. Mosby, Chicago
3. Currano G, Williams B (1985) Causes of congenital pulmonary hypoplasia: a study of 33 cases. Pediatr Radiol 115:15–24

4 Gastrointestinal Tract

Roentgenographic interpretation of a child's abdomen is a challenging experience, as there are many subtle clues to the nature of the disease process. Appropriate interpretation requires both knowledge of the technical aspects of how the film was made and a systematic approach.

Technical Factors

In the discussion of the chest we noted that observing gravitational effects is useful in assessing a film. This is also true in the abdomen, i.e., air always rises, fluid goes to the dependent area.

► *Reed's Rule No. 8:* The abdominal examination should include a minimum of three views: supine, prone, and erect.

One can think of the air in the abdomen as contrast medium; the purpose of obtaining three views is to move air into different loops of bowel so that the maximal quantity of bowel can be visualized. With the patient supine, what portions of the bowel are highest? The answer, of course, is the transverse colon and the body of the stomach. Therefore on the abdominal supine film air rises to these regions (Fig. 4.1). When the patient is prone, the highest portions of the bowel are ascending and descending colon, rectum, and fundus of the stomach. Therefore gas should rise to these areas (see Fig. 4.1). Remembering these facts can frequently help in distinguishing large from small bowel. Look carefully at the bones on the supine film. The iliac wings appear larger and more rounded than they do on the prone film (see Fig. 4.1).

The erect view is the last film in the series. (Decubitus is sufficient if the patient is too sick or unable to stand.) How do you know if the film is an erect view? Once again, remember the effects of gravity. There may be an air fluid level in the stomach. Similarly, if the bowel contains fluid, one sees multiple air fluid levels. Notice how most of the bowel falls into the lower abdomen and pelvis, while the gastric fundus remains fixed in the left upper quadrant. The colon is visible in the flanks, with the transverse segment extending from beneath the liver, across the abdomen below the stomach into the left upper quadrant.

The Radiologist's Circle and the ABC's

In a child with acute abdominal distress it is not uncommon to take sequential examinations of the abdomen. Therefore it is important to check the date and time of examination in the corner of the film. Progressing in our imaginary circle, the ABC's should be reviewed, but this time in the reverse order: chest, bones and soft tissues, and (in this instance) abdomen.

► *Reed's Rule No. 9:* On every abdominal examination, evaluate the chest as if you were looking at a chest film.

Chest

It is often easier to see basilar lung changes, fractures of the lower ribs, and pleural reactions on an abdominal film than on a chest film (Fig. 4.2). In addition, the chest film may not adequately show a low thoracic paraspinal mass, which is readily spotted on abdominal films. Remember, the posterior lung sulcus is located at the level of the 12th thoracic vertebra and the posterior diaphragm insert at L2. To find it, you must look *through* the liver density on the right and the gastric air bubble on the left.

Bones and Soft Tissues

The bones and soft tissues can provide extremely valuable information. In making our imaginary radiologist's circle, note whether there is swelling or edema of the soft tissues, as represented by a nonhomogeneous pattern. It is also important to identify the properitoneal fat line (Fig. 4.3). This radiolucent line is the lateral margin of the peritoneal cavity; the gas-filled ascending colon and frequently the descending colon

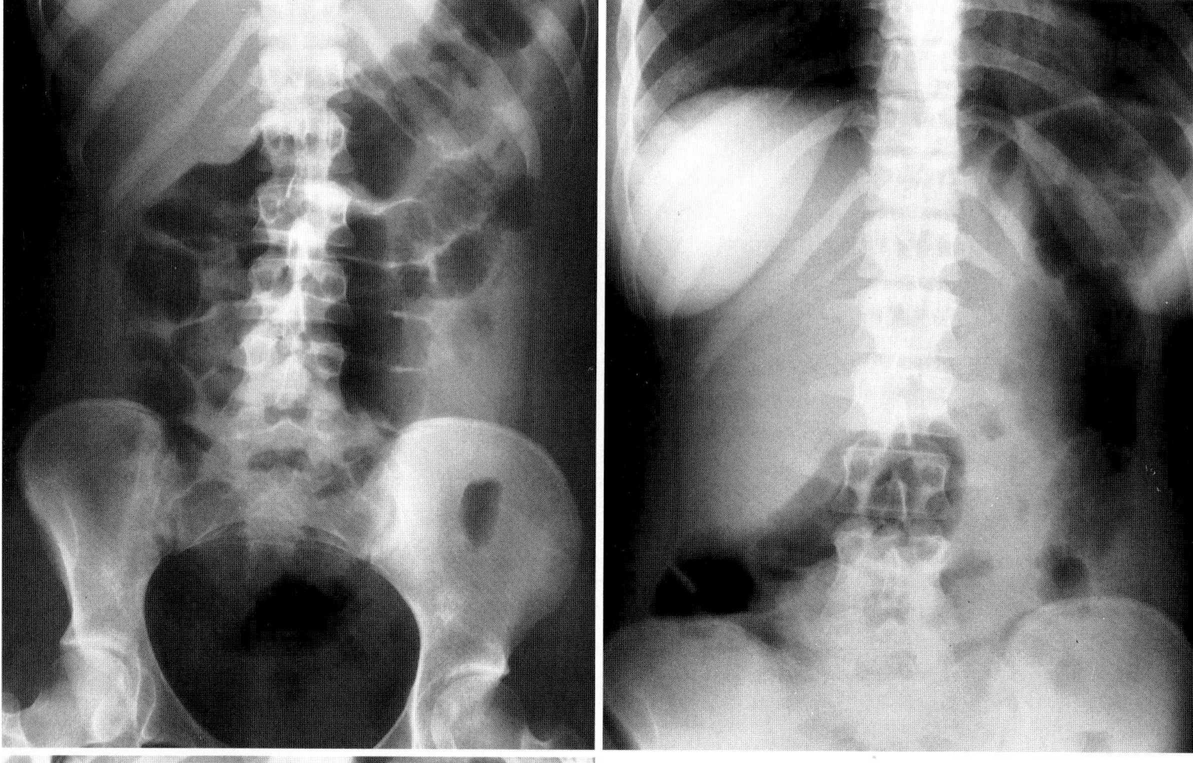

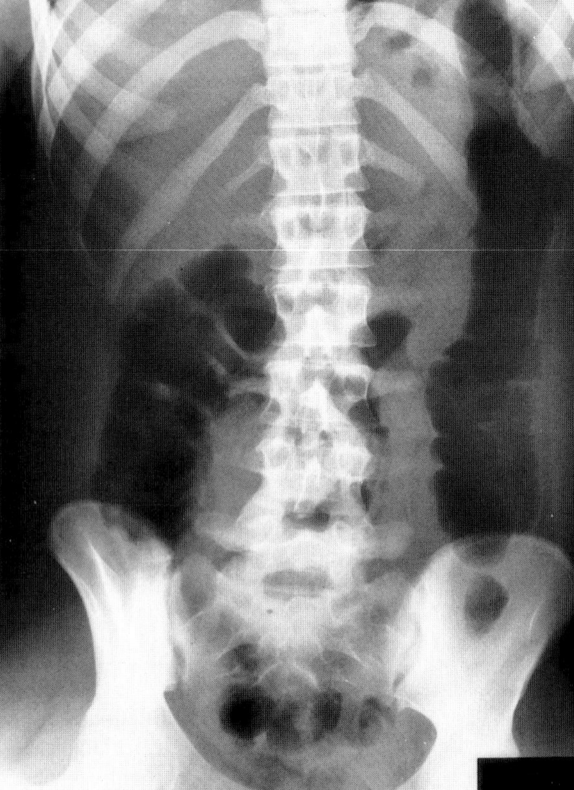

Fig. 4.1 a–c. The value of air as contrast media and utilizing three views: **a** Supine roentgenograph in this 15-year-old girl with abdominal pain reveals multiple loops of bowel in the midabdomen but little gas within the rectum. From this film it is not certain whether the air is in the large or the small bowel. **b** An erect film reveals that the base of the lungs is clear, and there is no free air under the diaphragm. There is gas in the hepatic flexure, transverse colon, and splenic flexure. **c** Prone examination reveals gas in the rectum, ascending and descending colon. The predominant pattern is that of colonic gas. The small bowel is not distended, and there is no evidence of obstruction

Fig. 4.2 a–d. On every abdominal film, examine the chest as if you were actually reading a chest film. **a** Supine view of the abdomen reveals a normal bowel gas pattern, but there is a suggestion of a density behind the liver on the right side. **b** On the erect film, notice how most of the bowel falls inferiorly into the lower abdomen, while the gastric fundus is fixed and filled with air. Above and lateral to the midliver there is a right lung density. **c** On the prone film, gas moves to the flanks. Note the right lung base. **d** The chest examination reveals pneumonia in the right lower lobe. Remember to look through the liver density on the right and the gastric air bubble on the left to see basilar infiltrates on any abdominal series ▶

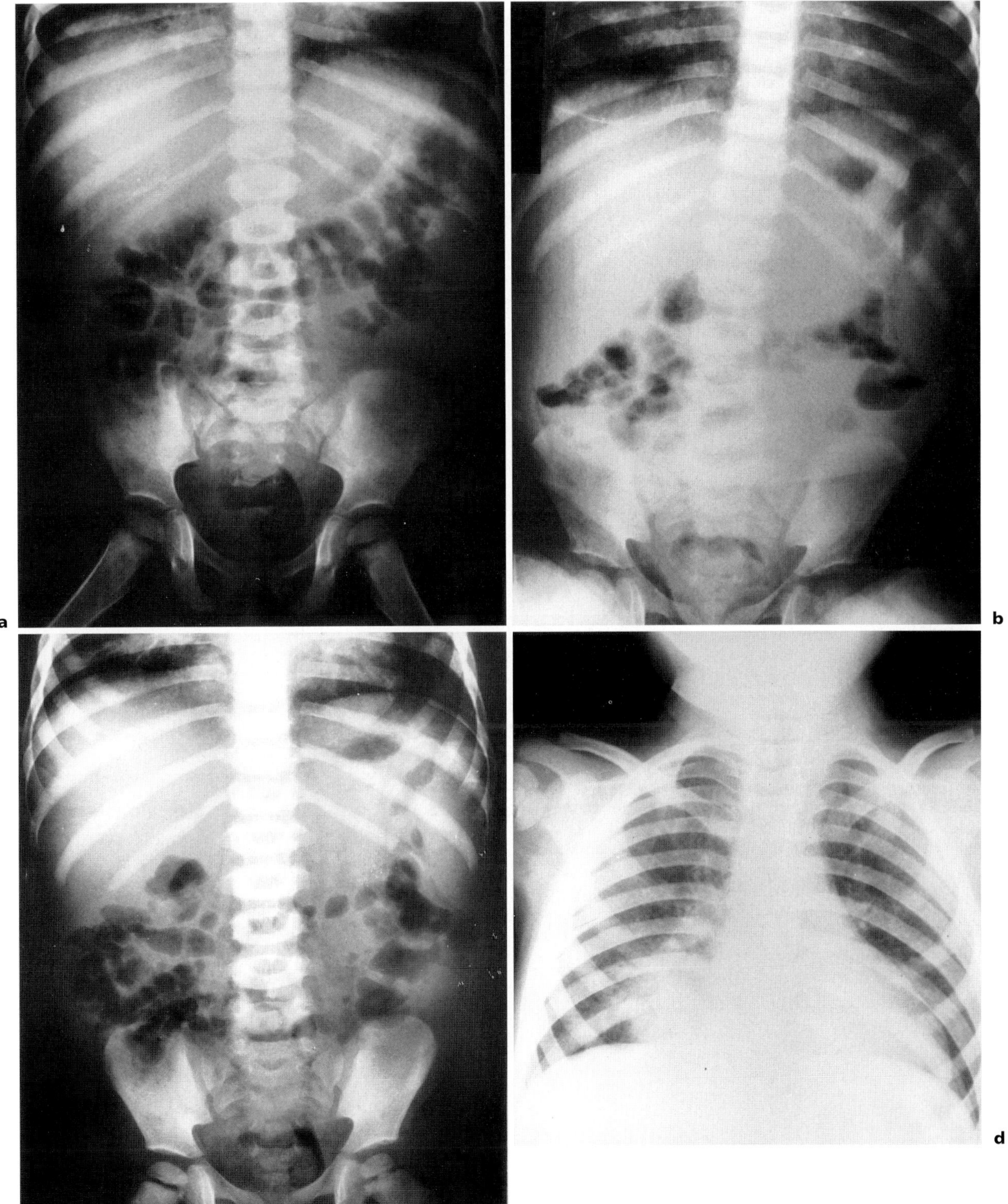
a
b
c
d

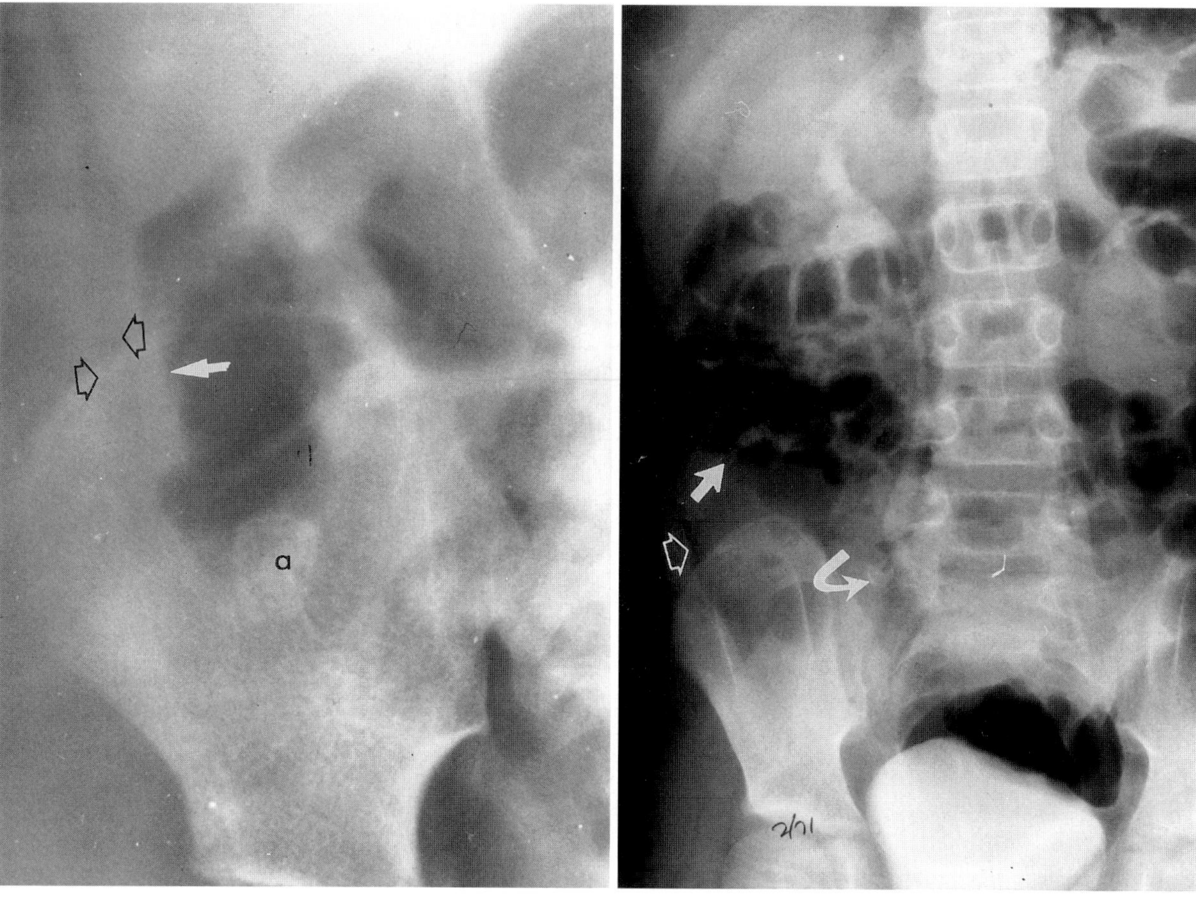

Fig. 4.3 a, b. Properitoneal fat line. **a** Close-up view of the right lower quadrant shows the dark, linear properitoneal fat line (*open arrows*), with the descending colon only a few millimeters away (*solid arrow*). Note the appendicolith (*a*). At this time the child was asymptomatic. **b** One month later the child became febrile and suffered right lower quadrant pain. Intravenous urogram shows the bowel (*solid straight arrow*) now displaced from the properitoneal fat line (*open arrow*). The appendicolith (*curved arrow*) is also displaced. A large appendiceal abscess was discovered at surgery

are within 1–2 mm of this line on the prone film. A separation between the properitoneal fat line and the colon on the prone film indicates the presence of fluid or possibly an intra-abdominal mass. Remember, this sign is useful only if the colon has air in it! (See Fig. 4.3.)

The lower ribs, spine, and pelvis are the major bones of concern on the abdominal film. Since specific abnormalities of these bones are discussed in Chap. 7, the major item of concern now is symmetry. Asymmetry must always be explained. Once again, abnormalities of bone should lead to careful searching of neighboring intra-abdominal contents, i.e., left lower rib fractures should suggest renal or splenic injury.

Abdomen

In the systematic approach, we look last at the area for which the film was requested. Therefore our approach to the intra-abdominal contents is to view the muscles, soft tissues, and viscera before examining the bowel gas pattern. Begin at the top of the film, most often

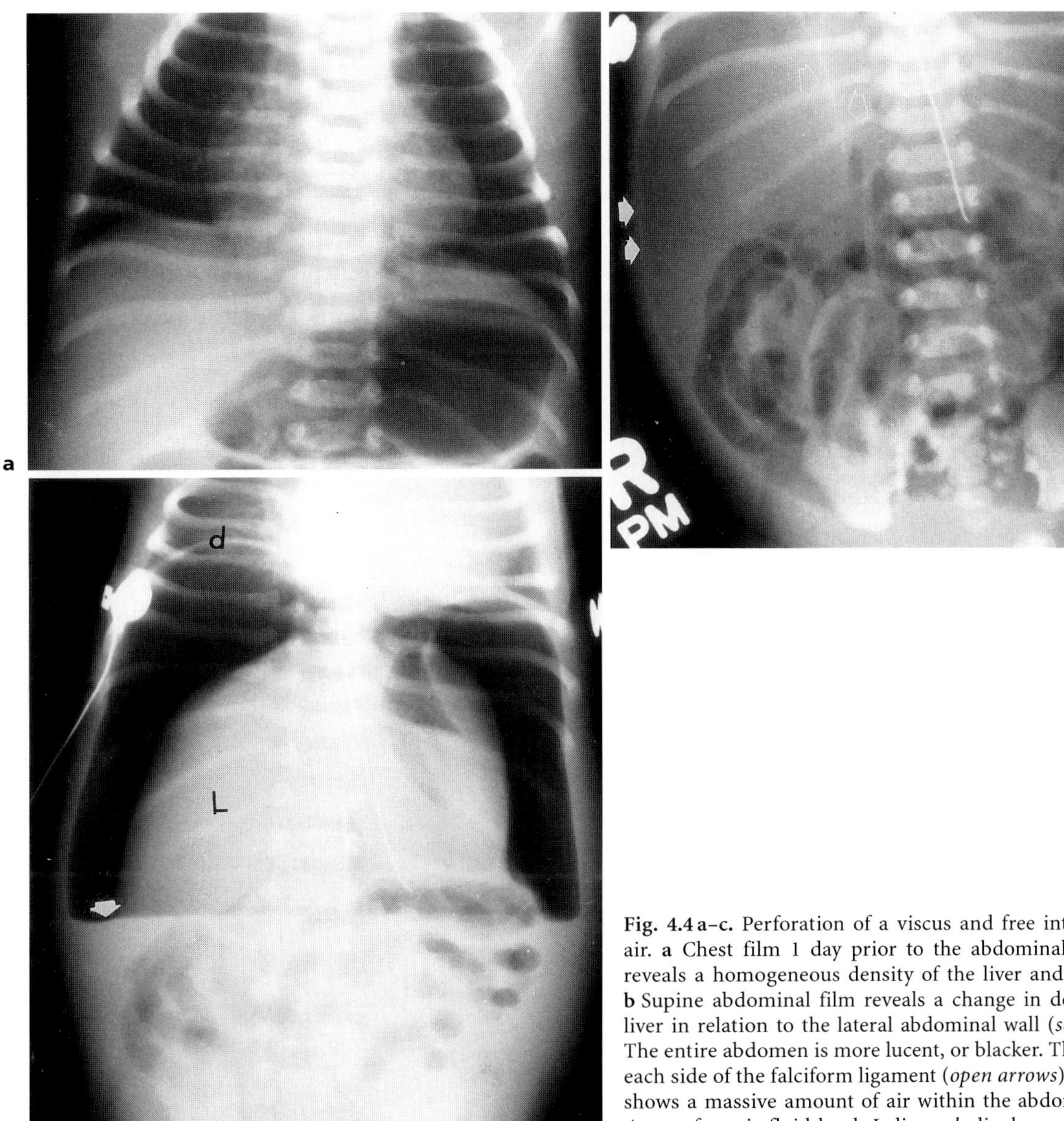

Fig. 4.4 a–c. Perforation of a viscus and free intraperitoneal air. **a** Chest film 1 day prior to the abdominal perforation reveals a homogeneous density of the liver and soft tissues. **b** Supine abdominal film reveals a change in density of the liver in relation to the lateral abdominal wall (*solid arrows*). The entire abdomen is more lucent, or blacker. There is air on each side of the falciform ligament (*open arrows*). **c** Erect film shows a massive amount of air within the abdominal cavity. *Arrow*, free air fluid level. *L*, liver; *d*, diaphragm

with the erect film, looking for signs of free intraperitoneal air. As can be seen in Fig. 4.1b, the diaphragm on the left is easily visible because of the stomach bubble. On the right the liver is directly beneath the diaphragm, and only the top margin – the thoracic margin – can be seen. Since air rises on the erect film, free air collects between the liver and diaphragm on the right and between the stomach bubble and the diaphragm on the left. On the supine film, however, air rises and fills the space above the viscera and beneath the umbilicus and the abdominal musculature. Free air is more difficult to see on this view but should nevertheless be recognized, as there is a subtle change in the soft tissue density of the abdomen (Fig. 4.4). The liver may be blacker than the adjacent soft tissues. Therefore, there are three densities, proceeding from the lateral aspect of the right side: (a) the soft tissue density, (b) the liver density, which is somewhat darker, and (c) the stomach density full of air, which is the darkest. Normally there are only two densities – the liver and soft tissues (which are of equal density) and the air in the stomach.

The falciform ligament is never normally visible; it can be seen only when surrounded by free intraperitoneal air. This ligament courses downward from its diaphragmatic attachment between the margin of the

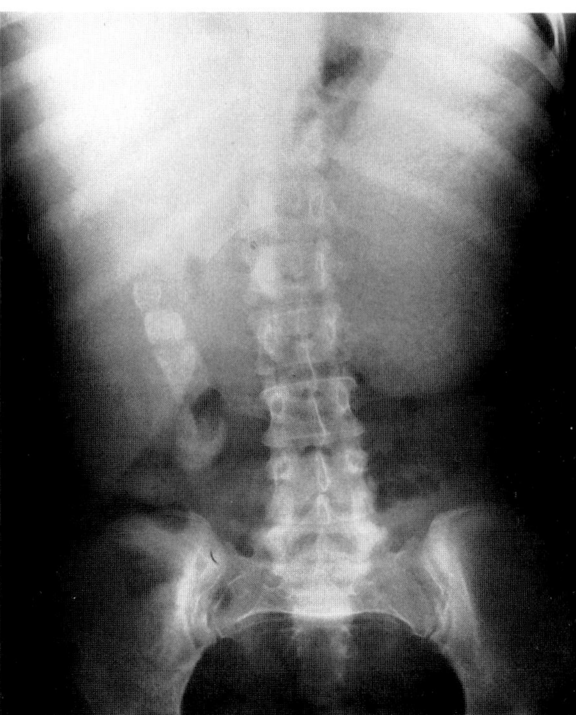

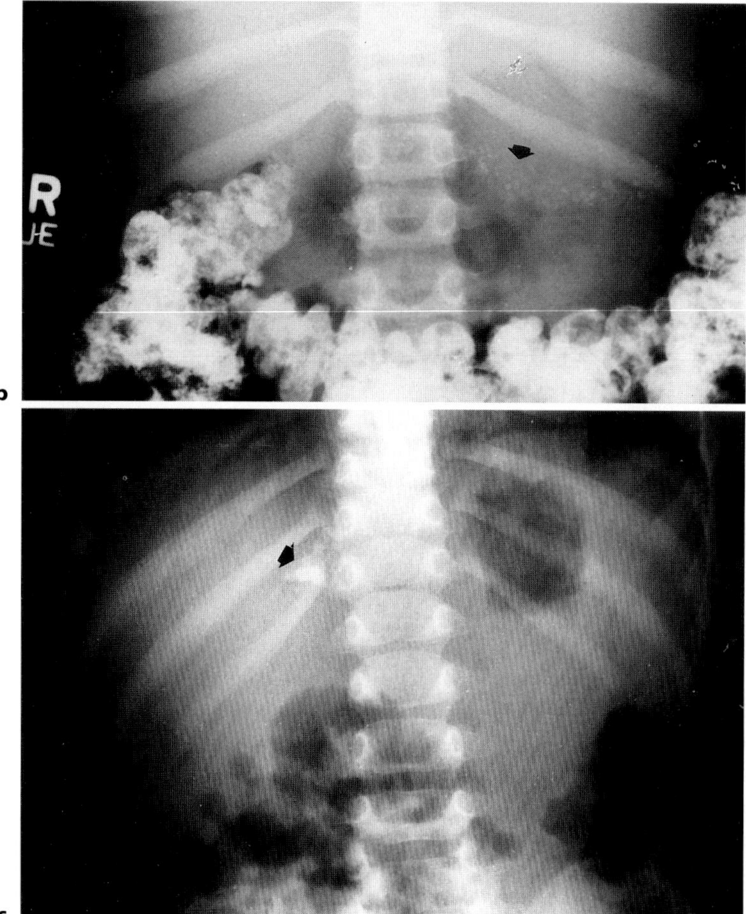

Fig. 4.5 a–d. Calcifications within the abdomen. **a** A 16-year-old with several areas of calcification. The first is a tubular density in the right midabdomen. This is a gallbladder which contained multiple radiopaque gallstones. The second is a large viscus in the left upper quadrant with punctate calcifications representing an enlarged spleen, which has undergone iron replacement secondary to multiple transfusions for hemolytic anemia (hemochromatosis). **b** This 15-year-old with cystic fibrosis and diabetes mellitus has calcifications in the region of the pancreas. A coned-down view from the barium enema shows that they extend the entire length, from the head to the tail, of the pancreas (*arrow*). **c** A 6.5-year-old child examined for urinary tract infection. At the 12th right rib there are coarse, triangular calcifications (*arrow*), which appear in the vicinity of the adrenal gland and are the end result of neonatal adrenal hemorrhage. **d** Appendicolith – calcification in the appendix often has multiple concentric calcific rings (lamina) that aid in their identification

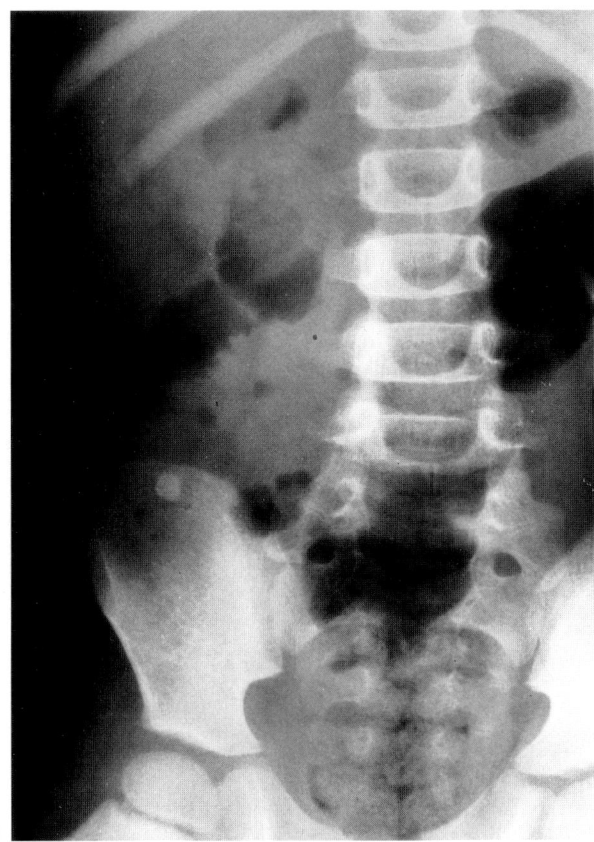
d

right and left lobes of the liver to the lowest aspect of the umbilical remnants. When there is free intraperitoneal air, the large bubble of free air assumes an oval configuration with the falciform ligament being central – the laces of a football – in the football sign (see Fig. 4.4).

Continuing with your appraisal of the film from the top down, look at the liver and spleen and assess their size, if possible (see Fig. 4.1). A radiologist measures liver size only infrequently; hepatic enlargement is usually an impression. The spleen is often obscured by bowel gas. Remember, a good inspiration pushes the liver down while a poor inspiration, in fact, lets it rise.

Determination of splenic size and position is usually possible by locating the inferior and medial margins. The stomach air bubble and gas in the splenic flexure of the colon lie immediately adjacent to the spleen; and both may be displaced, particularly if the spleen is enlarged. Since one can feel beneath the costal margin to palpate a spleen, reference of the splenic density to this margin helps determine whether it is actually enlarged. Ask yourself, "Could I palpate it?" If so, "How big does it feel?"

Proceeding inferiorly on the film, note the iliopsoas muscles attached to the spine at the upper lumbar vertebra, and proceed diagonally and laterally to the lesser trochanters of the femora. The lateral margins can usually be seen. The key to identifying pathology of the psoas margins is asymmetry. If a portion of the psoas muscle is not visible while the rest of the muscle and the opposite one are, abnormal soft-tissue densities in this region should be considered. The entire psoas margins sometimes cannot be seen on films of infants and children with abundant fecal material or bowel gas.

The kidneys are adjacent to the lateral margin of the iliopsoas muscles. This is discussed in more detail in Chap. 5.

Look specifically for calcifications in all areas of the abdomen. Stones in the gallbladder, urinary tract, pancreas, or appendix may occur if there is stasis or an inflammation (Fig. 4.5). Benign and malignant neoplasms can calcify. Once a calcification has been identified and anatomically located, characterize it. Is it sharply marginated and of uniform density? Is it laminated (Fig. 4.5 d)? Lamination indicates that it has been there for a long time, and that the chemical processes have varied, and thus different layers are formed. Is it well formed and flocculent, as found in adrenal calcifications; or is it punctate with poorly defined margins, representing irregular deposition in a necrotic, rapidly growing neoplastic process? What is the calcification doing to the system in which it resides? Is it producing obstruction, or is it ulcerating? Does it look "physiological"? A phlebolith in an infant is definitely abnormal but may be "normal" in an adult.

Continuing downward on the three views of the abdomen, evaluate the soft tissues of the pelvis for asymmetry. The bladder appears as a smooth and round soft tissue mass when distended. In infants it tends to extend up into the right lower quadrant.

Finally, look at the bowel-gas pattern. Figure 4.1 shows a normal bowel gas pattern in an older child, while Fig. 4.6 shows a normal bowel gas pattern in a neonate. Even though there is a large amount of gas in the neonatal abdomen, the bowel loops have a recognizable, polygonal pattern. In neonates with bowel distention, the loops become "sausage shaped"; it is frequently impossible to tell large from small bowel, but even here it helps to obtain the three views.

Observe the bowel gas pattern for position, contour, and size (distention). The bowel may be displaced by a mass (Fig. 4.7; see also Chap. 6). Comparing Figs. 4.1, 4.6, and 4.7, the presence of a soft tissue mass is striking. Free intraperitoneal fluid causes the bowel to move centrally and imparts a gray or hazy appearance to the abdomen (Fig. 4.8). The sharp liver angle (margin) is obscured by the fluid. Any fluid, be it lymph, blood, or pus, can give this appearance. Here again,

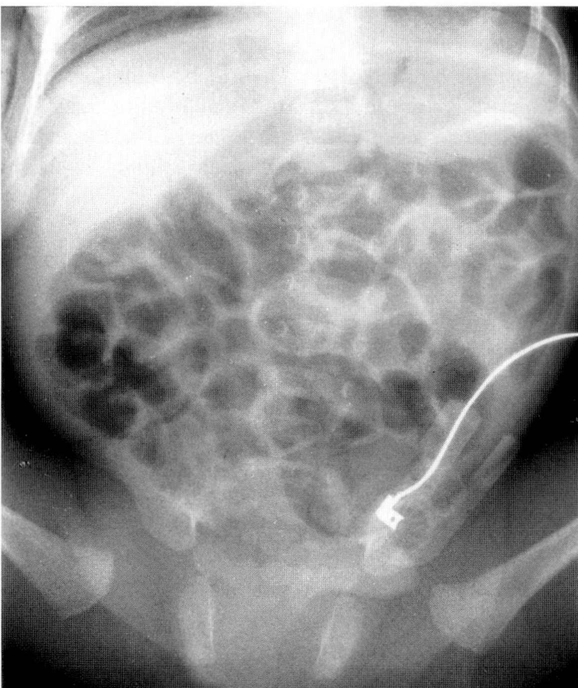

Fig. 4.6. Normal bowel pattern in a neonate. This supine abdominal film shows bowel loops that display a polygonal pattern. On this supine film gas is not seen in the rectum

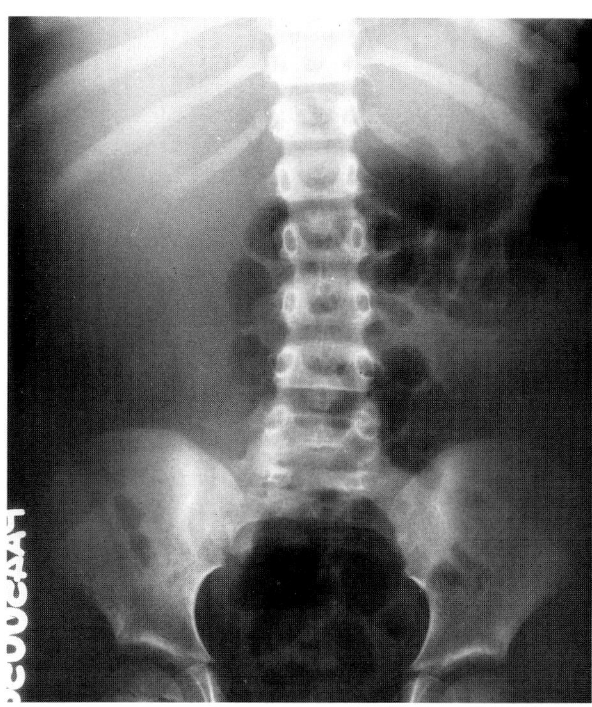

Fig. 4.7. Abnormal gas pattern. A supine film of a 4-year-old with a protuberant abdomen reveals a large, homogeneous density over the right and midabdomen. The bowel gas is pushed to the left. A sonographic examination confirmed the presence of a mesenteric cyst

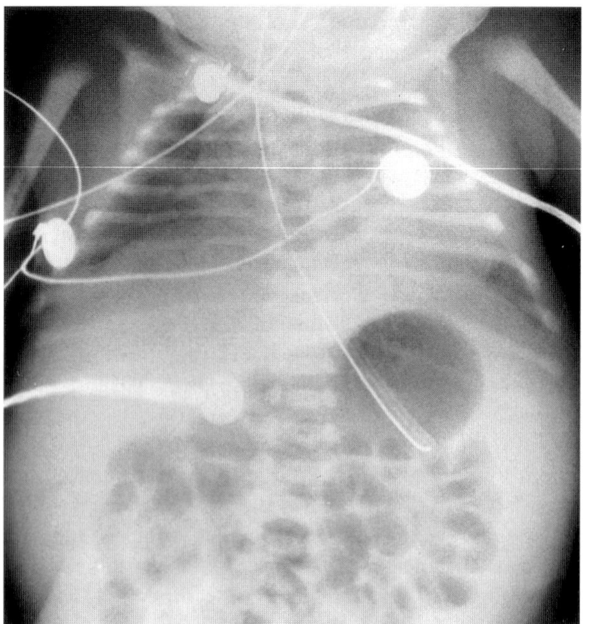

◀ Fig. 4.8. Ascites. On this supine radiograph of a 2-day-old male infant the bowel gas is pushed to the center, and there is a grayness to the flanks. The fluid moved appropriately on multiple views because it was free ascitic fluid, secondary to urinary obstruction and posterior urethral valves. Note how the bowel loops float centrally instead of being displaced to one side by a mass, as in Fig. 4.7

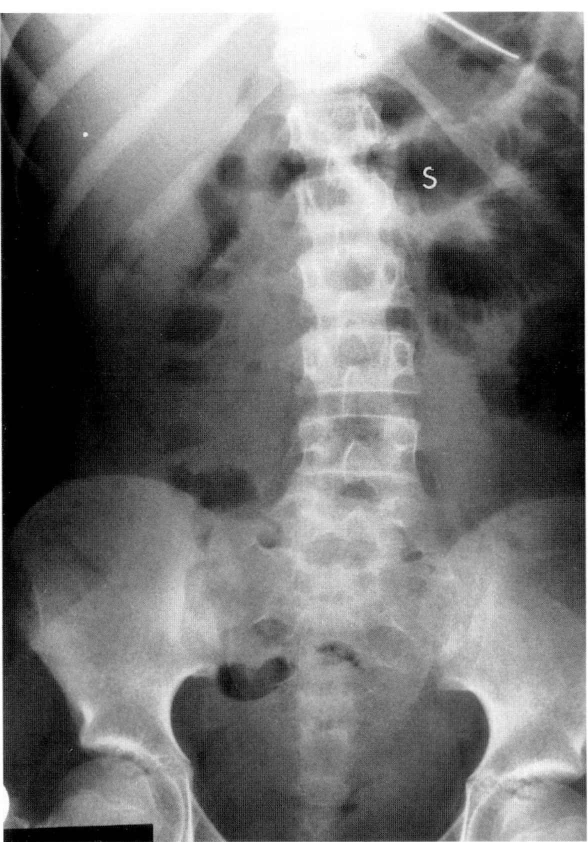

Fig. 4.9. Sentinel loop. On this supine film there is a localized distention of small bowel in the left upper quadrant (*s*). It is clearly identifiable as small bowel because of the valvulae conniventes (*parallel lines*). The sentinel loop remained in this region on multiple views. The child had blunt abdominal trauma, and the sentinel loop was anterior to an inflamed pancreas

however, we can use the effects of gravity to our advantage. Air in the bowel floats centrally, with the fluid in the dependent portions (see Fig. 4.8).

The contour of the bowel is discussed under "Contrast Examinations." However, we use air as much as possible because it is a good contrast agent. The bowel margins should be smooth, not ragged or irregular. The contour should change as position changes, implying pliability; it should not be rigid. If a space-occupying lesion – a mass – pushes on adjacent segments of bowel and changes the contour, the wall appears stretched as a result of the extrinsic pressure.

An increase in the size and amount of bowel distention is crucial to the diagnosis of intra-abdominal disease. Children normally have some small bowel gas or (on the erect film) even an occasional air fluid level in the colon. While *multiple* small bowel and colonic fluid levels are seen in mechanical bowel obstruction, they are also seen in infants as well as older children *without* obstructive bowel disease. Many of these children will have nothing more threatening than gastroenteritis. However, if you cannot see air in the colon or rectum, or if there is a *localized* distention of bowel, you should be very suspicious of underlying pathological changes. In crying children the stomach may be quite large without any pathology. However, localized distention of small bowel provides a valuable clue to the site of disease – a *sentinel loop* (Fig. 4.9). Remember:

► *Reed's Rule No. 2:* Knowledge of anatomy is the key to correct radiographic diagnosis.

What viscera are these sentinel loops near? What vessels are found in this area? What type of pathology commonly occurs in this quadrant?

Increase in bowel size (distention) may occur in both small and large bowel without obstruction, but there is a *recognizable pattern to the distention.* The small bowel is less distended than the colon, and there is gas in the rectum. This condition has been called paralytic (without peristalsis) ileus (distention). However, patients who have been given atropine derivatives, or who have dysmotility syndrome may have the same radiographic picture. Since the patient with gastroenteritis has normal to increased peristalsis, and the patient given atropine derivatives has decreased peristalsis, the term ileus is somewhat confusing. It is best to describe the pattern and allow the clinician to fit it into the patient's status.

A more *uniform*, generalized increase of all or parts of the small or large bowel along with multiple air fluid levels and no air in the rectum denotes mechanical bowel obstruction (Fig. 4.10). The site of obstruction is determined by how much bowel is distended. That is, many loops mean distal bowel obstruction, while a few distended loops mean proximal bowel obstruction (Fig. 4.11). In obstruction, the curvature or contour of the loops of distended bowel may be acute – hairpin turns – and the fluid levels may be uneven, i.e., a stepladder distribution (Fig. 4.10). Because of the hyperperistalsis the bowel beyond the obstruction is devoid of gas (assuming the process has been present for some time).

A helpful mnemonic for assessing plain film is: stones, bones, gas, mass!

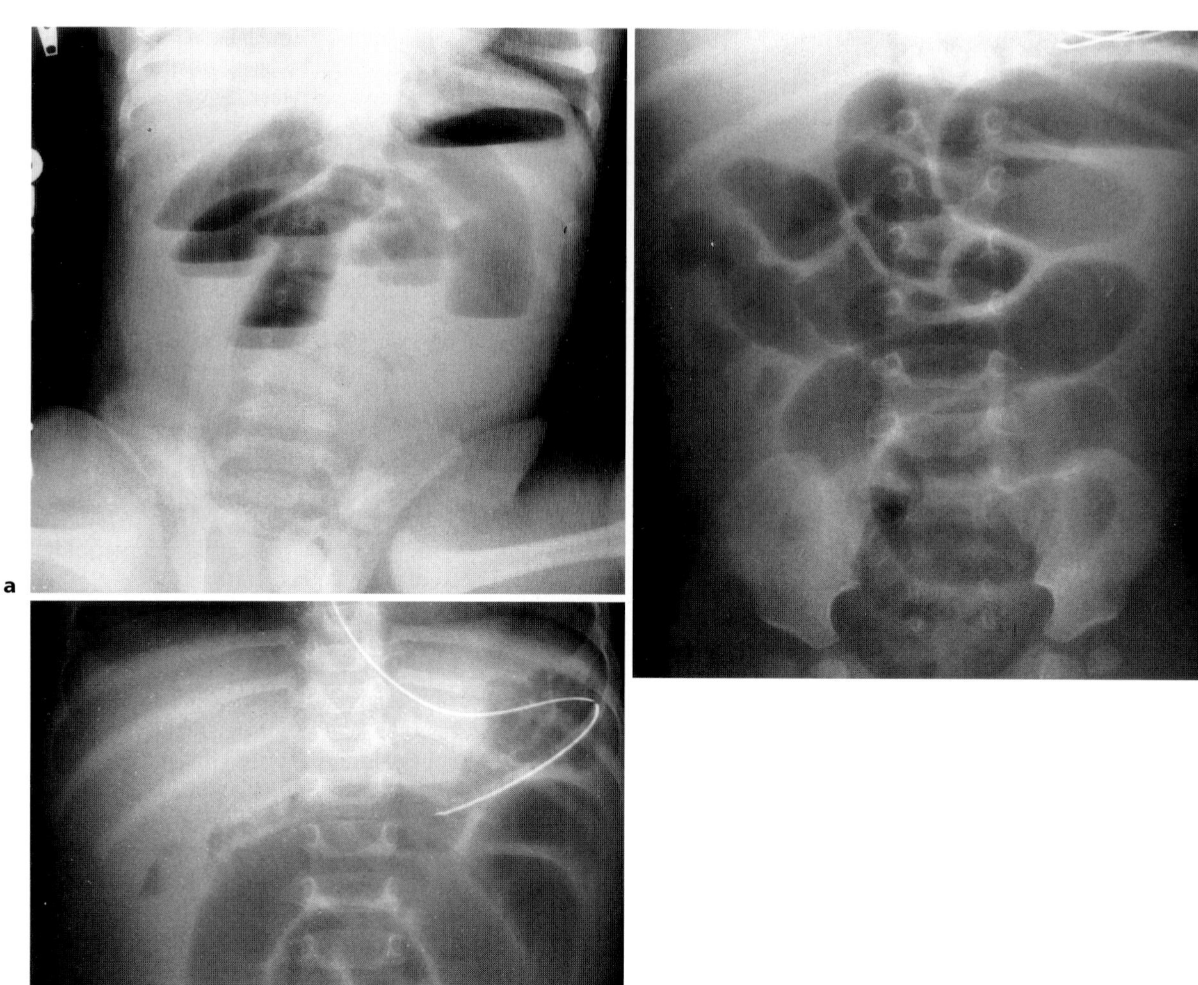

Fig. 4.10 a–c. Small bowel obstruction. This 1-year-old had an incarcerated inguinal hernia. **a** Erect film shows multiple air fluid levels in a stepladder pattern (uneven levels in each loop). When this occurs, it suggests obstruction rather than absence of peristalsis. **b** Supine radiograph shows large, distended loops in the midabdomen. **c** On the prone film, gas has not successfully shifted into the colon. The largest loops remain in the midabdomen. Small bowel obstruction is present

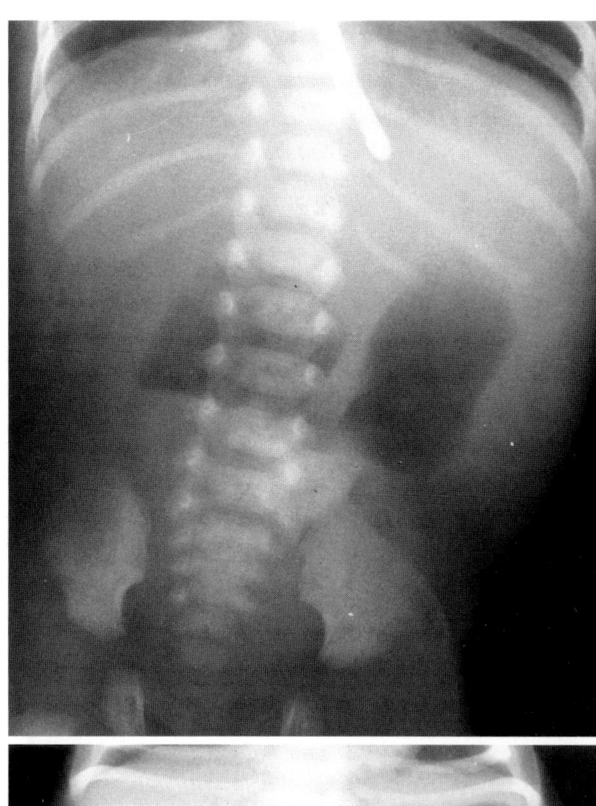

a

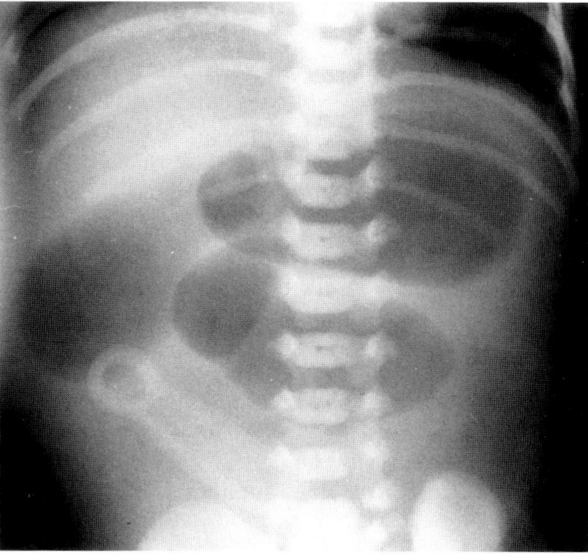

b

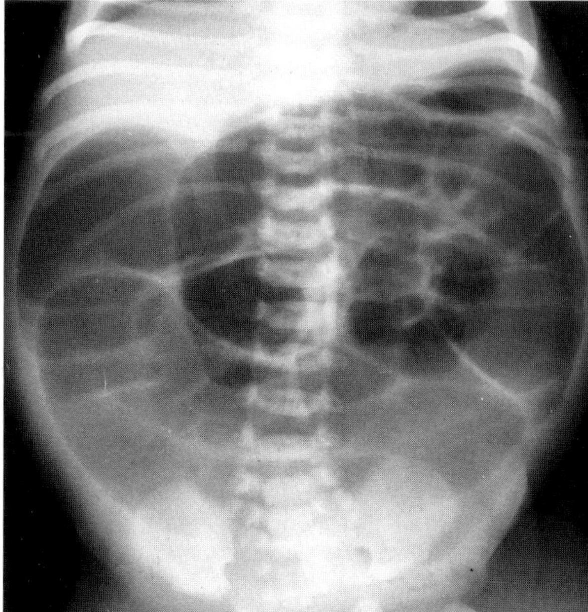

c

Fig. 4.11 a–c. Mechanical bowel obstruction at various levels of the Gl tract. **a** This neonate presented with vomiting. The radiographs of the abdomen reveal two air fluid levels (*double bubble*), one in the stomach and one in the duodenum. This child had a high obstruction which was shown to be duodenal atresia. **b** This 1-day-old presented abruptly with vomiting after feeding. Supine abdominal film reveals three air-containing structures: the stomach, duodenum, and jejunum. At surgery this child was found to have jejunal atresia. **c** This infant has multiple air-containing loops of bowel signifying a more distal obstruction. The diagnosis at surgery was ileal atresia

Routine Contrast Examinations

Barium sulfate is used to coat the *intraluminal surface* of the bowel in order to reveal mucosal, submucosal, and extrinsic masses impinging on or constricting the lumen. By filling the bowel under fluoroscopic control the radiologist can observe distensibility, pliability, and intraluminal content. Peristaltic activity, particularly in the upper gastrointestinal tract, is also observed. These features are important when one suspects neoplasm or inflammation. The intricacies of these radiological examinations are beyond the scope of this text. In general, the patient is placed in multiple positions while barium is introduced either orally or rectally under direct vision, i.e., fluoroscopic control. Films are obtained with the patient in many positions so that air and barium coat different portions of the bowel.

Esophagus

Evaluation of the upper gastrointestinal tract begins with an esophagram. (Fig. 4.12), and some of the indications for this procedure are discussed in Chap. 2.

▶ *Reed's Rule No. 5:* An esophagram must be performed in any child with unexplained respiratory disease.

Many abnormalities of the esophagus (foreign body, duplication, etc.) and disorders of the swallowing mechanism may lead to respiratory distress secondary to aspiration and/or compression of the airway. On an esophagram the entire nasopharynx, oropharynx, and hypopharynx, as well as the esophagus from its origin at the inferior margin of the hypopharynx to the diaphragm, should be seen (see Fig. 4.12). It is important to see that the nasopharynx is not filled with contrast. As with all examinations, it is crucial to look at adjacent structures, for example, the airway, to make sure there is no compression, displacement, or contrast material within the trachea. It is important to study the esophagus for position, contour, and size. The fluoroscopist evaluates the motility of the esophagus, but this is difficult to ascertain on plain films alone.

In evaluating the *position* of the esophagus note that in the lateral projection there should be no separation between the anterior wall of the esophagus and the posterior wall of the trachea. On frontal examinations the esophagus overlies the right side of the spine, passing through the intrathoracic portion until it crosses the spine distally. The esophagogastric junction is to the left of the spine.

The *contours* of the esophagus are smooth, with specific, normal indentations (see Fig. 4.12). The first is the cricopharyngeal muscle, a smooth posterior indentation in the cervical region at the C-5 level.

▶ *Reed's Rule No. 10:* In obstruction of a lumen there should be proximal distention.

It is unusual for the cricopharyngeal muscle to cause a problem, except in severe neurological impairment. The next two indentations on the barium column are seen on the frontal radiograph: the first at the level of the aortic arch and the next at the level of the left main-stem bronchus. Foreign bodies, when ingested, are usually found in these regions (see Fig. 4.13), as are vascular anomalies.

The *size* of the esophagus changes with peristalsis. The fluoroscopist sees a wave beginning above and proceeding uniformly through the esophagus until it empties its contents into the stomach. This is a stripping wave. Conditions with abnormal motility are usually detected at this time. On any single film one area of the esophagus may be more dilated or constricted than another, but this should be a transitory phenomenon. A specific area of normal intermittent widening is in the distal one-third of the esophagus, just above the gastroesophageal junction. This is a good place to detect esophageal varices or hiatal hernia.

The Upper Gastrointestinal Series

The upper gastrointestinal (GI) series (Fig. 4.14) includes visualization of the esophagus, as well as the stomach, duodenum, and ligament of Treitz. This ligament is the fibrous band that fixes the duodenal-jejunal junction to the posterior peritoneal wall to the left of the spine at a cephalic height equal to that of the duodenal bulb. The upper GI examination is useful for detecting ulcers or masses within the stomach, ulcers or obstruction of the duodenum, and malrotation, a condition in which the duodenal-jejunal junction is not properly affixed by the ligament of Treitz. Failure of this fixation often results in obstruction of the duodenum, either by peritoneal bands or twisting of the duodenum and subsequent midgut volvulus. An upper GI series can also detect masses within the epigastrium that may impinge on the duodenal sweep, as well as inflammatory bowel disease of the duodenum. Congenital anomalies of the stomach and duodenum can be seen. Direct visualization of the liver, gallbladder, and pancreas cannot be obtained by this method (see Chap. 5, sections "Ultrasound" and "Computed Tomography").

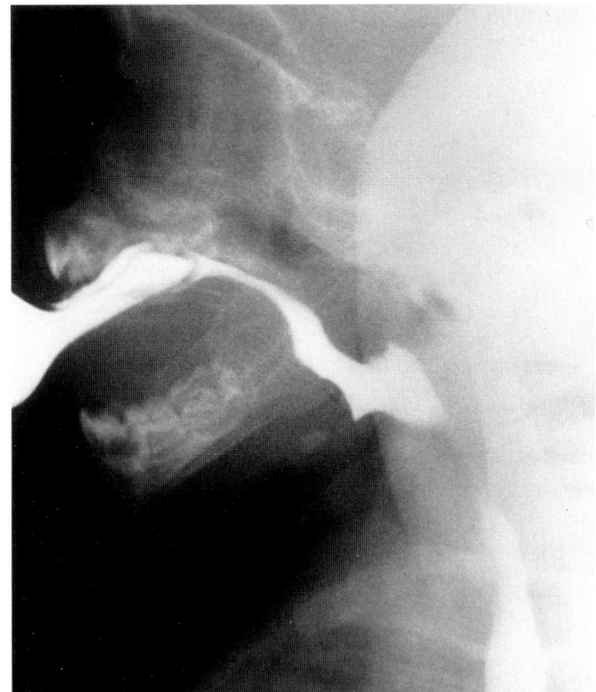

a

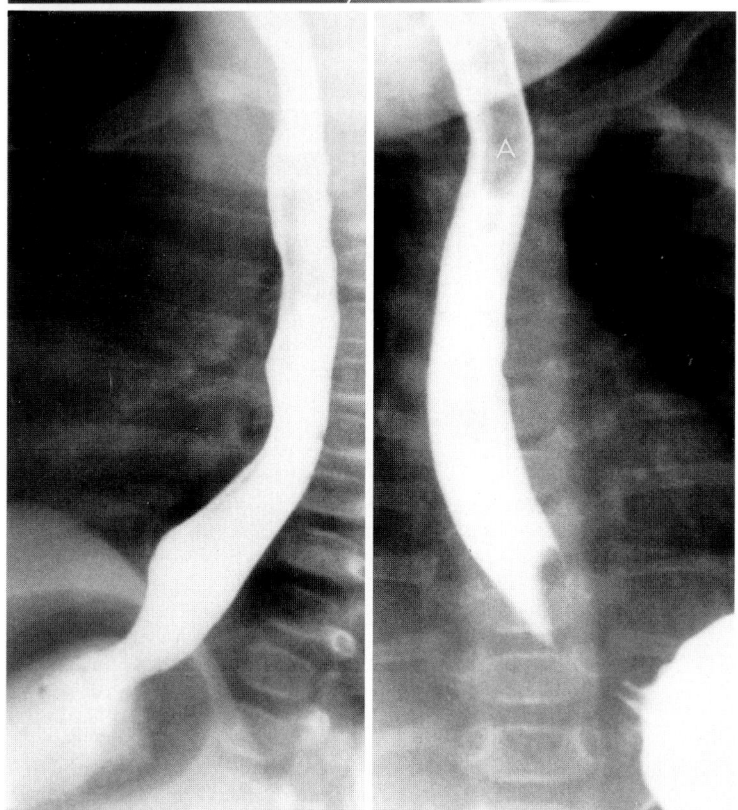

b c

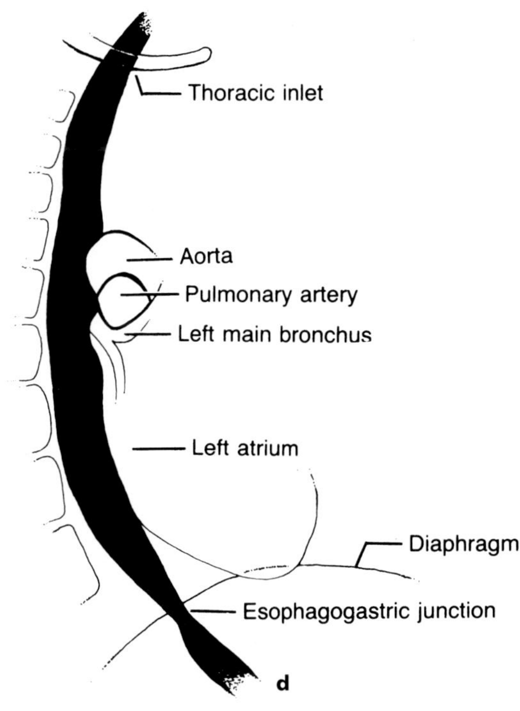

Fig. 4.12 a–d. The normal esophagram. **a** Films are taken routinely in the frontal and lateral projections. In this lateral view the swallowing mechanism is observed, and the contrast is noted in the oropharynx, hypopharynx, and proximal esophagus. There is no nasal reflux. Barium in the nasopharynx indicates swallowing dysfunction. **b** The entire esophagus is visualized, as well as the esophagogastric junction. The walls are smooth and undulate gently. There are no mass impressions upon the esophagus. **c** Frontal view reveals a distended esophagus and some air bubbles in the esophagus (*A*). **d** Drawing of the lateral view of the barium-filled esophagus with the normal physiological areas of narrowing

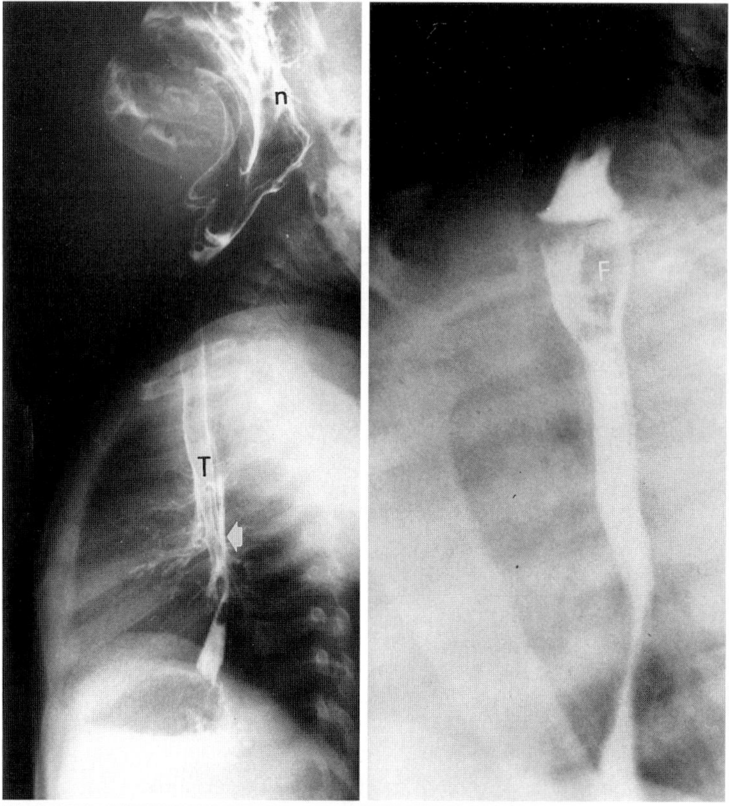

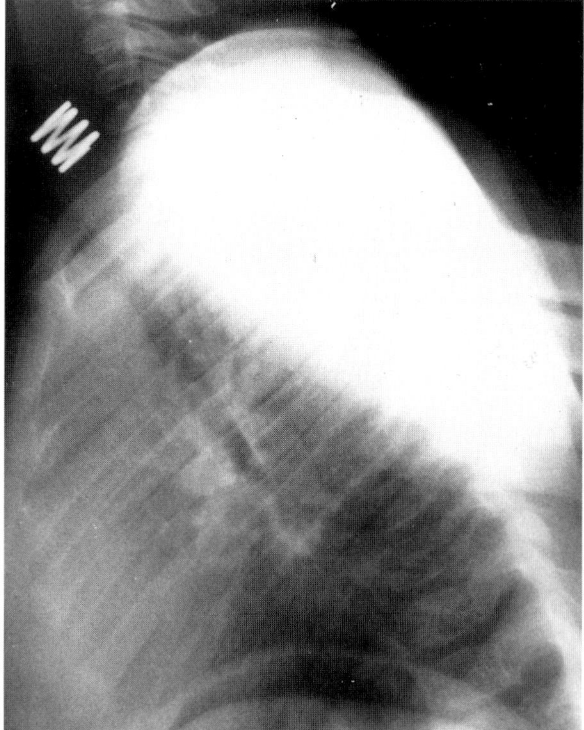

Fig. 4.13 a–c. Esophageal abnormalities. **a** This infant has swallowing difficulty and nasal reflux (*n*). The infant choked and aspirated the contrast, which is now seen in the esophagus posteriorly (*arrow*) and in the tracheobronchial tree (*T*) anteriorly. **b** This 16-month-old had a radiopaque spring in the cervical esophagus. The cricopharyngeus muscle at C5 is one of the areas of physiological narrowing. Children with esophageal foreign bodies frequently present with airway symptoms due to impingement on the trachea. **c** The aortic arch is another site of physiological narrowing. When this food substance (*F*) was removed, no stricture was found. If a foreign body is stuck at an area other than a normal site of narrowing, a stricture should be suspected. Note the distension of the esophagus above the level of the aortic arch

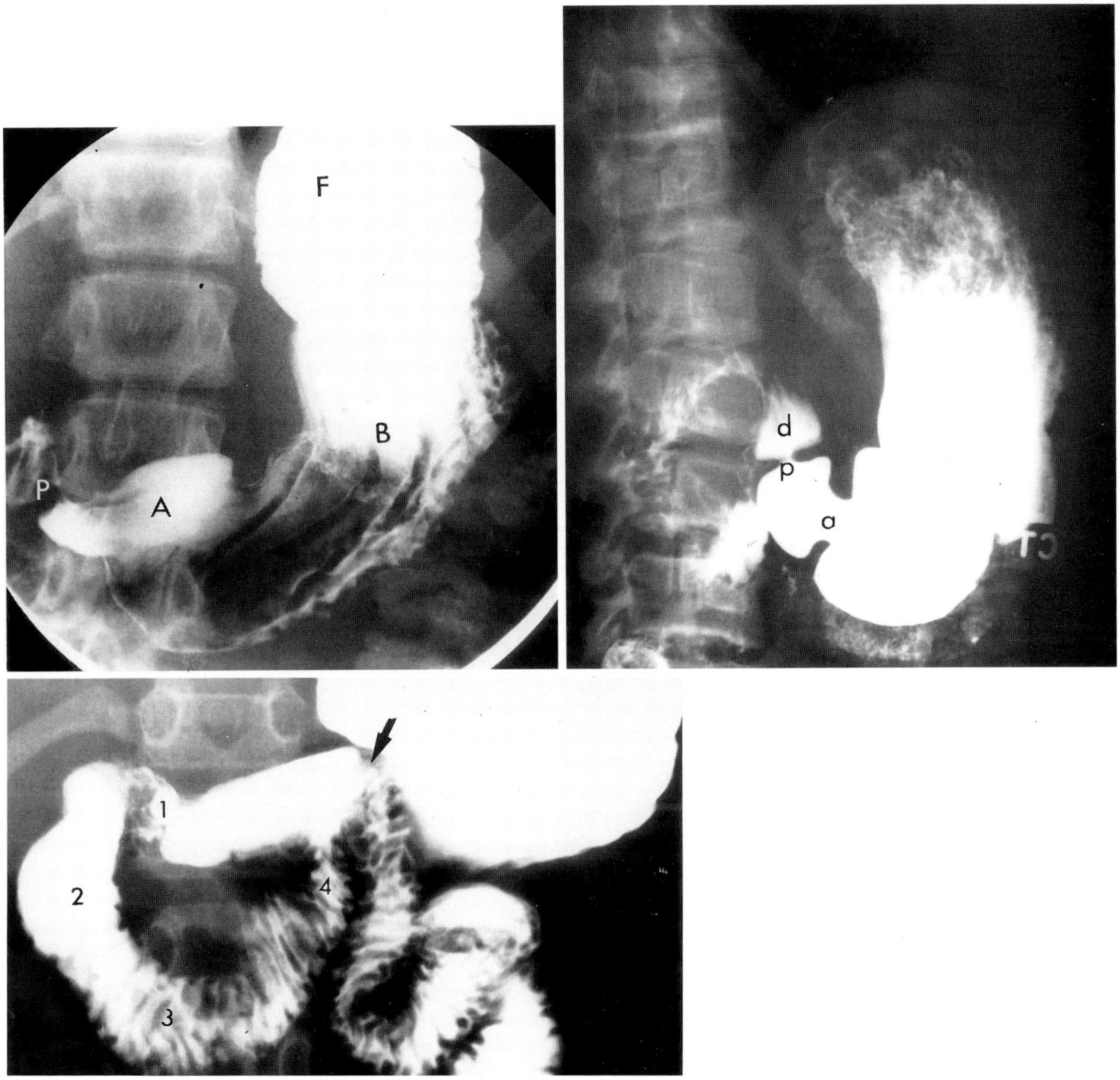

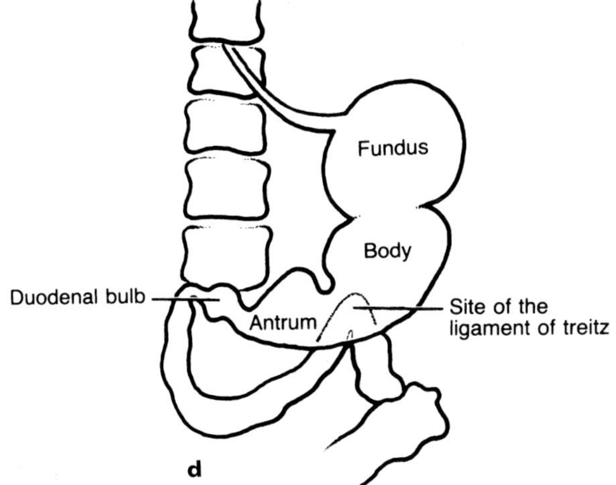

Fig. 4.14 a–d. The upper gastrointestinal series. **a** The stomach is visualized in multiple positions so that contrast is moved through the fundus (*F*), body (*B*), antrum (*A*), and pyloric region (*P*). The mucosal pattern is smooth and regular without any disruptions. Peristaltic waves can be deduced by the various shapes of the stomach, noted on multiple films as well as at fluoroscopy. **b** Oblique view shows to advantage the contraction at the antrum (*a*) and the pyloric channel (*p*). The duodenal bulb (*d*) is triangular and smooth. The duodenum is partially filled. **c** Further along in the study, the duodenum is entirely visualized, and the ligament of Treitz (*arrow*), behind the stomach, is at the level of the duodenal bulb. Note the four portions of the duodenum (*1*, *2*, *3*, *4*). The jejunal pattern appears feathery and unobstructed. **d** Drawing of the proximal stomach to the jejunum

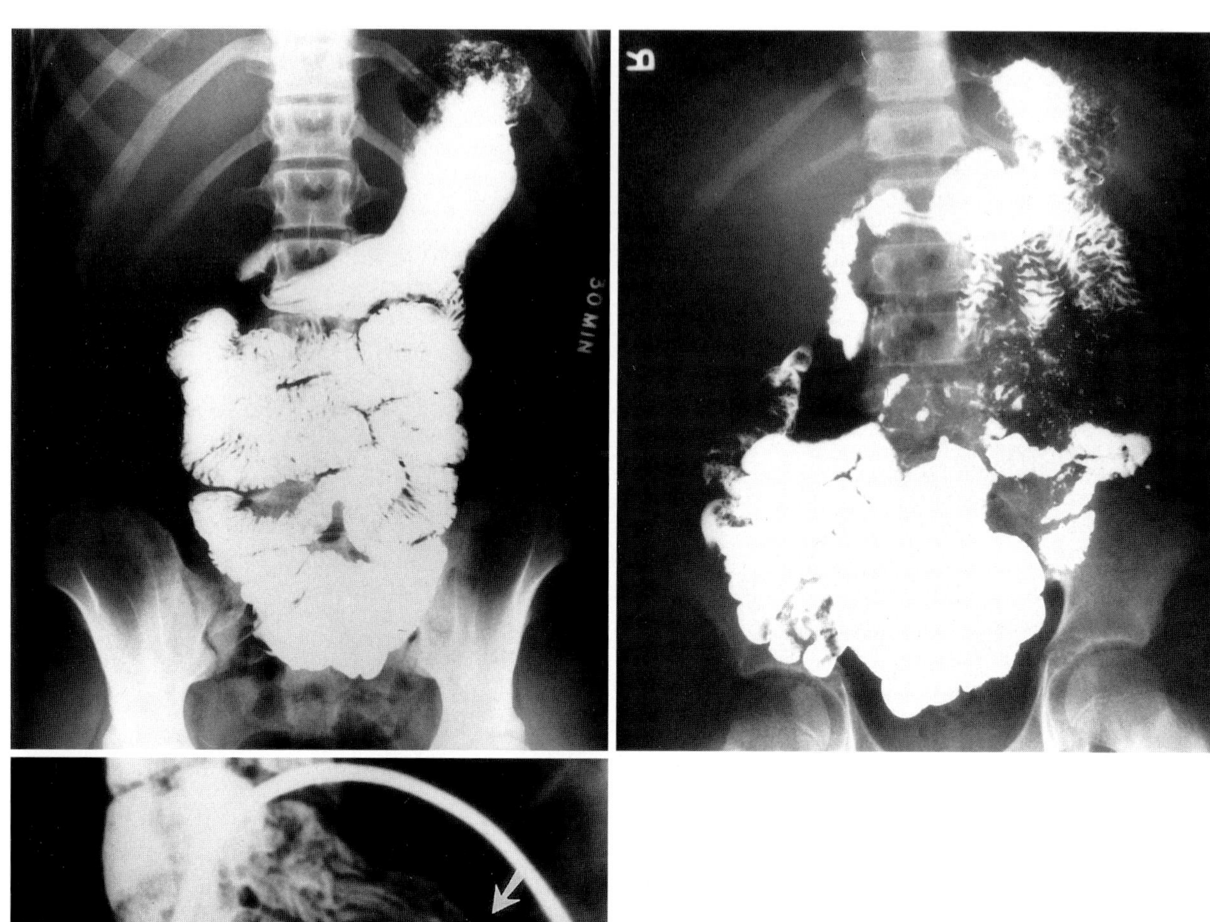

a

b

c

Fig. 4.15 a–c. Small bowel follow-through. **a** A film taken 30 min after the upper portion of the gastrointestinal tract was viewed reveals that the proximal half of the small bowel is now filled. The demarcation between the jejunum and ileum is difficult to see, but bowel is filled on both the right and left sides of the midline. The loops are not significantly separated. **b** The 2-hour film shows that contrast has advanced into the right ascending colon; the feathery pattern of the jejunum is still visible. **c** The terminal ileum (*arrows*) is best demonstrated by compressing it with a balloon paddle and taking a spot film. This method helps evaluate the cecum, ileocecal valve, and terminal ileum

The stomach is then studied in its entirety by placing the patient in various positions and using the effects of gravity to move the liquid barium and air content from one area to another. The mucosal pattern is formed by the gastric rugae throughout the fundus, body, and antrum of the stomach. The *contours* of the stomach are smooth, and the stomach narrows in an expected manner at the pyloric channel which readily opens into the duodenal bulb (see Fig. 4.14). It is important to recognize the normal pyloric channel, as this is the site of pyloric stenosis in young infants.

The duodenum is divided into four parts: the bulb, vertical portion, transverse portion, and ascending portion (see Fig. 4.14). The vertical and horizontal portions form the C loop and are the retroperitoneal portions of the duodenum. The medial margin of the duodenum is adjacent to the head of the pancreas, while the lateral margin is adjacent to the liver and gallbladder. It is important to note the contours and position of the duodenum, as masses or abnormalities in adjacent structures affect the duodenum and cause distortion. It is also important to view the duodenum in frontal and lateral projections to detect anterior or posterior deviation. The horizontal portion of the duodenum crosses the spine from right to left, and the ascending portion ends at the ligament of Treitz to the left of the spine and assumes a position at the height of the duodenal bulb (see Fig. 4.14).

Small Bowel Follow-Through

This study (Fig. 4.15) includes visualization of the esophagus, upper GI tract, and small bowel to the ileocecal valve. It is the examination of choice in children with suspected inflammatory bowel disease such as Crohn's disease. The study is also useful in defining partial distal small bowel obstruction. Immediately beyond the ligament of Treitz, the jejunum begins in the left upper quadrant and runs from left to right. The jejunal-ileal junction is *not* a clearly defined landmark. The mucosal pattern of the small bowel has been described as feathery. This is caused by the valvulae conniventes – Kerckring's folds. In contrast to the colon, these are transverse, circular muscles that convolute the mucosa (see Fig. 4.15).

The terminal ileum has a nodular appearance in children due to the lymphoid tissue of Peyer's patches. This is normal and not, as in an adult, associated with an immune-deficient state.

In a small bowel series it is important that all loops be filled at some point, and that adjacent loops not appear unduly separated when filled. The feathery mucosal pattern of the valvulae should have no irregularity or ulceration. Once the barium is swallowed, it takes between 30 min and 2 hour to reach the ileocecal valve in most children, depending on the rate of gastric emptying and bowel motility.

Barium Enema

In this study (Fig. 4.16), contrast is introduced through the rectum until the entire colon is filled. By coating the intraluminal surface of the colon, polyps, diverticula, as well as ulcerations and fistulous tracts, inflammatory bowel disease, ulcerative colitis, or Crohn's disease can be diagnosed. Masses, both intraluminal and extraluminal, may be detected.

Let us begin with the barium enema and go through the regular film-viewing pattern. The emphasis is on the normal anatomy and the method of looking at the examination. As with other films, use the parameters of position, contour, and size when evaluating the colon. The position of the rectum and sigmoid can be noted on the filled films. The rectum is in the midline on the frontal view, and the posterior wall lies immediately adjacent to the inner curve of the sacrum on the lateral view (see Fig. 4.16). The sigmoid colon extends into the right lower quadrant and then swings laterally to the left lower quadrant. The distal descending colon is seen at this level, with the proximal portions in the left flank and the left upper quadrant. Because of its contiguity with the spleen the highest curve is noted as the splenic flexure. The transverse colon hangs from the mesentery in the midabdomen, suspended at the hepatic and splenic flexures. As mentioned above, this is an anterior structure. The hepatic flexure is in the right upper quadrant and more caudad (inferior) than the splenic flexure. It lies just below the liver. The ascending colon is in the right lateral gutter, and its most proximal portion is the cecum. It can be recognized by detecting either the appendix or the ileocecal valve or by the reflux into the terminal ileum. The cecum is normally in the right lower quadrant overlying the iliac crest; when it lies between the iliac crest and the hepatic flexure, it may be mobile due to a loose fixation of the mesentery. However, when the cecum is not in the right lower quadrant, suspect the congenital abnormality malrotation or malfixation of the midgut. By definition, the midgut extends from the ampulla of vater to the splenic flexure, with the foregut being all bowel proximal to this and the hindgut distal to the midgut (Fig. 4.17).

The *contours* of the bowel lumen should be smooth and devoid of irregularities. When irregularities are present, they may be due to either poor preparation (retained fecal material) or pathological conditions such as ulcerations of inflammatory bowel disease (Fig. 4.18; compare Fig. 4.16). The colon is normally

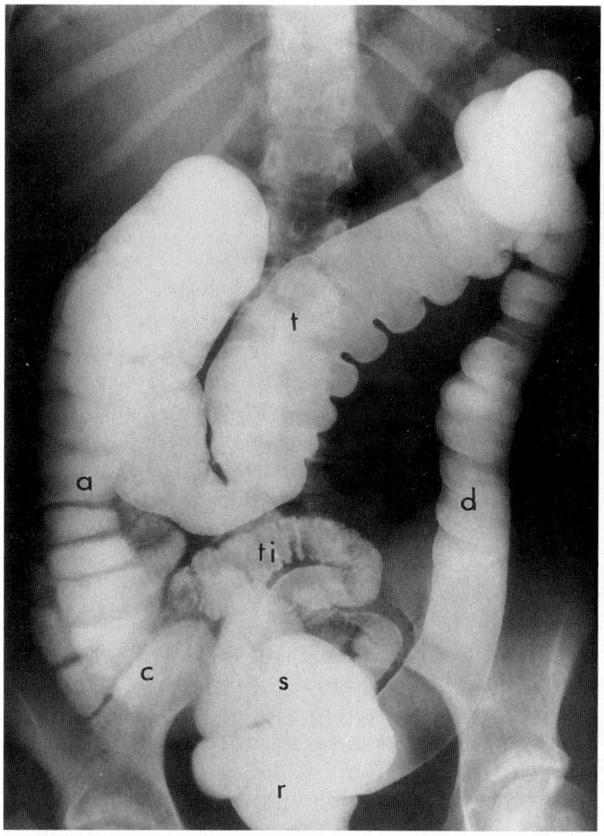

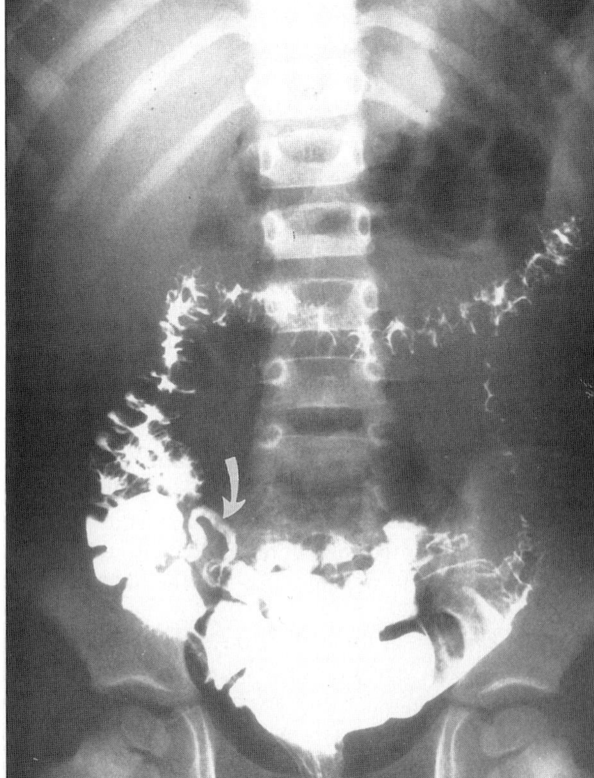

Fig. 4.16 a–c. Normal barium enema. **a** Frontal view of the barium-filled colon shows the midline rectum (*r*), tortuous sigmoid (*s*) and rather smooth-walled descending colon (*d*). The haustrated transverse colon (*t*), ascending colon (*a*), and the cecum (*c*) are also identified. Reflux into the terminal ileum (*ti*) is present. **b** Lateral projection affords a good view of the rectum and its proximity to the sacrum. **c** Postevacuation film shows the bowel almost totally collapsed, with no filling defects. The thin, tubular, barium-filled appendix is seen in the right lower quadrant (*arrow*)

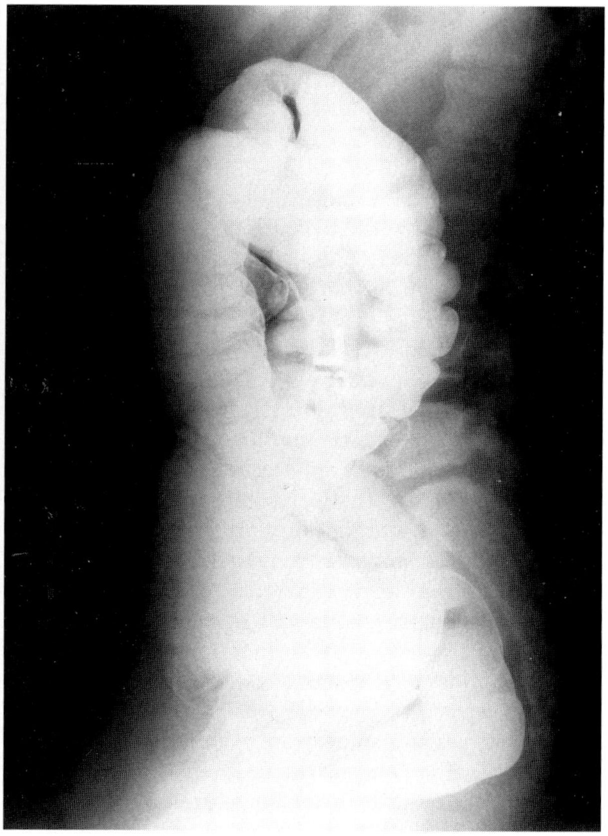

Fig. 4.17 a–d. Malrotation of midgut. **a** Plain film of the abdomen in this 5-year-old, who had been vomiting, reveals a cluster of small bowel to the right of the spine, a very "soft" finding. Frequently, the plain film is entirely normal. **b** A film after barium was given by mouth shows the jejunum entirely to the right of the abdomen. The ligament of Treitz is absent (see Fig. 4.14 c). **c** Spot film of the duodenum shows that the barium never goes to the normal location of the ligament of Treitz but forms a "corkscrew" pattern around the superior mesenteric artery (which is not visualized), typical of malrotation. If the duodenum gets twisted (volvulus), bowel ischemia results. **d** An evacuation film following a barium enema in another patient reveals the cecum high in the right upper quadrant (*c*). This is another sign of malrotation ▶

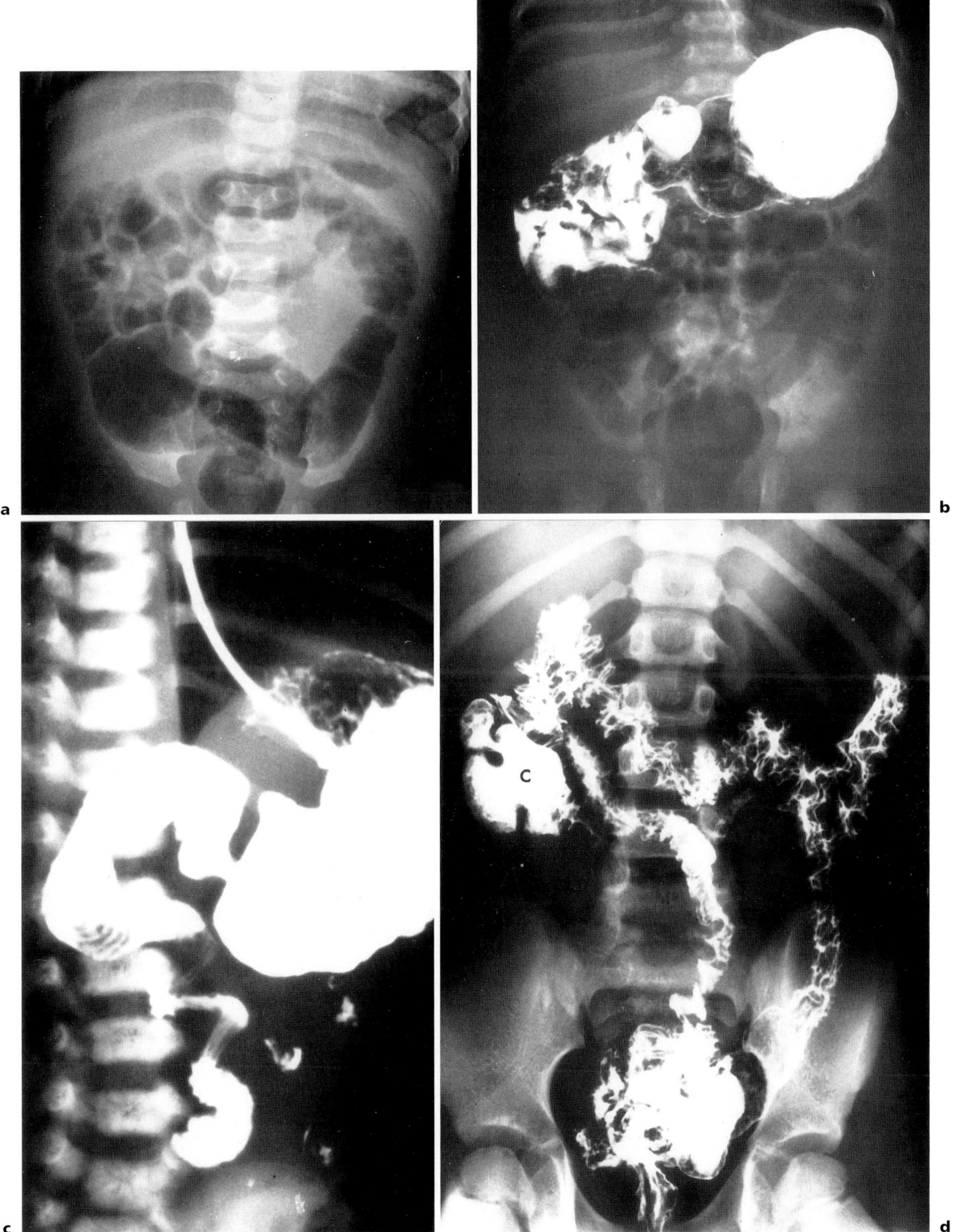
a
b
c
C
d

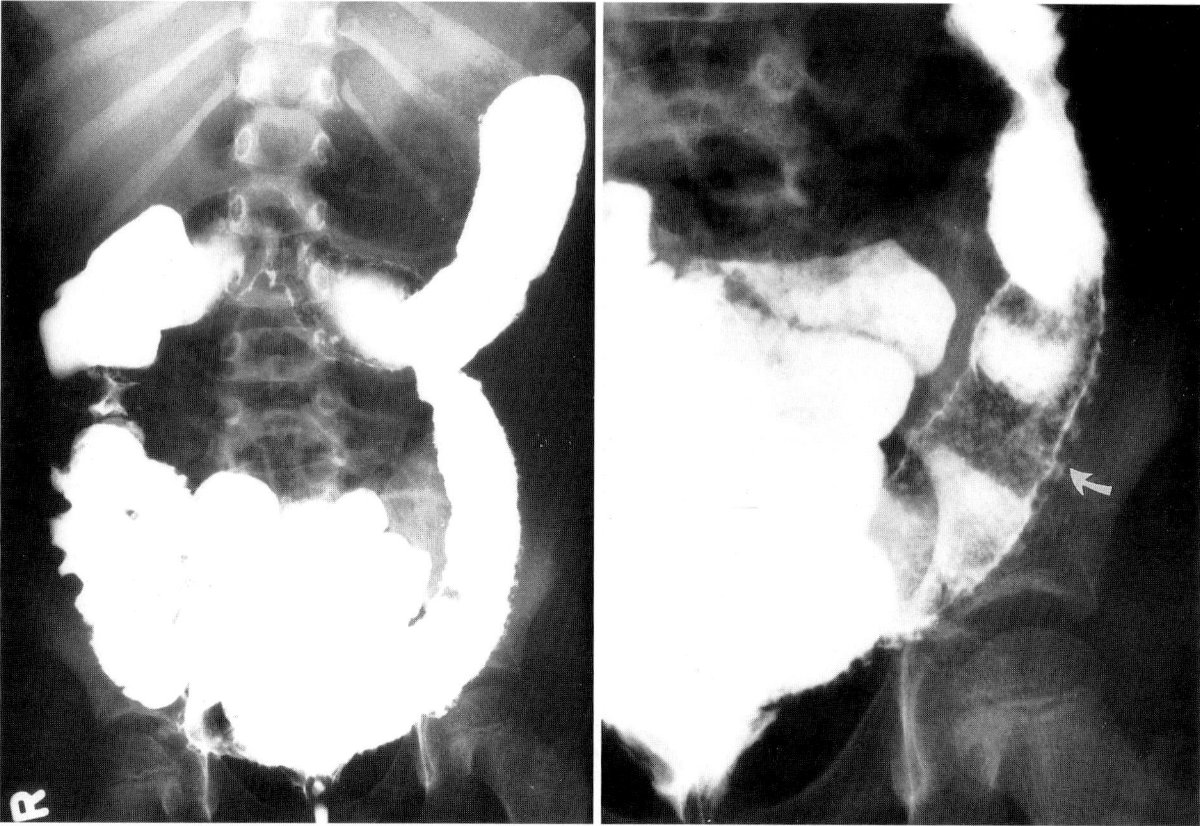

Fig. 4.18 a,b. Ulcerative colitis. a Frontal film from a barium enema reveals contrast material outside the lumen and in the wall, particularly evident in the descending colon. Note "collar-button" ulcerations. b Close-up shows the "collar-button" (*arrow*) ulcerations to advantage. The key to diagnosis in this case is the abnormal contour of the bowel

indented at intervals by haustra or sacculations, which are smooth indentations caused by the longitudinal muscular band on the surface of the colon that compresses it like an accordion. The muscles of the longitudinal band are called taeniae coli. Normally, there are fewer haustral markings in the left colon than in the right.

After the colon has been filled and appropriate films taken, the patient is allowed to evacuate the contrast, and several postevacuation films (see Fig. 4.16) are obtained to evaluate the mucosal pattern. On these films, the mucosa is feathery, and any mass within the colon, such as a polyp, disrupts this fine, regular, feathery pattern (Fig. 4.19).

The *size* of the colon is greatest at the rectum and cecum. The left colon may be slightly smaller than the rest of the colon.

The search for intraluminal filling defects is mandatory at fluoroscopy and also on filled and postevacuation films. Since these may represent polyps, look for a stalk. The most common intraluminal filling defect in children is fecal material, but the most common pathological intraluminal defect is that of a juvenile polyp (see Fig. 4.19).

Since it is easier and faster to evacuate the contrast from the colon, the barium enema precedes the upper GI series when both are ordered for a gastrointestinal work-up. A delay of several days may be involved if the upper GI is examined before the enema. If ultrasound, CT, or radionuclide examination is indicated, these examinations should also precede the barium study.

The gastrointestinal tract can also be evaluated by CT. Thickening of various portions of the esophagus, stomach, small intestine, and colon is readily seen and is usually due to inflammation or edema (Fig. 4.20).

The child drinks a dilute water-soluble contrast mixture so that the bowel can be positively identified and the bowel wall evaluated by noting the distance from the contrast to serosa thickness. Ideally, the GI tract should be full of opaque contrast or air. Any fluid collection that does not contain air or opaque contrast must be outside the GI tract, and thus an abscess or

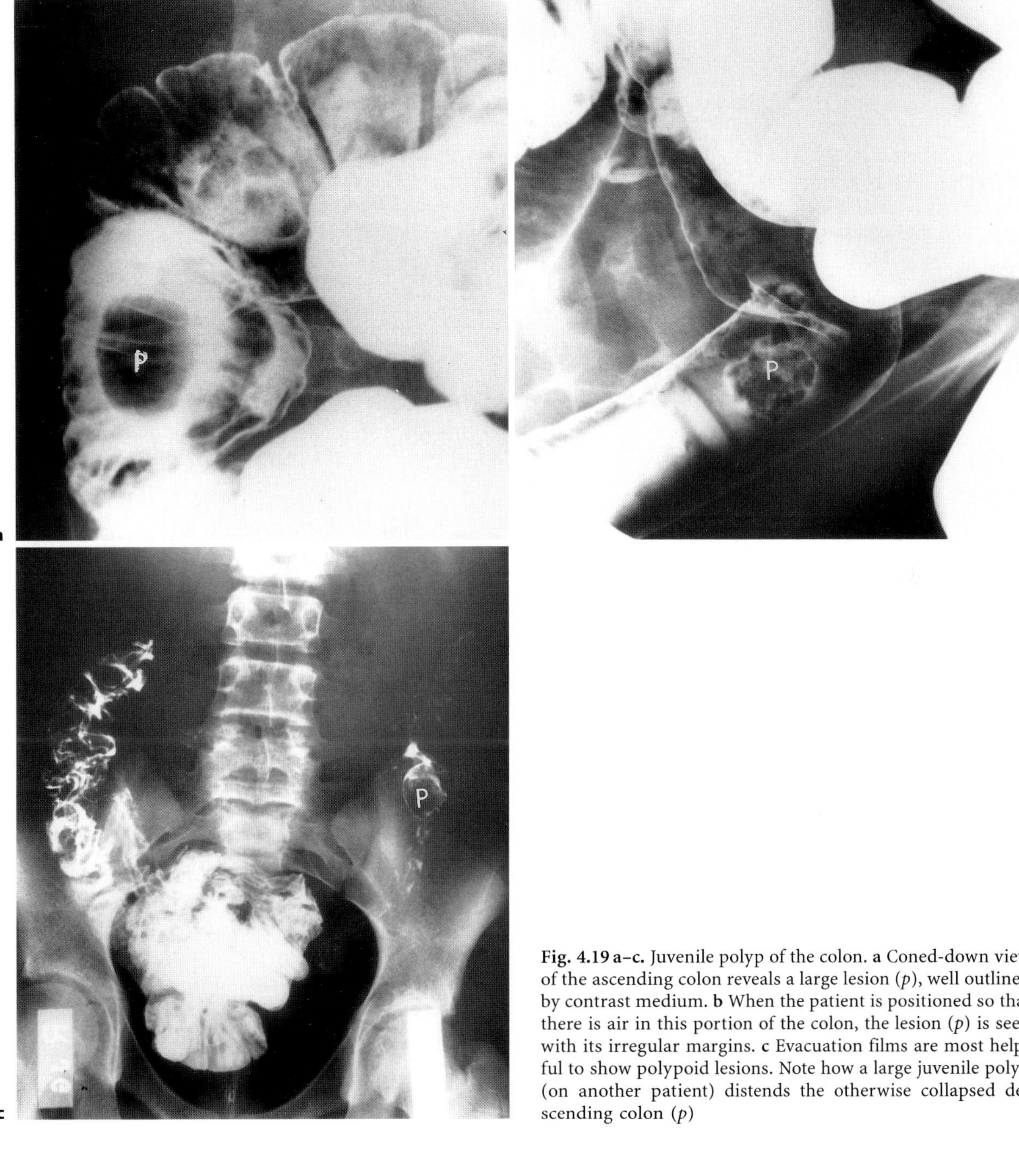

Fig. 4.19 a–c. Juvenile polyp of the colon. **a** Coned-down view of the ascending colon reveals a large lesion (*p*), well outlined by contrast medium. **b** When the patient is positioned so that there is air in this portion of the colon, the lesion (*p*) is seen with its irregular margins. **c** Evacuation films are most helpful to show polypoid lesions. Note how a large juvenile polyp (on another patient) distends the otherwise collapsed descending colon (*p*)

cystic mass can be identified (Fig. 4.21). Contrast-enhanced CT (intravenous contrast as well as oral contrast) is useful in evaluating the mesenteric and pericolonic spaces. Contrast-filled vessels are very easily distinguished from lymph nodes anywhere in the abdomen and pelvis.

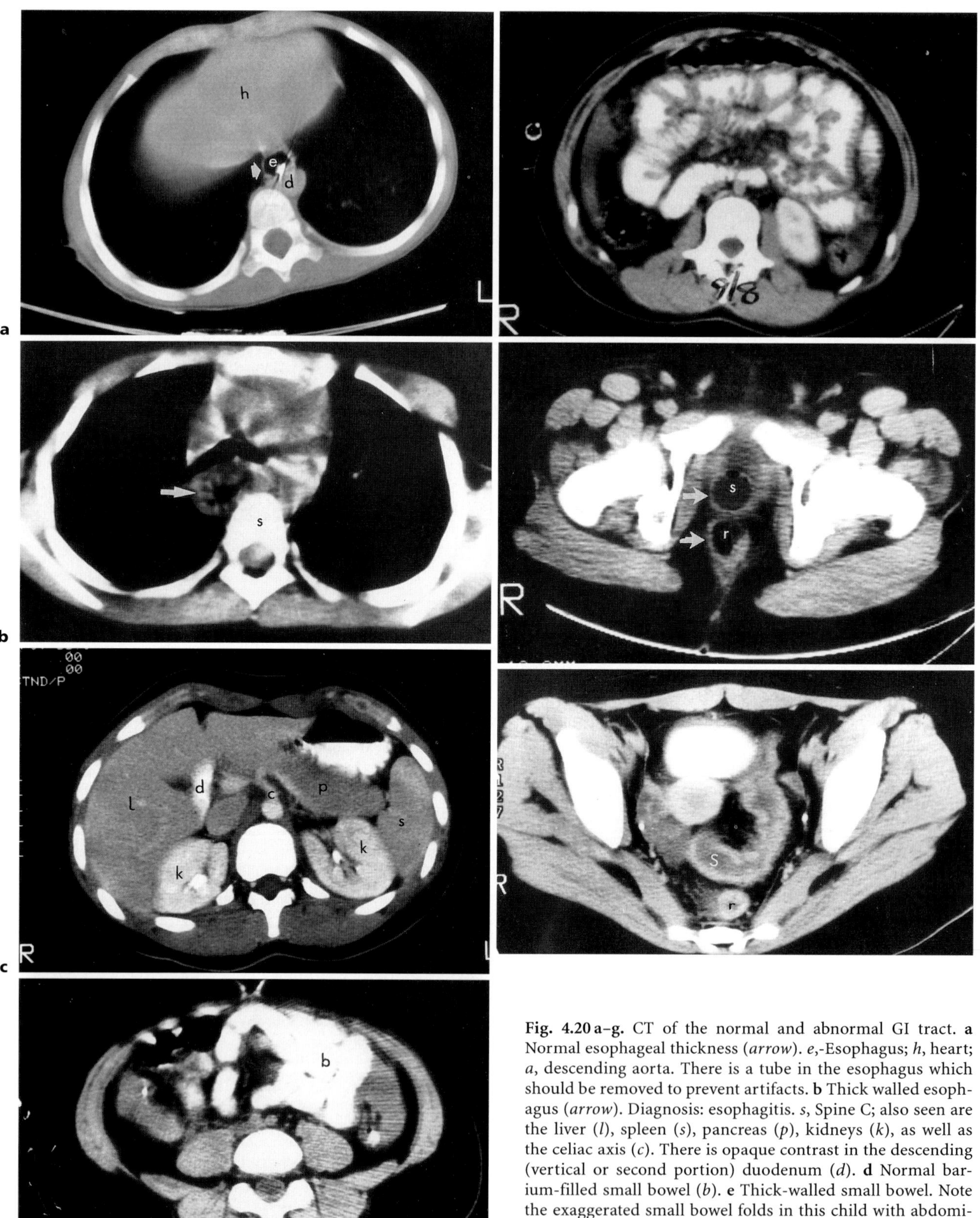

Fig. 4.20 a–g. CT of the normal and abnormal GI tract. **a** Normal esophageal thickness (*arrow*). *e*,-Esophagus; *h*, heart; *a*, descending aorta. There is a tube in the esophagus which should be removed to prevent artifacts. **b** Thick walled esophagus (*arrow*). Diagnosis: esophagitis. *s*, Spine C; also seen are the liver (*l*), spleen (*s*), pancreas (*p*), kidneys (*k*), as well as the celiac axis (*c*). There is opaque contrast in the descending (vertical or second portion) duodenum (*d*). **d** Normal barium-filled small bowel (*b*). **e** Thick-walled small bowel. Note the exaggerated small bowel folds in this child with abdominal trauma and subsequent edema. **f** Normal sigmoid and rectal wall thickness (*arrows*). **g** Thick-walled rectum and sigmoid. Diagnosis: colitis. *r*, Rectum; *s*, sigmoid

a

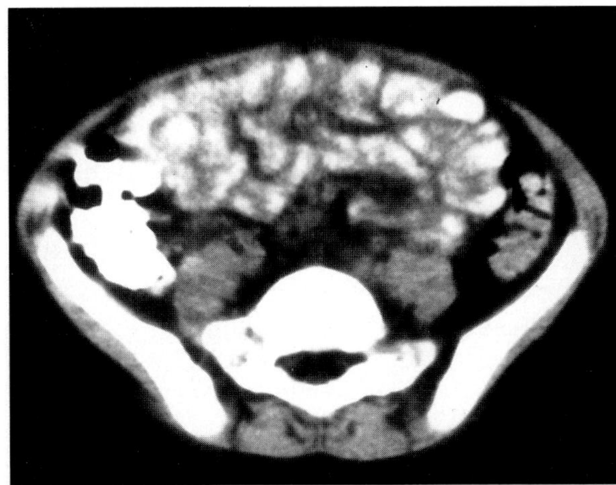

b

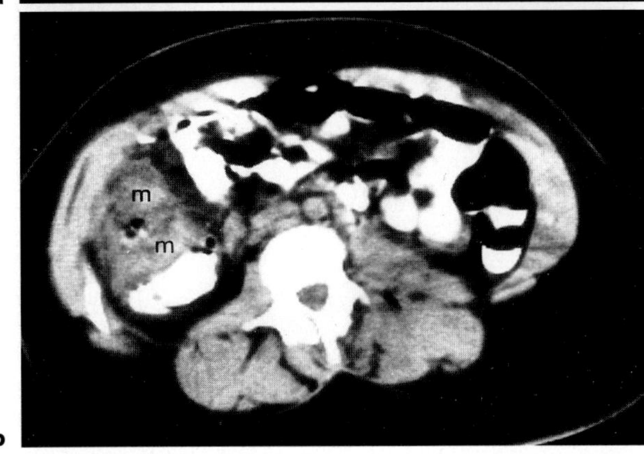

Fig. 4.21. CT of appendiceal abscess. **a** Normal lower abdomen. **b** Appendiceal abscess. Note how there is a large void of contrast in the right lower quadrant. The fat is less black (inflammation), and there is an inhomogeneous soft tissue mass in the right lower quadrant (*m*)

Evaluation of Other Organ Systems Within the Abdomen

Liver and Biliary System

Liver size will already have been noted on the plain film, and whether there is a mass arising from the liver determined indirectly by displacement of the stomach and duodenum. Calcifications will have been sought within the liver and gallbladder. A more specific evaluation of the liver and biliary system would involve any of four newer noninvasive imaging modalities: ultrasound, radionuclide imaging, CT, or MR. The least invasive procedure is ultrasound; we therefore discuss it fully. Ultrasound, CT, and MR examinations provide precise anatomical information, while the radionuclide study gives only *gross* anatomical information but *precise* functional information (see Chap. 1). Remember, ask the proper question (function or anatomy) before ordering a study!

Ultrasonic evaluation usually visualizes the liver in transverse and longitudinal sections. Transverse ultrasonic sections of the abdomen (as well as CT transverse sections) are oriented with the patient's right on the viewer's left; the superior aspect of the scan is the abdominal surface with the patient supine (Fig. 4.22). In the longitudinal sections, the patient's head is oriented to the viewer's left.

Each organ has its own reproducible parenchymal architecture. The lack of echoes or anechoic regions suggests a fluid-filled structure, such as a blood vessel or gallbladder. They appear black and are easily defined by color Doppler when there is any question as to whether a structure is a blood vessel (fills with color) or a cyst. It is not the purpose of this text to review the interpretation of ultrasonic scans, but rather to portray the anatomy of the hepatobiliary system (see Fig. 4.22). It is fair to say, however, that ultrasonic evaluation of the gallbladder is the best method for demonstrating gallstones.

The CT scan has the same orientation as the transverse sonographic study. More precise anatomical information is obtained, but at some "cost." The young patient must be sedated, contrast medium must be injected for enhancement, bowel contrast must be utilized to opacify bowel loops for abdominal scans, and the study a priori uses radiation (see Fig. 4.21). The diseases most suitable for diagnosis by CT in the GI tract are the following:

- Visceral abnormalities (liver, spleen, pancreas, kidney)
  - Inflammation or tumors
  - Congenital lesions
  - Traumatic lesions
- Lymphadenopathy
- Masses
- Incidental lesions easily seen on CT performed for other reasons
  - Bowel obstruction
  - Foreign body
  - Calcifications (gallstones, pancreatic stones, etc.)
  - Free fluid
  - Bony abnormalities

An isotope scan of the liver is usually performed with technetium (a radioisotope) bound to compounds taken up by either the reticuloendothelial system (technetium sulfur colloid) or hepatocytes (technetium iminodiacetic compounds). Sequential scans are obtained so that function can be properly assessed (Fig. 4.23).

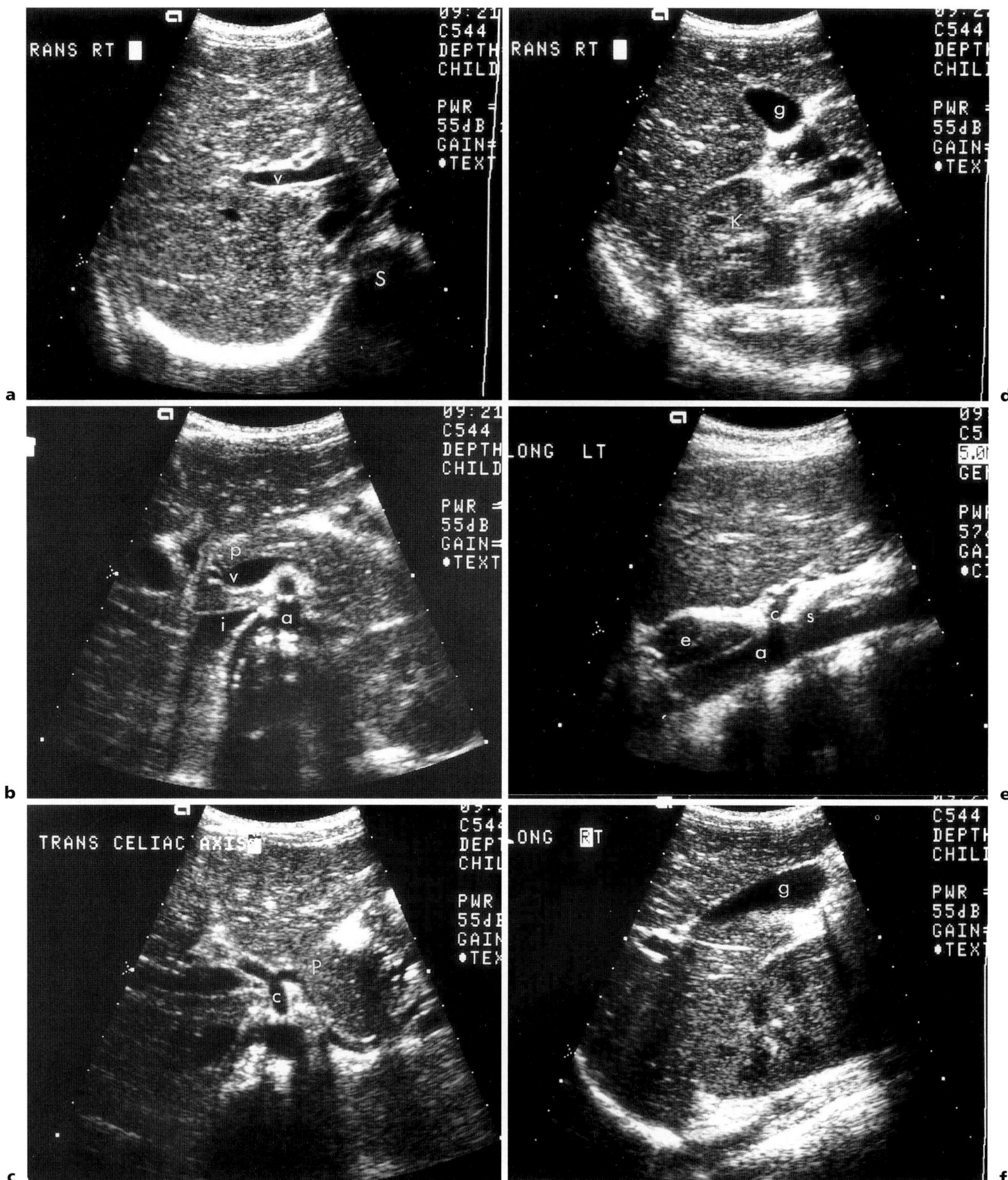

Fig. 4.22 a–f. Normal ultrasound. **a** Transverse section through the liver showing portal vein (*v*); *s*, spine. **b** Transverse section through the head of pancreas (*p*) and portal vein (*v*). The inferior vena cava (*i*) and aorta (*a*) are noted; *s*, spine; *c*, transverse section at the level of the celiac artery; *p*, tail of pancreas. **d** Transverse section showing gallbladder (*g*), kidney (*k*), and renal vein and inferior vena cava. Note there is fluid in the duodenum. **e** Longitudinal section through aorta (*a*), celiac artery (*c*), and superior mesenteric artery (*s*). The esophageal gastric junction is just anterior to the aorta (*e*). **f** Longitudinal section through the gallbladder (*g*) and right kidney

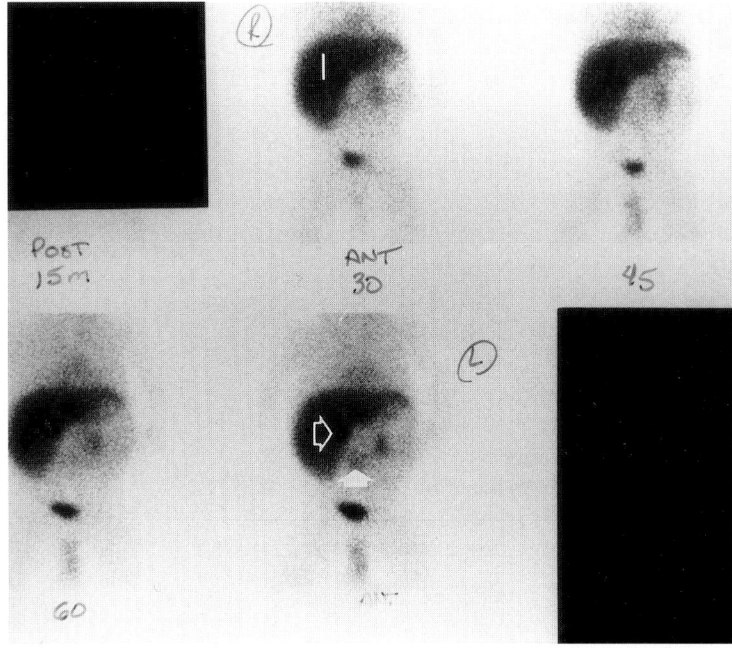

Fig. 4.23. Liver scan with technetium iminodiacetic compound, PIPIDA. Sequential scans show the isotope being taken up by the hepatocytes of the liver (*l*), excreted into the gallbladder (*open arrow*), and eventually into the Gl tract (*solid arrow*). The liver intensity gradually diminishes

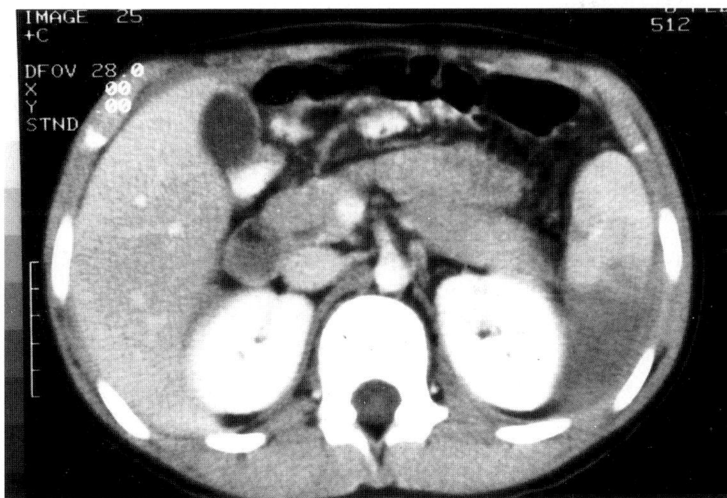

Fig. 4.24. Ruptured spleen (compare Fig. 4.21). Contrast-enhanced CT shows the spleen has two densities, the normal anterior portion (*upper*) and fluid density inferior margin – the laceration

Pancreas

Ultrasound is an excellent way of visualizing the pancreas. It is identified by finding some important anatomical landmarks (see Fig. 4.22). CT also demonstrates this area quite well (see Fig. 4.21). There are no comparable radionuclide studies.

Spleen

The spleen can be seen by any of these three imaging modalities. However, contrast-enhanced CT is preferred, particularly in cases of trauma (Fig. 4.24).

Common Clinical Problems

Vomiting

Vomiting is extremely common during childhood and is so nonspecific that history and physical examination are crucial to diagnosis. The character of the vomitus as well as the age of the child play an important role in the differential diagnosis. In the neonate to 2 months of age this may be:

- Nonbilious
  - Chalasia
  - Pyloric stenosis
- Bilious
  - Midgut volvulus
  - Small bowel obstruction
  - Bowel atresia in newborn
  - Hirschsprung's disease

In infants aged 2 months to 2 years the possibilities are:

- Nonbilious (rarely an organic cause other than chalasia)
- Bilious
  - Midgut volvulus
  - Small bowel obstruction
  - Intussusception

In children over 2 years old:

- Most causes not related to GI tract abnormalities

From age 1 day to 2 months the most common cause of nonbilious vomiting is chalasia – gastroesophageal reflux. Immaturity of the esophagogastric junction results in food substances (or contrast during an esophagram) flowing back from the stomach into the esophagus. This obviously is imaged best with nuclear scintigraphy (best sensitivity) (Fig. 4.25). It also can be detected during the fluoroscopy phase of the esophagram or upper GI examination. The diagnosis can also be made on the delayed film if there is contrast in the esophagus long after the patient has been given the barium. In most children this is not accompanied by a hiatal hernia and is a self-limiting disorder. The best nonimaging technique is the pH monitor – a probe placed at the end of a feeding tube. It is positioned in the distal end of the esophagus and the patient is monitored for 24 hours. When reflux is the primary consideration, a nuclear scan may suffice. When there are other considerations, a radiographic contrast study is indicated.

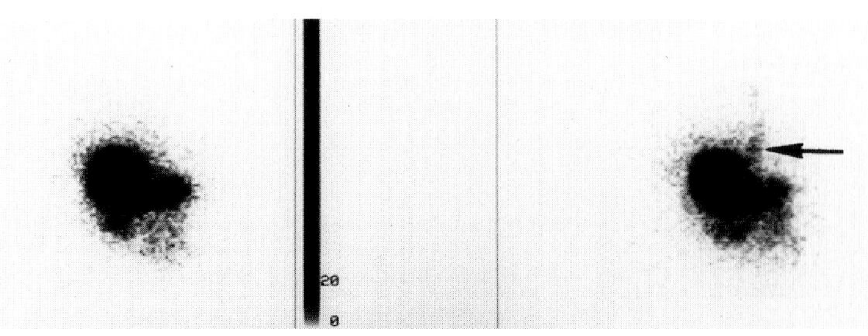

Fig. 4.25. Gastroesophageal reflux study. The patient was given Tc-sulfacolloid in formula. Posterior imaging was done at 1-min intervals. The stomach is seen without reflux (*left*) and with esophageal reflux (*right, arrow*)

Another common cause of nonbilious vomiting in this age group is pyloric stenosis (Figs. 4.26, 4.27). These children usually have projectile, nonbilious vomiting. If it persists for some time, the child stops gaining weight, and electrolyte abnormalities (alkalosis with low chloride) become apparent. On careful physical examination the hypertrophied pyloric muscle can be palpated and feels somewhat like an olive. Most pediatric surgeons feel confident enough with this finding to operate and to perform an imaging examination only in those patients in whom the finding is absent. When one is quite certain of the diagnosis of pyloric stenosis but would like imaging confirmation, an ultrasound can be performed. Reliable criteria have been worked out for the hypertrophied pylorus (4 mm muscle thickness and 18 mm pyloric length; Fig. 4.26).

When one is less certain of the diagnosis and is concerned about other anomalies, an upper GI is the correct procedure. The upper GI series defines the elongated, upturned, curved pyloric canal with the "railroad track" sign (see Fig. 4.27).

In the neonate and infant up to 2 months of age bilious vomiting strongly suggests obstruction distal to the entrance of the common bile duct into the duodenum. In the first days of life midgut volvulus and atresias of the small bowel are suspected. By using air as a contrast medium, the level of obstruction can be

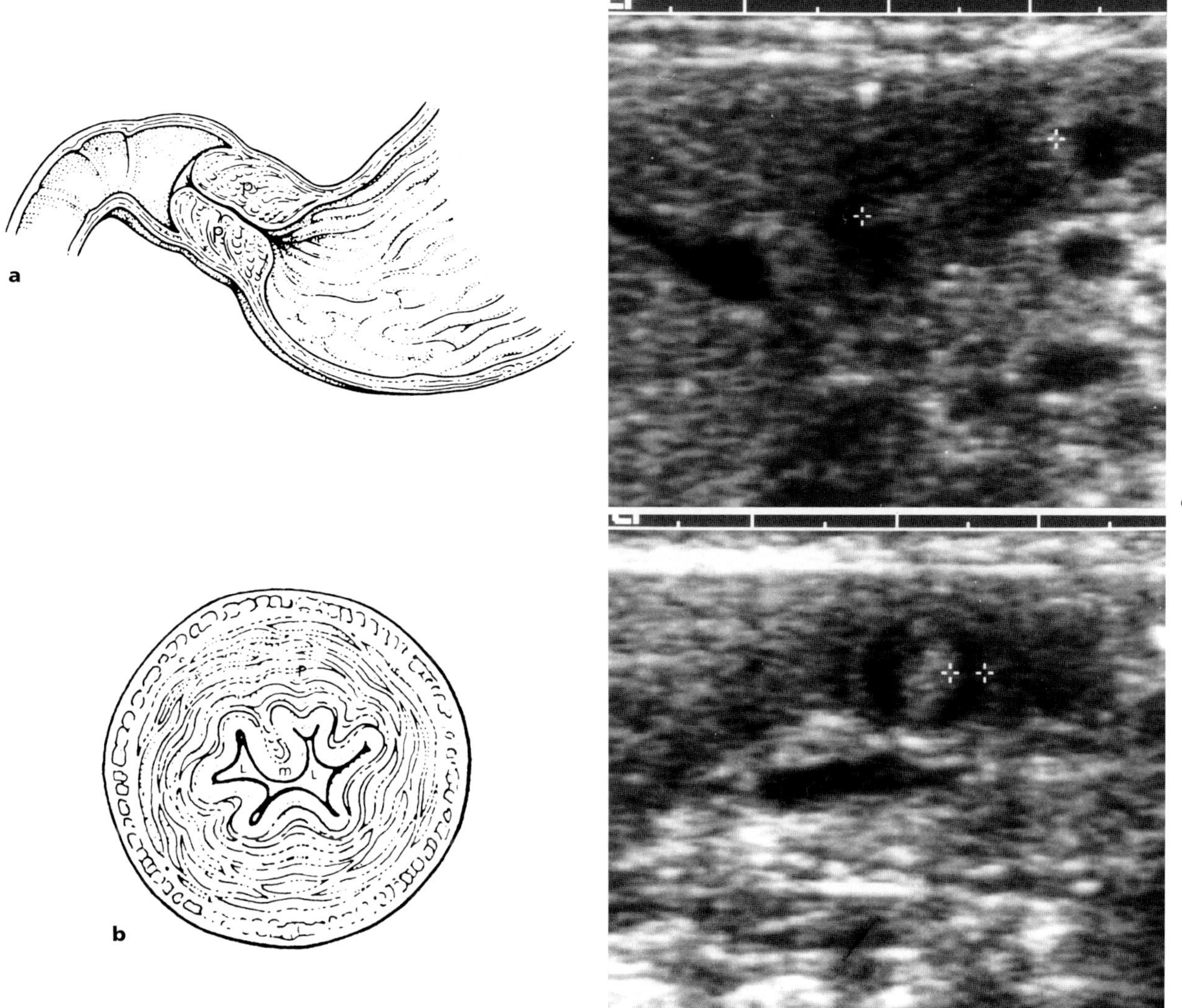

Fig. 4.26 a–d. Pyloric stenosis ultrasound diagnosis. **a** Drawing of longitudinal section through hypertrophied muscle (*p*). **b** Drawing of transverse scan through thickened pylorus. *p*, Pylorus; *m*, mucosa; l, lumen. **c** Longitudinal sonogram corresponding to **a**, cursors delineate length of pylorus. **d** Transverse ultrasound corresponding to **b**, cursors delineate muscle thickness. (From [1])

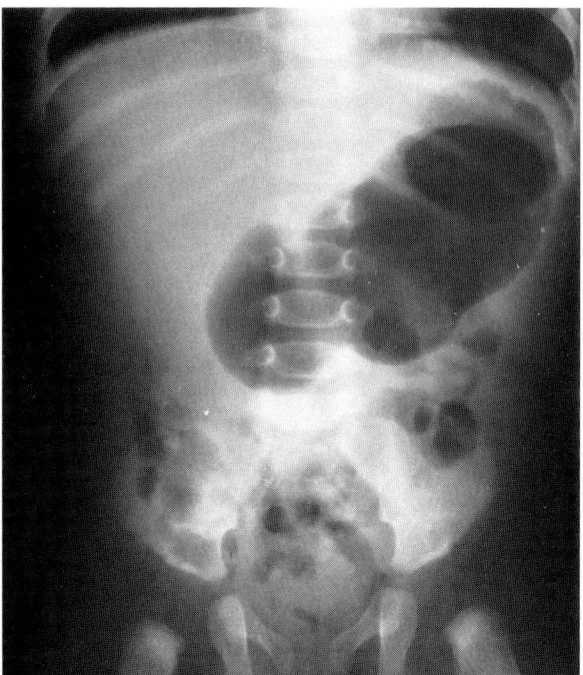

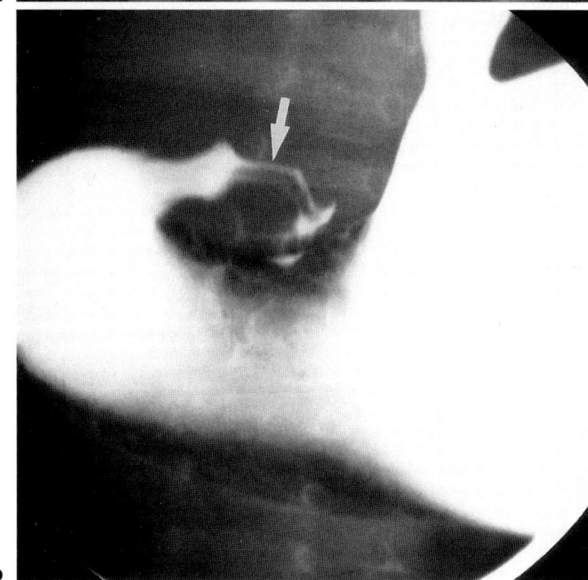

Fig. 4.27 a, b. Pyloric stenosis. **a** Supine film of the abdomen reveals distention of the stomach. Multiple peristaltic waves (contractions) are visible. This is one of the plain film findings of gastric outlet obstruction. **b** Upper GI reveals the elongated, upturned pyloric channel (*arrow*). Note there are two contrast-filled tracts (railroad track) because of asymmetric hypertrophy of channel of the muscle

diagnosed by the number of air-filled, distended loops of bowel seen on the plain film (see Fig. 4.11). Midgut volvulus is the most important emergent condition to consider. In these situations there is developmental abnormality of rotation and fixation of the midbowel from the ligament of Treitz to the splenic flexure. The ligament of Treitz is absent. Lack of proper fixation provides the mechanical basis that permits the bowel to twist (volvulus), leading to vascular compromise (superior mesenteric vessels). Initially, venous return is occluded, followed by arterial obstruction involving the superior mesenteric artery (see Fig. 4.17).

Causes of more distal abdominal obstruction presenting in the newborn include ileal and colonic atresia and aganglionosis (Hirschsprung's disease). In the latter, there is extensive dilatation of bowel loops indicating low obstruction. When a barium enema is performed, a discrepancy between the *dilated proximal ganglionic portion* of bowel and the abnormal aganglionic distal portion of bowel is seen. The transition zone, together with the child's failure to satisfactorily evacuate the barium after 24 h, confirms the presence of mechanical bowel obstruction proximal to the malfunctioning colon segment.

Between 2 months and 2 years of age the major cause of *nonbilious vomiting* continues to be chalasia (gastroesophageal reflux). *Bilious vomiting* in this age group suggests malrotation, small bowel obstruction, or intussusception. Intussusception occurs when small bowel invaginates into small bowel or colon, causing obstruction and eventual ischemia of the telescoped portion of the bowel – the intussusceptum (Fig. 4.28). Most often, intussusception is manifest clinically by acute, colicky abdominal pain (see below) and in late stages by bloody diarrhea and signs of intestinal obstruction. The obstruction often results in bilious vomiting.

In children over 2 years of age most causes of vomiting are not related to GI tract anomalies, although certainly small bowel obstruction, midgut volvulus, and intussusception do occur.

Abdominal Pain

This is an extremely common complaint in the pediatric age group. It can be separated into acute and chronic abdominal pain. In chronic abdominal pain most clinicians have found radiographic studies (upper GI series and barium enema) to be futile when pain is the *only* complaint. However, when this symptom is coupled with weight loss, diarrhea, and/or blood in the stool, inflammatory bowel disease is frequently found. The term "inflammatory bowel disease" includes regional enteritis and ulcerative colitis

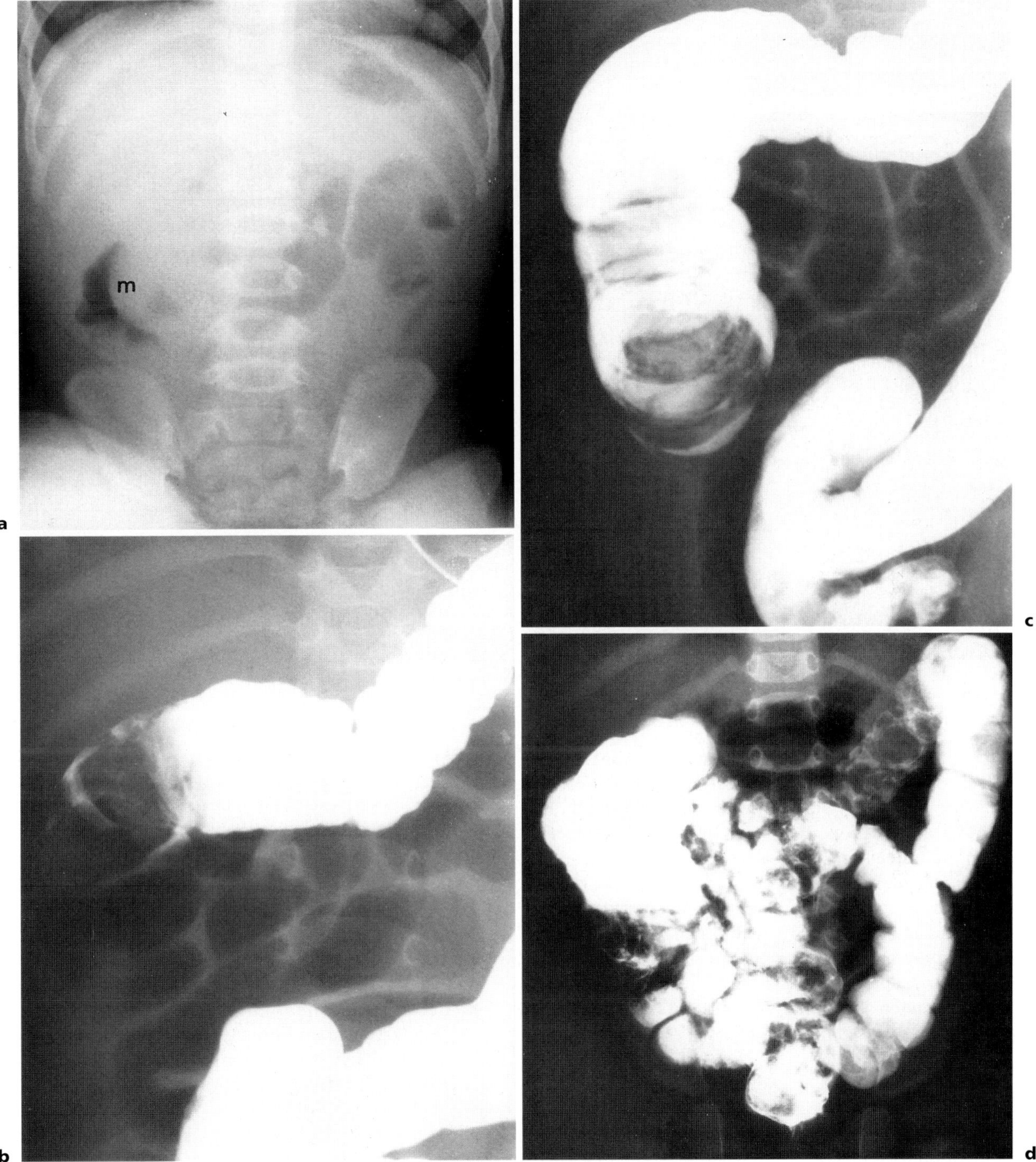

Fig. 4.28 a–d. Intussusception. **a** Upright abdominal film in this 8-month-old with acute, colicky abdominal pain reveals a mass in the region of the hepatic flexure (*m*). This finding was consistent on all films. **b** A barium enema was performed, and a large filling defect is seen in this region. **c** This mass was pushed back to the cecum by barium enema. **d** There was abundant small bowel reflux and the mass is no longer visible

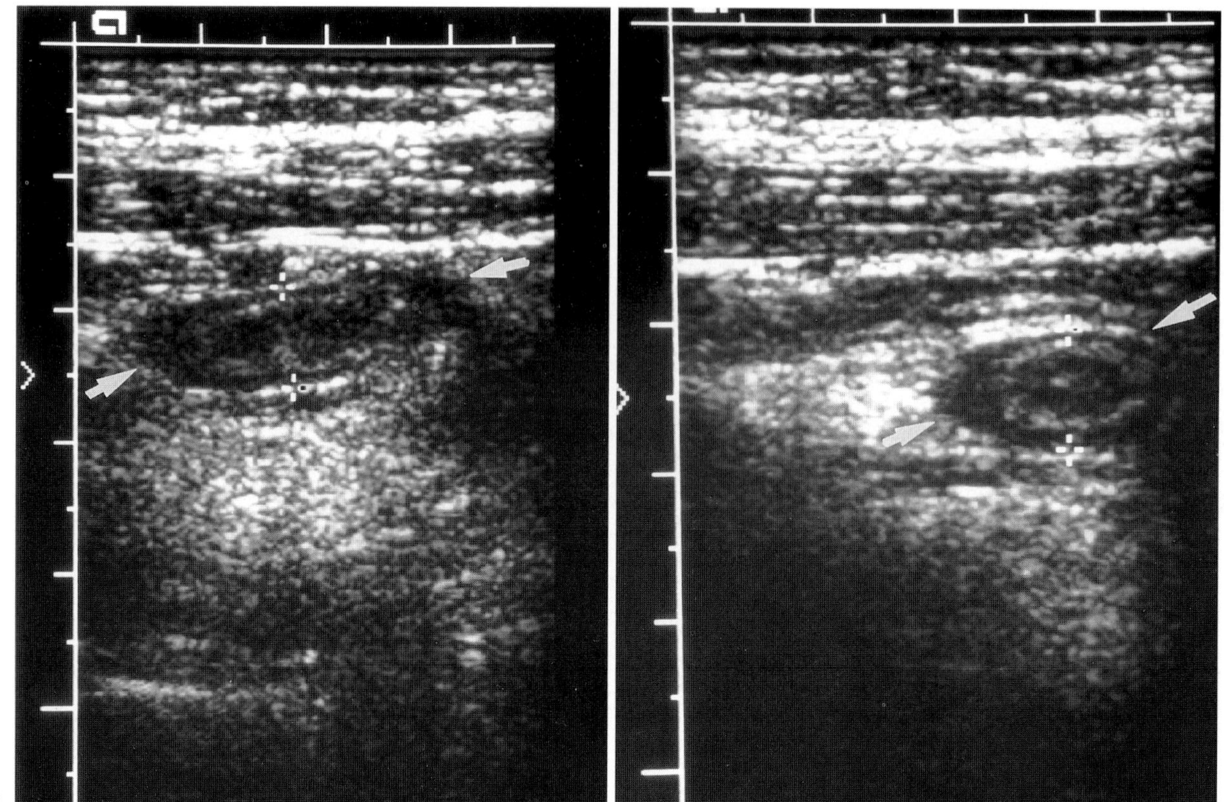

and can be diagnosed by various investigations of the upper and lower gastrointestinal tract (see Fig. 4.18).

Acute abdominal pain in children is most often due to medical conditions such as gastroenteritis. However, the radiologist must be alert for surgical causes of abdominal pain, the most common of which are appendicitis, incarcerated inguinal hernia, and intussusception (see Figs. 4.3, 4.10, 4.28). While routine plain radiography may be indicated when any of these conditions is suspected, only with an intussusception is the barium enema done. The radiographic signs of these three disorders are as follows:

- Appendicitis
  - Appendicolith
  - Free fluid in the cecal area or elsewhere within abdomen
  - Sentinel loop of small bowel
  - Absence of psoas margin
  - Scoliosis, with concavity toward side of disorder
  - (In appendicitis, radiographic signs are found in only 50% of cases examined.)
- Inguinal hernia
  - Signs of intestinal obstruction
  - Bowel gas in inguinal canal or lower

Fig. 4.29 a, b. Ultrasound of appendicitis. **a** Longitudinal scan of right lower quadrant. An inhomogeneous mass is seen. It is not compressible and is the inflamed appendix (*arrows*). **b** Another somewhat oblique view of the appendix (*arrows*)

- Intussusception
  - Mass
  - Signs of obstruction
  - Coiled-spring appearance on barium enema
  - (A negative plain film should not deter one from doing a barium enema in a child with a clinical picture of intussusception.)

While sonography has long been used to diagnose the complications of appendicitis, such as periappendiceal abscess, it has only been in the last decade that sonography has been reliably used to diagnose the nonperforated, uncomplicated, inflamed appendix. Using criteria worked out by numerous investigators for width and size and compressibility of the appendix and with the addition of color Doppler (flow may be increased in the inflamed appendix), appendicitis can be readily diagnosed (Fig. 4.29).

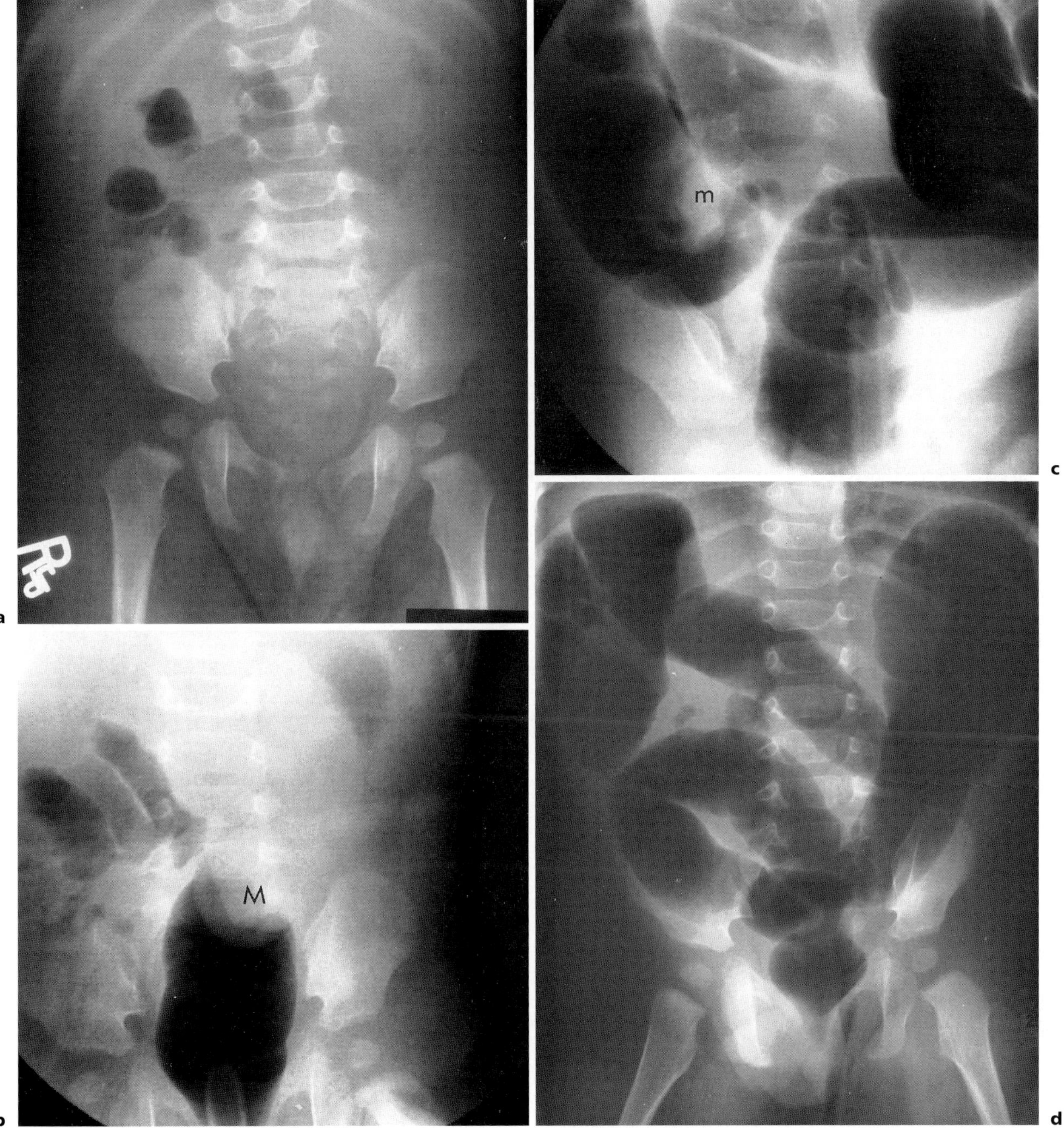

Fig. 4.30 a–d. Attempted air reduction of intussusception. **a** Vague suggestion of a mass in the lower midabdomen and pelvis in this stable 10-month-old. **b** Air enema shows mass (*M*) impinging on sigmoid gas. **c** The intussusception was pushed to ileal-cecal region but is still present (*m*). **d** Despite repeated efforts there is no small bowel reflux. At surgery the intussusception was seen in the region of the ileal-cecal valve

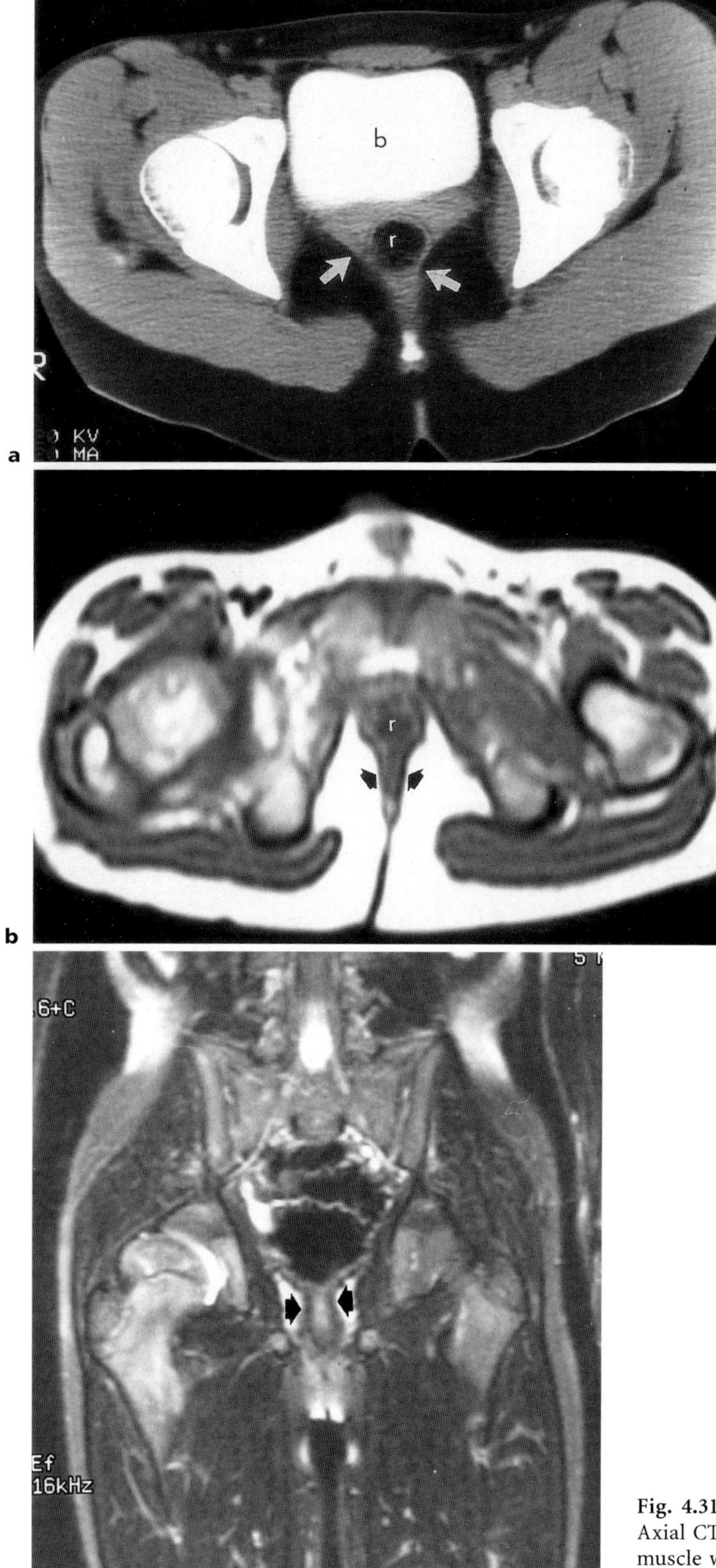

Fig. 4.31 a–c. Normal CT and MR of the levator muscles. **a** Axial CT reveals the air-filled rectum (*r*) and normal levator muscle wall thickness (*arrows*). Note contrast is in the bladder (*b*). **b** Similar axial MR section. **c** Coronal MR section shows muscles to advantage (*arrows*)

Occasionally, CT is utilized to diagnose the inflamed appendix but should be reserved for equivocal cases.

The diagnosis and reduction of intussusception can be performed with either opaque contrast or air. This pneumatic method uses air as the contrast agent under controlled pressure (Fig. 4.30). Air contrast obviates the risk of barium peritonitis should there be a perforation demonstrated during the procedure.

Anal-Rectal Malformations

In the past the invertogram (holding the baby upside down so that colonic gas rises and estimating how close the distal rectum comes to the anal dimple) was used to assess the level of imperforate anus. However, this technique was always unreliable, as meconium can block air from going distally. Prone cross-table lateral films are probably more reliable. Now, however, with the advent of MR we can depict the anal canal and distal rectum with much greater accuracy. Visualizing the levator muscle is key to successful operative repair of this anomaly and is rendered easy with CT and even better with MR (Fig. 4.31). MR also allows the visualization of associated renal and spinal anomalies (10% of imperforate anus cases). Postoperatively, the rectal pull-through procedure is nicely assessed with MR as well.

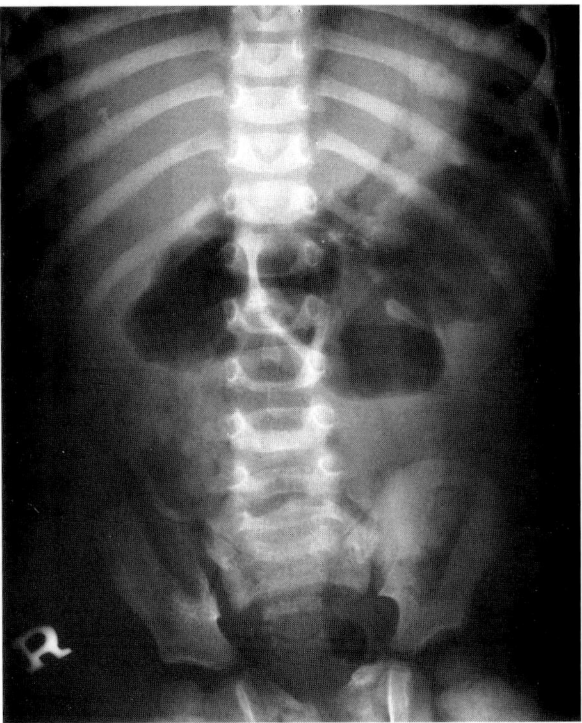

Fig. 4.32. This child presented to the emergency room with abdominal pain. On this supine film the bowel pattern shows air in the transverse colon. But the astute radiologist picked up something else. Do you see it? Look at the healing left posterior rib fracture at T8. This child was battered

Blunt Abdominal Trauma

Plain films of the abdomen may be extremely valuable in blunt abdominal trauma because free air, free fluid, sentinel loops, as well as fractured ribs, and transverse processes of the spine can be found. Remember the radiologist's circle and ABC's (Fig. 4.32).

CT has become well established as routine in the diagnosis and management of children with blunt abdominal trauma. Diagnostic peritoneal lavage is usually not necessary, especially in children who are hemodynamically stable. Visceral injuries are treated medically in most centers, and there has been a reduction in the need for exploratory laparotomy. The beauty of CT is that it allows the detection, localization, and characterization of hepatic, splenic, adrenal, and renal injuries. Mesenteric lesions and bowel injury are noted less well. With the trend toward nonoperative management of many of these visceral injuries, CT has been invaluable in the management of these children.

Constipation

Late onset of symptoms, particularly after toilet training has begun, suggests a functional basis for this disorder. Plain film studies reveal a dilated rectum and colon distended with stool. The barium enema confirms the presence of a large, capacious rectum, and postevacuation studies show *no lower segment* of narrowing, i.e., transition zone between dilated and nondilated bowel. However, if the patient has had a history of constipation from birth, one must consider a diagnosis of Hirschsprung's disease (Fig. 4.33). The barium enema differentiates the findings of chronic mechanical obstruction from those of a malfunctioning *distal aganglionic segment*. This may be seen most graphically on the postevacuation films, where the caliber disparity is striking. Since the examination attempts to show not only anatomical abnormality but also pathophysiology, the usual rigorous colonic emptying, i.e., purgatives and enemas, should be omitted.

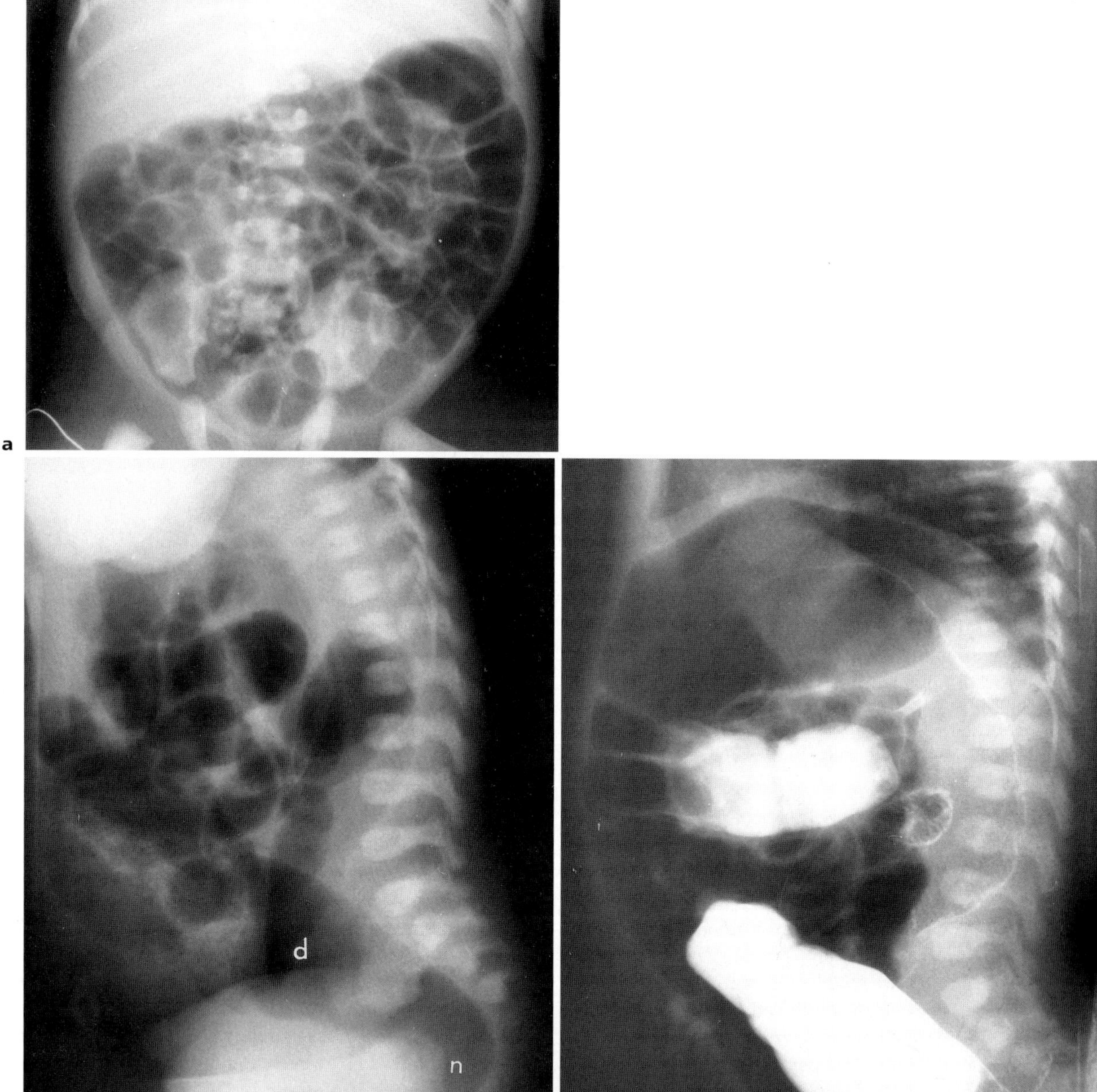

Fig. 4.33 a–c. Hirschsprung's disease. **a** Abdominal film in a 5-day-old reveals considerable distention of the bowel, with gas all the way down into the pelvis. **b** On lateral films the rectum is considerably smaller than any portion of the colon, and there is a transition zone between the nondilated (*n*) and dilated (*d*) portions of the bowel. **c** Lateral postevacuation film reveals that the rectum is not the most dilated portion of the colon. *Arrows*, transition zone between the nondistensible, aganglionic distal colon and the dilated, ganglionic proximal colon. Note how much of the colon is dilated. The rectum is nondistensible

Table 4.1. Rectal bleeding

Suspected causes	Kind of bleeding	Procedure of choice
Peptic ulcer	Melena	Endoscopy and/or upper Gl
Anal fissure	Blood-streaked stool	None; physical examination
Polyps	Red blood mixed with stool	Endoscopy and barium enema
Intussusception	See abdominal pain and vomiting in text	Enema with air or opaque contrast reduction
Meckel's diverticulum	Voluminous, bright-red blood	Technetium radionuclide study
Inflammatory bowel disease	Bright red blood and/or streaking in stool	Endoscopy, upper GI with small bowel follow-through, barium enema
Necrotizing enterocolitis	Variable	Plain films; radiographic signs in newborns dilated bowel loops, pneumatosis intestinalis (air out of bowel lumen but in wall of the bowel), portal venous gas free air

Rectal Bleeding

Rectal bleeding varies from guaiac positive stools to frank bright red blood. There are many causes, and the proper approach is determined by the suspected etiology in each case. Table 4.1 outlines the procedures.

Jaundice

In the newborn, *prolonged* jaundice is most commonly due to either neonatal hepatitis or biliary atresia. None of the imaging procedures satisfactorily separates these two entities. However, ultrasonic examination is the initial procedure of choice, as it reveals any masses in the porta hepatis, such as a choledochal cyst and intrahepatic biliary dilatation. The second imaging procedure of choice is a radionuclide investigation (DISIDA) for the patency of the biliary system. It seems that most children with prolonged jaundice undergo liver biopsy. If the results of this biopsy show signs of obstructive liver disease, an exploratory laparotomy follows.

In older children with jaundice, the most common diagnosis is viral hepatitis. These children do not need roentgenographic evaluation except when their course is atypical or recurrent. In these instances ultrasound is an excellent, noninvasive method. Both gallstones and masses in the porta hepatis can be diagnosed. Intrahepatic biliary ductal obstruction with enlarged biliary radicals is easily seen. In the atypical case procedures such as radionuclide study, CT scanning, percutaneous transhepatic cholangiography, and endoscopic retrograde duct catheterization may be necessary.

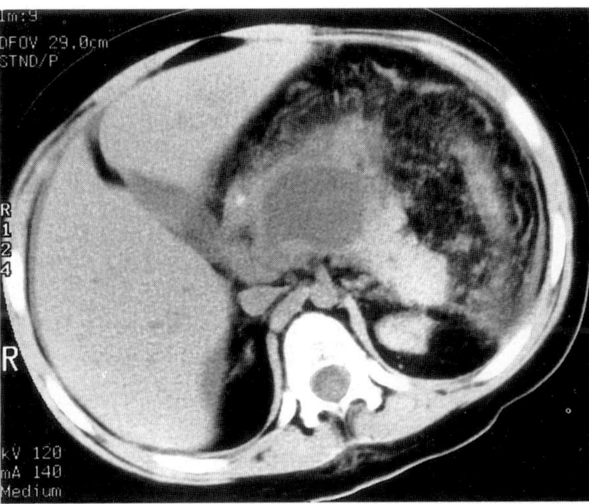

Fig. 4.34. Nine-year-old with abdominal pain 3 weeks after falling off his bike. Amylase was elevated (see "Appendix 2")

Figures 4.34–4.37 are presented as "unknowns." The history is given with each figure, and you are to make the correct diagnosis.

Reference

1. Haller JO, Cohen HL (1986) Hypertrophic pyloric stenosis: sonographic evaluation. Radiology 161:335–339

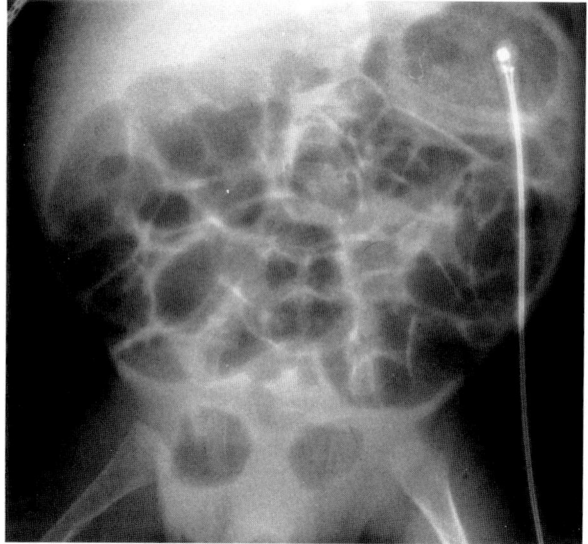

Fig. 4.35. An infant with abdominal distention (see "Appendix 2")

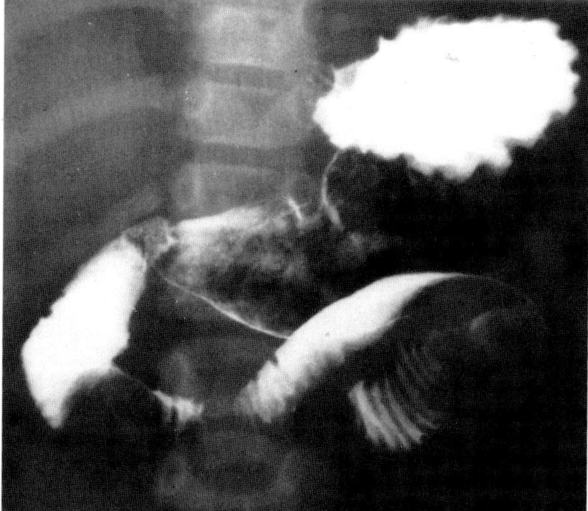

a

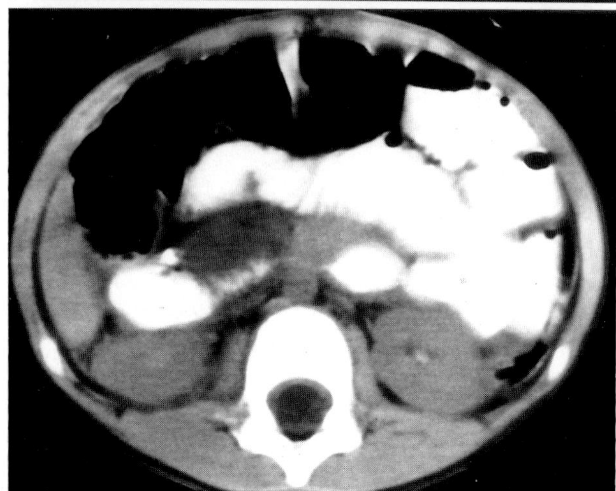

b

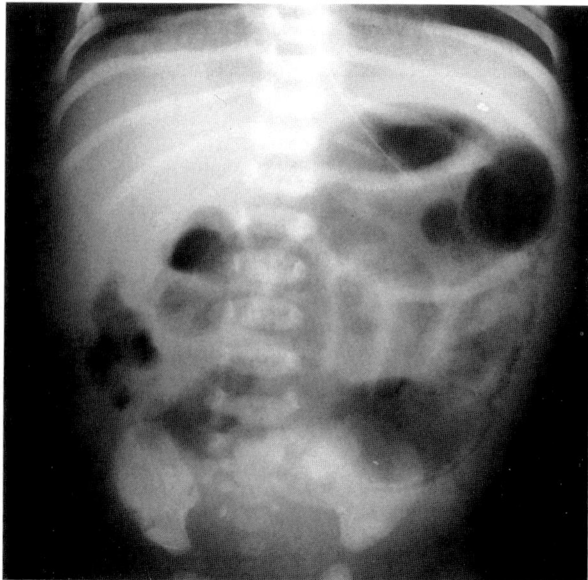

a

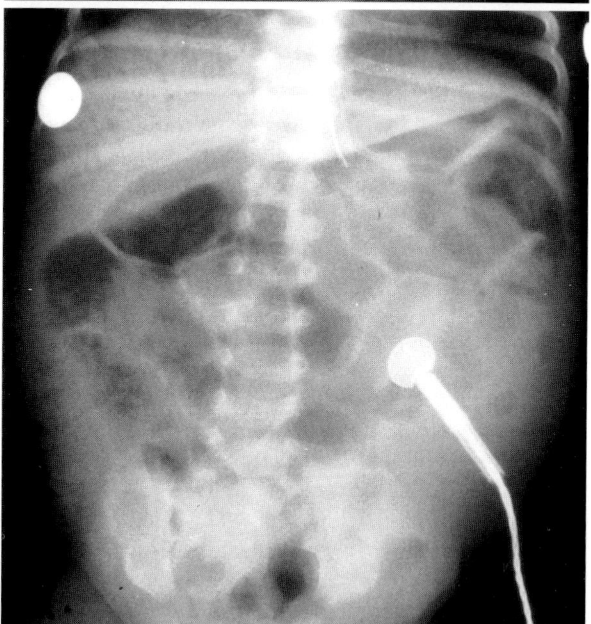

b

Fig. 4.37 a, b. Two neonates with abdominal distentions (see "Appendix 2")

◀ Fig. 4.36 a, b. Abdominal pain after trauma (see "Appendix 2")

5 Urinary Tract

Imaging of the urinary tract can be performed by many of the modalities already discussed. Depending on the signs and symptoms, the upper (kidney and ureter) or lower (bladder and urethra) urinary tract may be studied first. In this chapter we discuss the methodology of each modality (beginning with the plain film) and then precise indications for imaging.

Plain Film

Evaluation of the urinary tract begins with a plain film (see Chap. 4), which must show the diaphragm as well as the pubic bones. If this film does not include the entire abdomen, valuable information may be lost (Fig. 5.1). The systematic approach described in previous chapters should be used to evaluate this film. If calcification is seen, it is imperative to decide whether this is within the urinary system. Oblique radiographs can facilitate the decision, since once contrast material is injected, calcific densities may be obscured and precise localization difficult.

Renal size can often be estimated from the plain film. A rough guide to appropriate size is that the length from the top to the bottom of the kidney should be no greater than 4–4.5 vertebral bodies. The left kidney is usually slightly larger than the right (no greater than 1.5 cm difference). A kidney longer than 5 vertebral bodies is enlarged. The lower limits of normal are not as precise, but a kidney less than 3 vertebral bodies in length is abnormally small.

Cystogram

Radiographic Voiding Cystourethrogram

The purposes of the radiographic voiding cystourethrogram (VCU) are (a) to study the bladder and urethra for abnormalities of size, position, and contour, (b) to screen for vesicoureteral reflux (retrograde flow of contrast material into the ureters and/or kidneys), and (c) to evaluate pelvic abnormalities that impinge or invade the bladder.

If the VCU is to be performed alone, no preparation is necessary. The patient is asked to void, and then a small catheter (either a feeding tube or straight catheter) is passed into the urethra and bladder. Residual urine is drained and the amount recorded. This is important because bladder dysfunction or distal obstruction can lead to retention after voiding. Contrast material is then instilled through the catheter into the bladder until it is filled to capacity.

The bladder appears as a round, opaque density, symmetrically situated in the pelvis. The inferior margin of the filled bladder should be seen at the top of the pubic symphysis on a well-centered film. The bladder wall is smooth, and there should be no filling defects within the bladder. Irregularity of the wall may indicate mucosal edema or diverticulum formation. Contrast seen in the ureters signifies incompetence of the ureterovesical junction and reflux (Fig. 5.2). When the catheter is removed, the patient voids, allowing for visualization of the urethra. This is much more crucial in a male, as significant pathology may exist in the posterior urethra, which is between the bladder neck and the urogenital diaphragm (see Fig. 5.2). This part of urethra is arbitrarily divided into the prostatic urethra and membranous urethra. In the male the prostatic and ejaculatory ducts terminate in the verumontanum, located on the posterior wall of the prostatic urethra. The membranous urethra is shorter, beginning at the inferior margin of the verumontanum and extending downward to the urogenital diaphragm. The anterior urethra extends from the urogenital diaphragm distally to the urethral meatus and is divided into the bulbous and penile portions. When there are abnormalities such as posterior urethral valves, there is marked discrepancy between the anterior and posterior urethral caliber (Fig. 5.3).

In the female the urethra is shorter and is infrequently the site of significant pathology (Fig. 5.4). Voiding in the recumbent position often causes vaginal filling, which is not pathological.

During fluoroscopy, the upper abdomen is viewed to make sure there is no evidence of reflux of contrast material from the bladder to the kidneys (see Fig. 5.2). This is important because reflux is one of the causes of pyelonephritis and parenchymal changes, frequently

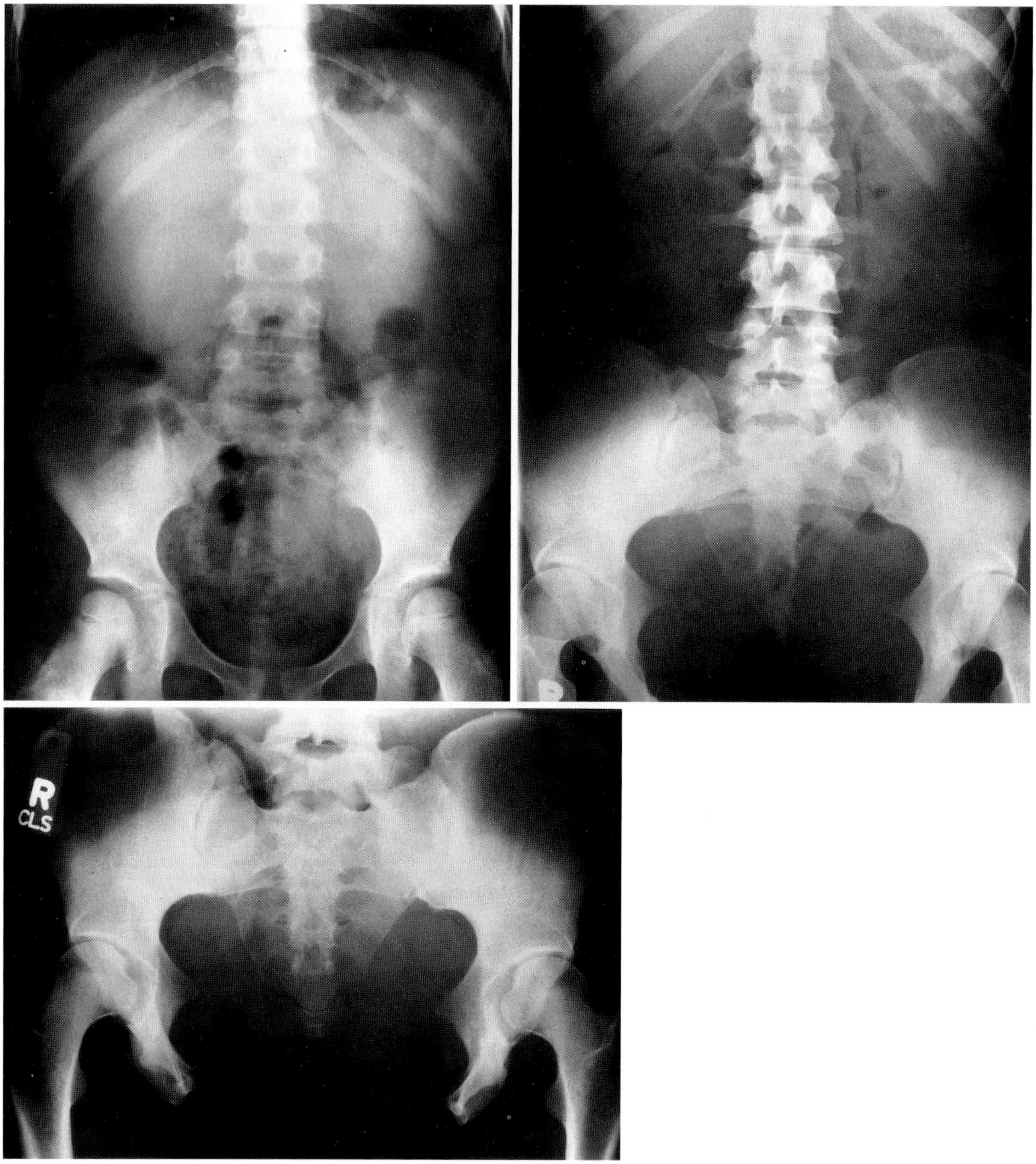

a b

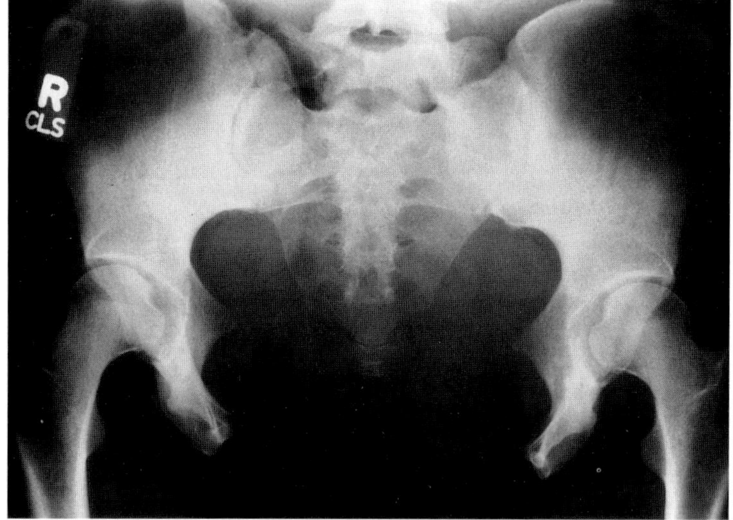

c

Fig. 5.1 a–c. Preliminary films. **a** Normal supine radiograph includes the bases of the lungs, the diaphragm, and the pubic bones. As the ABC's of the film are evaluated, note renal size. **b** Preliminary film of a 12-year-old girl. Is it adequate? **c** Pelvis of the young lady who has widespread pubic bones and exstrophy of the bladder. Did you see the findings in **b**? **b** includes neither the diaphragm nor the pubic bones

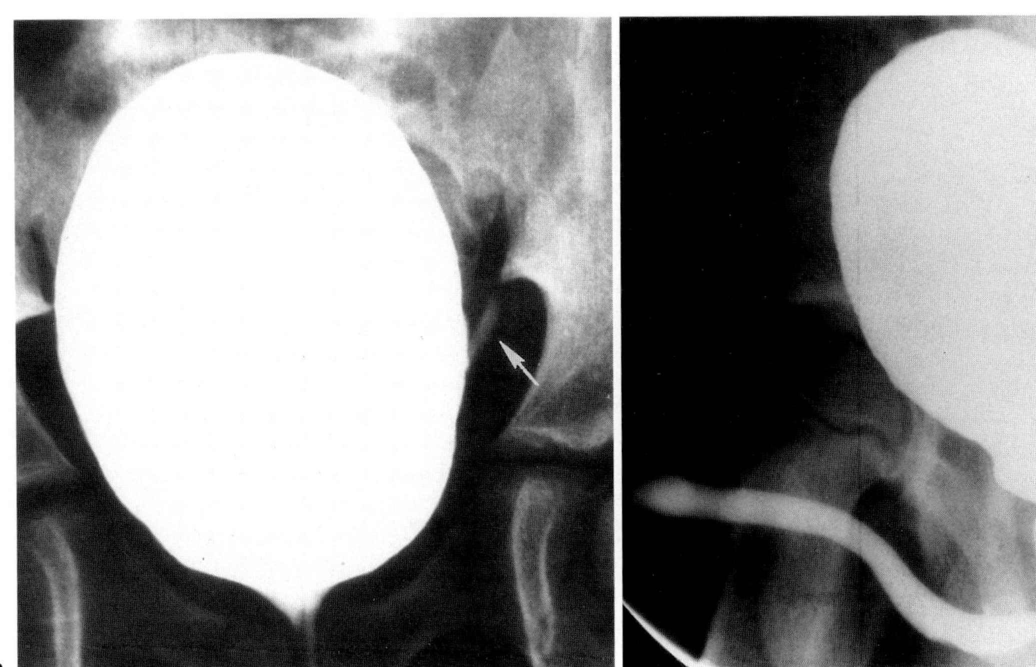

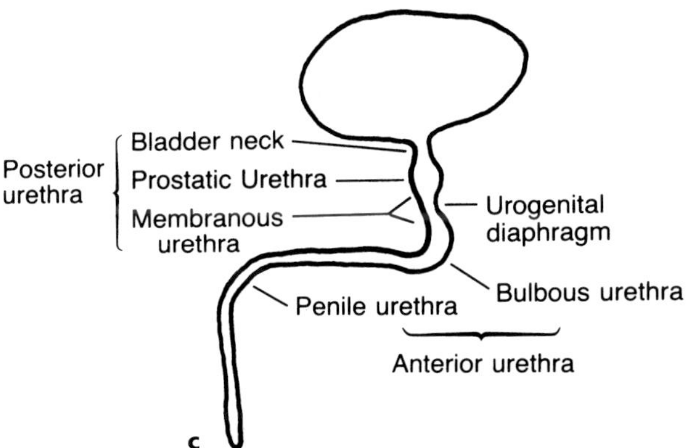

Fig. 5.2 a–c. VCU in a boy. **a** Filled bladder. The inferior margin is adjacent to the pubic bones, and the bladder is in the center of the pelvis. There is no mass impression on the bladder. Contour and position are smooth and normal. Incidentally noted is a small amount of refluxed contrast in the distal left ureter (*arrow*). **b** Patient is placed in the oblique position, and the reflux into the left ureter is noted (*arrows*). As patient voids, the entire posterior urethra is easily seen; in this instance the anterior urethra is seen as well. Slight irregularity at the base of the bladder posteriorly is expected during voiding. **c** Drawing of the male urethra

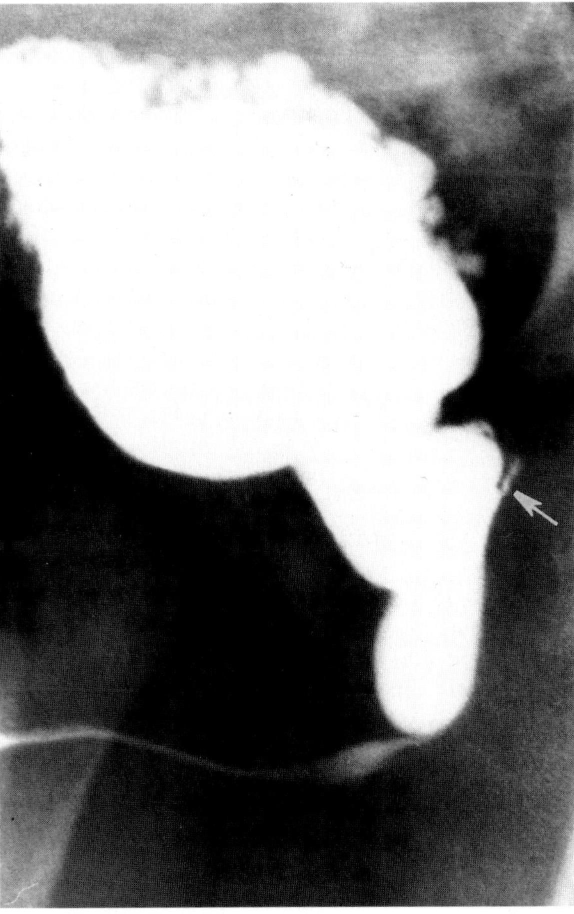

Fig. 5.3. Posterior urethral valves. This single oblique view ▶ during a VCU reveals the irregularity of the bladder wall. Large collections of contrast in saccules are due to bladder obstruction. The posterior urethra is quite dilated when compared to the anterior urethra. Note that the opening between the anterior and posterior urethra is located quite posteriorly and, of course, is narrowed (see normal urethra in Fig. 5.2). Reflux into the ejaculatory ducts is also present (*arrow*)

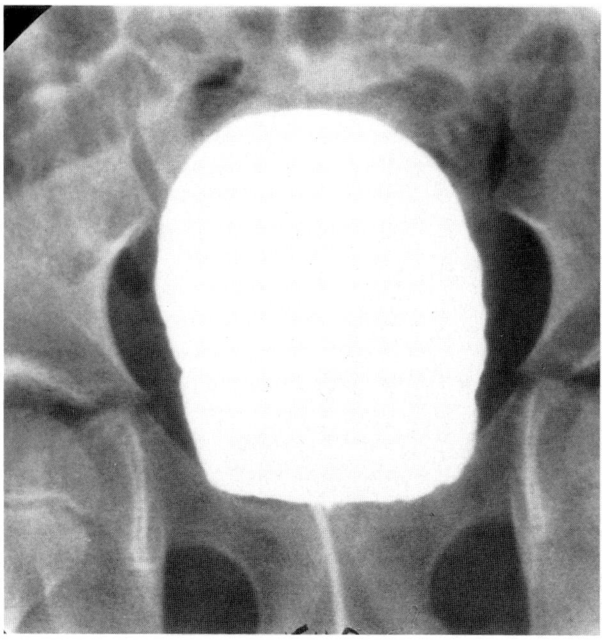

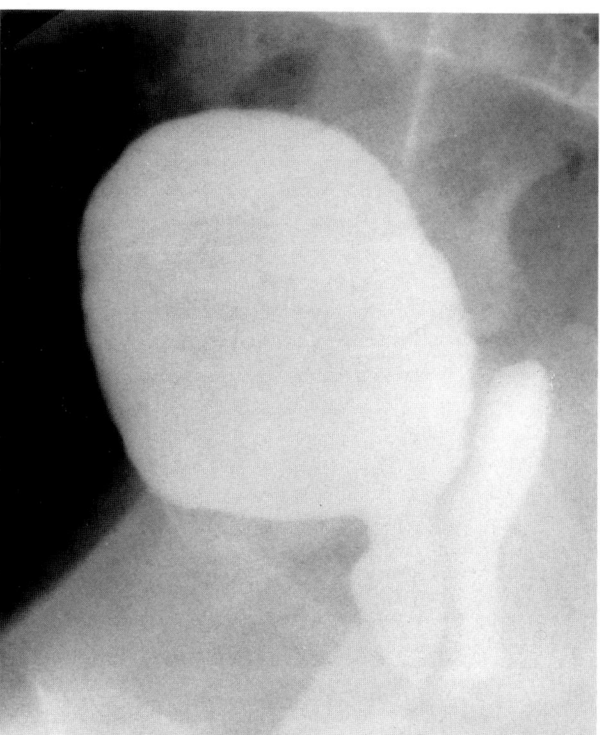

most marked in the polar regions. A postvoiding film is obtained to assess whether the bladder empties completely (see below, "Urinary Tract Infection").

In instances of trauma to the pelvis the possibility of urethral disruption must be considered. The anterior portion of the urethra is best seen when a small catheter is placed within the urethral meatus and retrograde injection is made. If the urethra is intact, the catheter is passed into the bladder and a conventional VCU is performed to visualize the posterior urethra.

What abnormalities are visible in Fig. 5.5? (Answer in "Appendix 2.")

Nuclear Cystogram

In the case of the nuclear cystogram, as with the VCU, a small catheter or feeding tube is placed into the urethra and into the bladder. The bladder is drained and normal saline with 1 mCi technetium pertechnetate added is infused into the bladder. The volume given varies with the child's age. The nuclear camera continually records during filling and voiding. Since there is continuous monitoring, this is a very sensitive test (Fig. 5.6). There is considerably less radiation to the gonads, particularly in females, from a nuclear cystogram than from a radiographic cystogram.

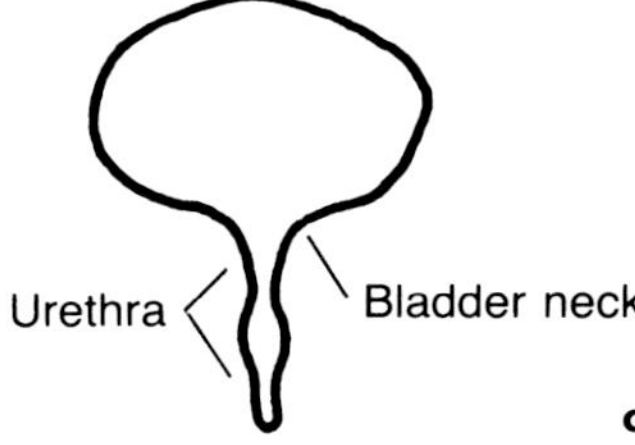

Fig. 5.4 a–c. The female urethra. **a** Filled bladder with catheter in place again reveals the central position of the bladder without any mass impinging on its wall. **b** On voiding, as seen on this oblique view, the posterior aspect of the bladder becomes slightly irregular. The urethra is much shorter in a female and often displays a "carrot-top" or "spinning-top" deformity (*arrow*). There is often reflux into the vagina when the patient voids in the recumbent position (*star*). **c** Drawing of the female urethra

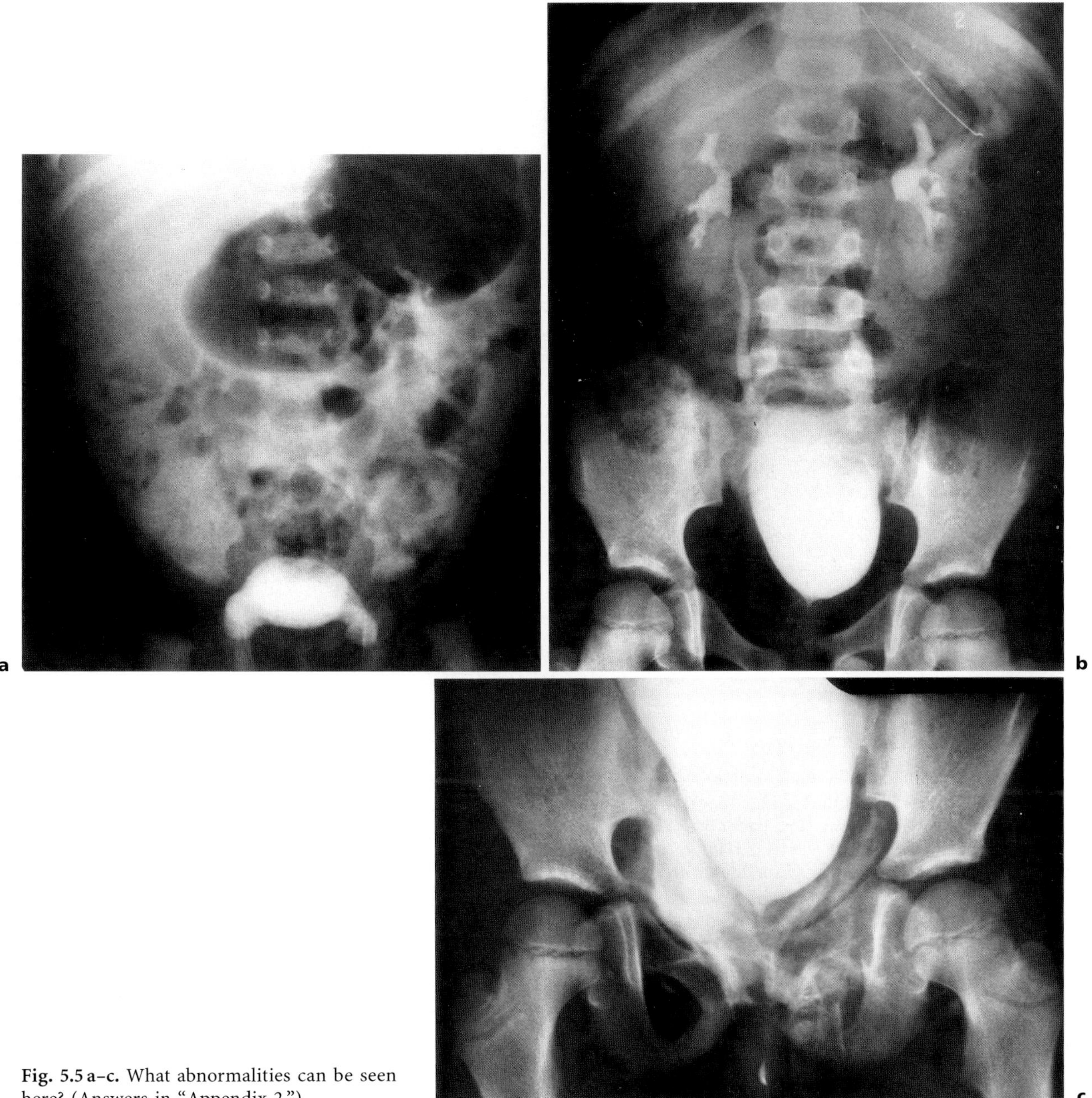

Fig. 5.5 a–c. What abnormalities can be seen here? (Answers in "Appendix 2")

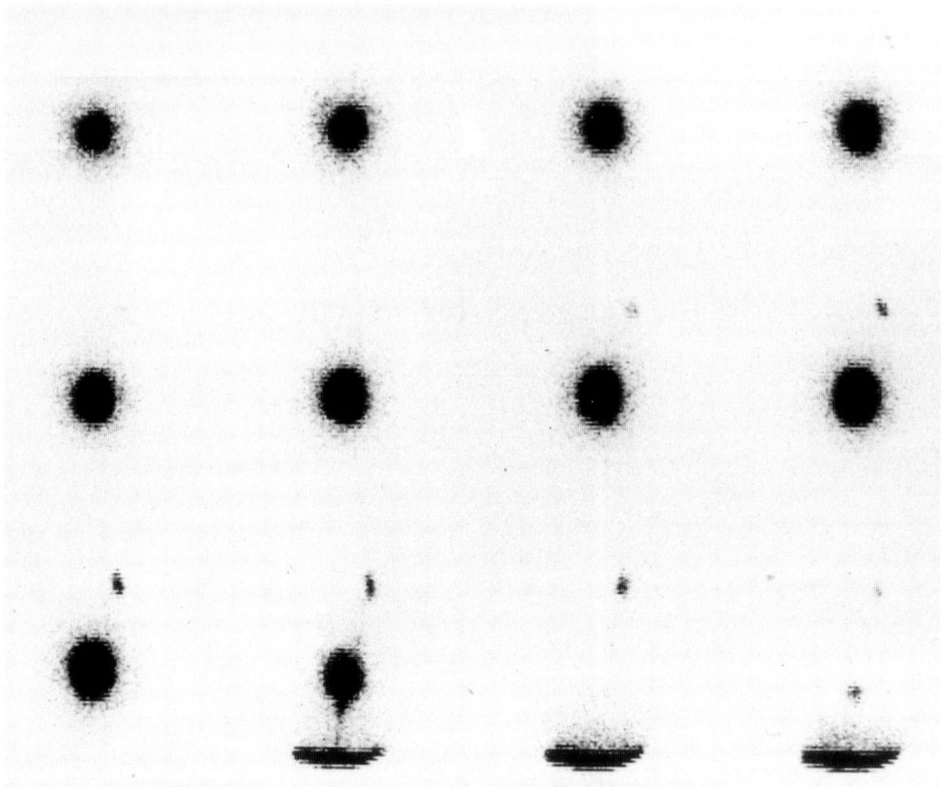

Fig. 5.6. Nuclear voiding cystogram. The viewer's top *left* image is the earliest film of the bladder. Progressing from left to right, the bladder is filling. The patient is being scanned from behind; therefore, the viewer's *right* is the patient's right. There is reflux into the right kidney with voiding

Indications for Upper Urinary Tract Evaluation

Patients with any of the following conditions should have an upper urinary tract work-up:

- Urinary tract infection
- Abdominal mass (see Chap. 6)
- Hematuria of unknown etiology
- Renal or bladder trauma; pelvic bone fracture
- Recurrent abdominal pain with clinical evidence of urinary tract disease
- Conditions that predispose to renal tumors (tuberous sclerosis, hemihypertrophy, Beckwith's syndrome, aniridia)
- Failure to thrive
- Meningomyelocele
- Malformations associated with a moderate to high degree of renal anomalies (unusual development of the ears, imperforate anus, anomalies of the reproductive system, unexplained or refractory pneumomediastinum or pneumothorax in the newborn, fetal alcohol syndrome)

Studying the Upper Urinary Tract

The upper urinary tract can be studied in many different ways. The examinations include ultrasound, nuclear medicine, excretory urogram (or intravenous pyelogram,), CT, MR, and angiography. (The following section is taken in part from [1].)

Ultrasound

Ultrasound is a noncontrast tomographic study that in most instances requires no special patient preparation or sedation. There is no ionizing radiation and the examination can easily be performed portably. This study is tomographic in that thin slices of the kidney can be obtained, and the study can be performed in almost any plane. Since the examination is operator dependent, it is important that all members of the ultrasound team perform the study in the same systematic fashion. The usual planes of study are transverse and longitudinal with the transducer placed on the patient's abdomen; these are followed by transverse and longitudinal views with the transducer placed on the patient's side (coronal views) as well as prone views (Fig. 5.7). All examinations may be recorded on videotape or as multiple images on film.

The sonogram has several distinct advantages over the excretory urogram (see below). Multiple viscera, vessels, and the peritoneal cavity are seen as part of the examination (see Chap. 4). The three compartments (pararenal, perirenal, and renal) of the retroperitoneum are visualized. Because the examination is carried out with high-frequency transducers and real-time technique, the examiner is able to see exquisite intrarenal detail, vascular pulsations, and dilated fluid-filled structures such as the ureters. With the use of color Doppler ultrasound, renal veins and arteries are easily seen. Unlike the excretory urogram (below), however, ultrasound cannot detect subtle loss of parenchyma. Ultrasound also has the disadvantage of being hindered by bowel gas.

The internal architecture of the kidney also changes with age (Fig. 5.8). The reason for the different sonographic appearances is that the neonatal kidney is anatomically different. In the full-term neonate the maximum number of glomeruli are present in the cortex, but there are relatively few tubules (the cortex grows primarily by way of tubular growth). Thus in the neonate the glomeruli are crowded together in a volumetrically small cortex. Although quantitatively at a maximum, the neonatal glomeruli are qualitatively different from those seen later in life. The basement membrane in the neonate is much more cellular than the older child. Therefore it is not surprising that the neonatal renal cortex is echogenic and approximates or occasionally exceeds the echogenicity of the liver. The renal medullae (the renal pyramids) are of greater relative volume now than it will ever be again, and the echo-free collecting ductules are visualized in striking relief against the echogenic cortex. There is little fat in the neonate, and therefore the characteristic central sinus echogenic fat seen in the older child is not present. At all ages the renal pelvis and calyces can be seen if they are distended. It has been suggested that in well or overly hydrated patients the collecting system is seen more frequently. With a full bladder the renal pelvis can be quite distended; however, with voiding the system returns to normal size.

Duplex Doppler imaging allows vascular evaluation of the kidney. The image is obtained, a cursor is insonated in the appropriate vessel, and flow characteristics are evaluated. The major vessels (the main renal artery and vein) as well as smaller arcuate vessels can be insonated by the cursor and assessment of flow velocities and wave characteristics follows.

Nuclear Medicine Techniques

The applications of nuclear medicine techniques to evaluate the pediatric urinary tract are probably more varied than those of any of the other modalities. Radionuclide imaging procedures have been developed to assess function of the kidneys by measuring effective renal plasma flow, glomerular filtration rate, and renal transit time. In addition, anatomic information such as cortical integrity can be shown in exquisite detail.

Little patient preparation is necessary for nuclear medicine examinations. It is crucial, however, that barium procedures do not precede the radioisotope or ultrasound examinations. In most instances the patient is catheterized, and in all cases intravenous injection of radiopharmaceutical is necessary.

Renal imaging depends predominantly on technetium-labeled compounds. These compounds differ in the manner by which they are eliminated by the kidney. ^{99m}Tc-labeled diethylenetriamine pentaacetic acid (^{99m}Tc-DTPA) is eliminated by glomerular filtration without any adherence to the renal tubules, whereas ^{99m}Tc-labeled glucoheptonate (^{99m}Tc-GH) and ^{99m}Tc-labeled dimercaptosuccinate (^{99m}Tc-DMSA) are to some extent bound to the tubular epithelial cells.

Tubular-bound chelates are used for evaluation of the renal cortex in such clinical conditions as renal infection, renal infarction, renal abscess or lobar nephronia, and acute tubular or cortical necrosis. The excretory phase is evaluated with ^{99m}Tc-DTPA.

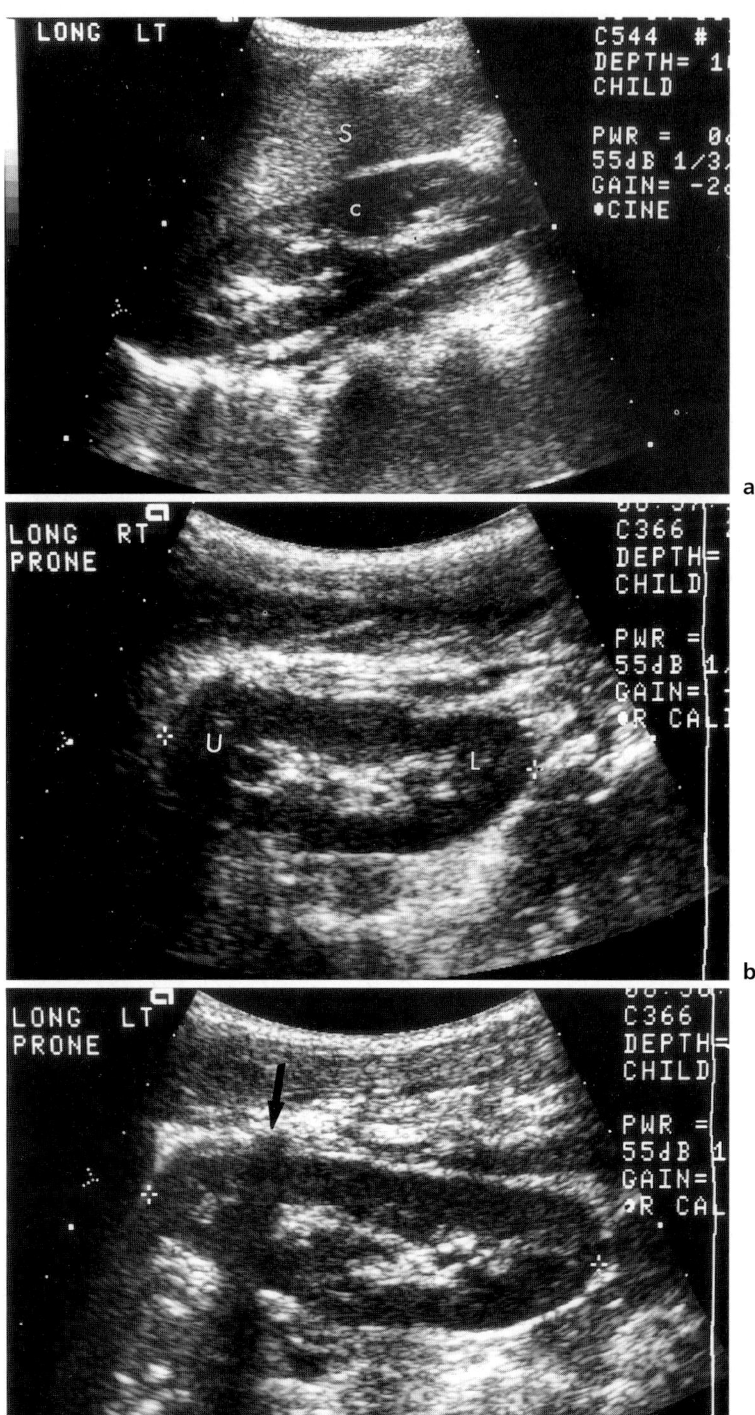
LONG LT
C544
DEPTH=
CHILD
PWR =
55dB
GAIN=
CINE
S
c
a
LONG RT
PRONE
C366
DEPTH
CHILD
PWR =
55dB
GAIN=
R CA
U
L
b
LONG LT
PRONE
C366
DEPTH
CHILD
PWR =
55dB
GAIN=
R CA
c

◀ **Fig. 5.7 a–d.** Ultrasound of kidney in a 6-year-old. **a** Longitudinal supine view of the normal left kidney. The spleen (*s*) is seen anteriorly. The cortex (*c*) is less echogenic (*fewer white dots*) than the spleen. The fat in the central sinus and around the kidney (*f*) is white. **b** Prone longitudinal examination of the right kidney shows both upper (*u*) and lower (*l*) poles. **c** Prone longitudinal view of the left kidney demonstrates lack of echo because of overlying rib (rib artifact; *arrows*). **d** The ultrasound examination always includes the bladder. Longitudinal view of the bladder (*b*) shows it to be filled with clear liquid (urine) and is rendered black. The wall is thin

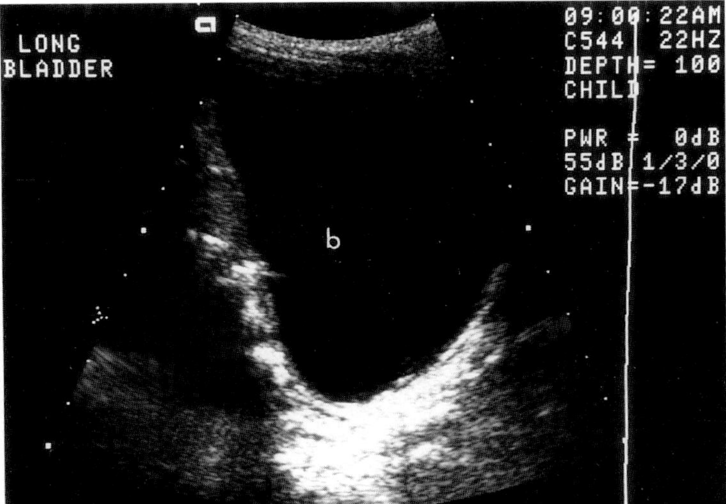

5.7 d

Fig. 5.8 a, b. Neonatal kidney. **a** Supine longitudinal view of the kidney reveals the almost anechoic medullary pyramids (*p*) arranged around the center of the kidney. There is no central sinus fat. The cortex is almost as echogenic as the liver. *c*, Cortex; *l*, liver. **b** Supine longitudinal view in another neonate shows how large the normal medullary pyramids can be

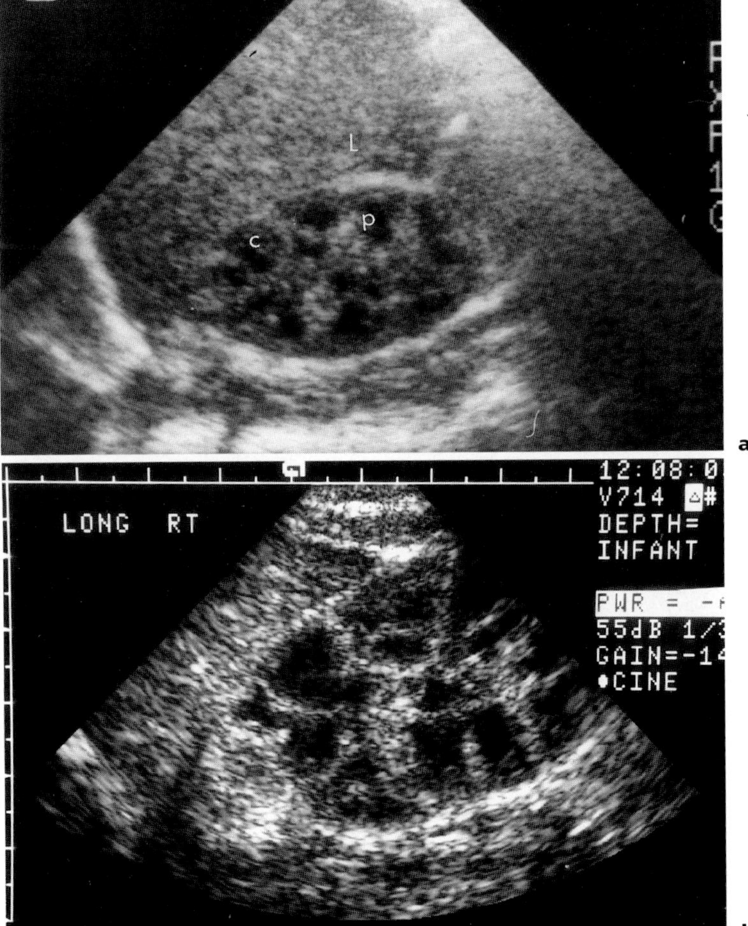

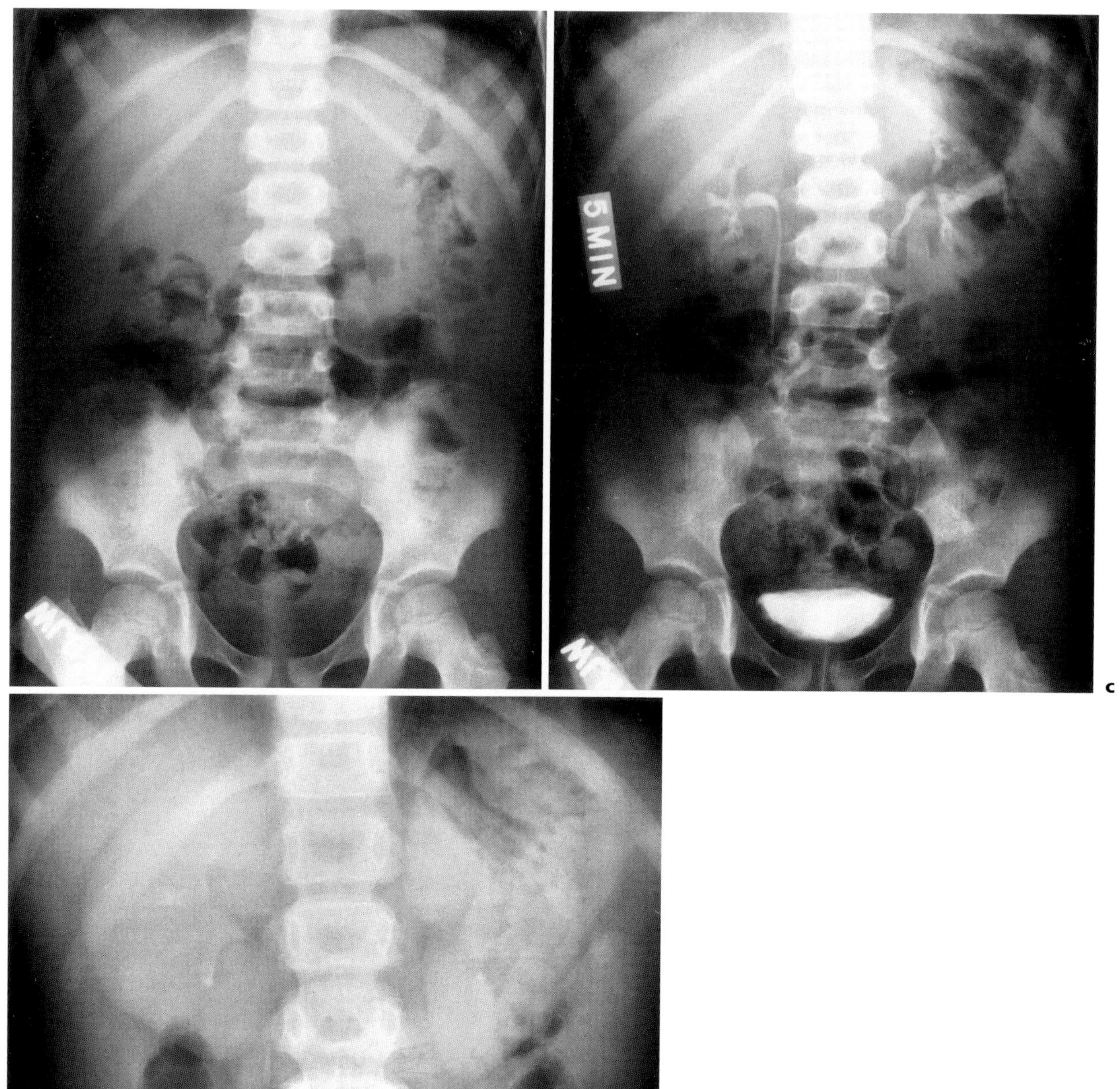

a
b
c

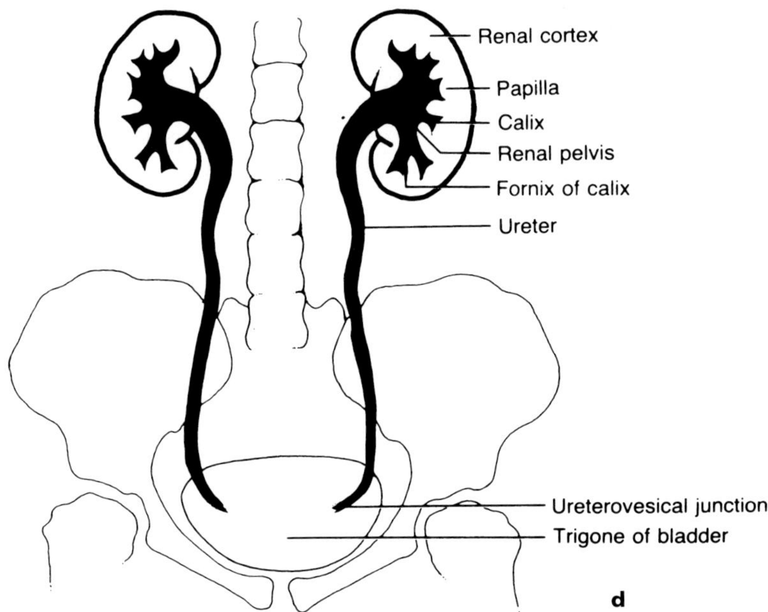

▲

◀ **Fig. 5.9 a–d.** The normal IVU. **a** Film of the abdomen, including both the diaphragms and pubic bones. Use the systematic approach to evaluate this film! **b** Prone coned-down view shows a nephrogram effect. The kidneys are homogeneous at this point, and there is very little contrast material in the collecting systems. Occasionally such a film is taken several minutes after injection; the collecting systems are then seen to better advantage. On this initial film the renal axis is noted with the upper pole being closer to the spine than the lower pole. The renal contours are evaluated and should be smooth without scarring or indentations. **c** This 5-min film reveals the renal collecting systems, calices, and infundibulum leading to the renal pelvis. Any deviation or blunting of the collecting system is seen at this time. The renal pelvis then tapers into the ureter. The ureters pass inferiorly, crossing the margins of the transverse processes. The bladder is separate from the pubic bones because it is partially filled. A 10-min frontal film is usually obtained to view the entire system to see if there has been any change secondary to osmotic load. **d** Drawing of the normal intrarenal anatomy as seen on the IVU

Excretory Urogram

A scout film of the abdomen is obtained prior to performing the excretory urogram to ascertain proper radiographic technique. The scout film allows detection of calculi that may be obscured after contrast injection as well as evaluation of the position and size of the viscera. Evaluation of the spine is important as well (to identify defects, pedicle erosion, and so on). The scout film should include the entire abdomen from the diaphragm to the pubic bone (Fig. 5.5).

The exact sequence of the films taken after injection of the contrast agent varies according to the indications for the study and the bias of the radiologist.

There are two kinds of contrast agents: the older high-osmolar ionic contrast agents and the newer low-osmolar nonionic agents. The incidence of minor reactions is reduced tremendously with the low osmolar agents, and there is less motion allowing for more optimal imaging. Many centers for children use these new agents exclusively. Most pediatric radiologists, however, obtain a 1-min coned-down prone radiograph of the kidneys – the total body opacification film, which shows the parenchyma most advantageously (Fig. 5.9). The use of this precise nephrogram film is predicated on the principle that the peak plasma level of contrast agent is obtained immediately after a bolus injection. This vascular phase film shows the renal parenchyma very well because of the high renal blood flow (which includes 25% of cardiac output) and rapid removal of contrast agent by the glomeruli. Films in this phase also show avascular structures such as cysts or masses as negative defects. It is important to note that in the neonatal period, renal blood flow is considerably reduced compared with that in the older child, and therefore that the parenchymal phase is delayed.

The differential diagnosis relative to size of kidney on intravenous urography (IVU) includes the following:

- Single large kidney
  - Tumor
  - Renal vein thrombosis

  - Pyelonephritis
  - Abscess
  - Hematoma
  - Obstruction
- Two large kidneys
  - Polycystic disease
  - Hydronephrosis due to neurogenic bladder, posterior urethral valves, or other obstruction
  - Glycogen storage disease
  - Amyloidosis
  - Bilateral Wilms' tumor
  - Acute glomerulonephritis

In the case of small kidneys:
- Single small kidney
  - Chronic renal disease
  - Congenital hypoplastic kidney (renal artery stenosis)
  - Postinfectious nephropathy
  - Reflux
- Two small kidneys
  - Chronic renal insufficiency
  - Reflux
  - Postinfectious nephropathy

In the nonvisualized kidney:
- Congenital absence of the kidney
- Surgically removed kidney
- Ectopic kidney with abnormal function
- Multicystic dysplastic kidney
- Renal artery thrombosis
- Renal vein thrombosis
- Tumor

The 5-to 15-Min Films

By this time, the contrast material has filtered from the vascular system, through the glomeruli, and into the renal collecting systems. The delicate fornices of the calix and the infundibula are seen leading to the renal pelvis. An outline drawn of the lateral aspect of the kidney and a line connecting the tips of the fornices of each calix should show two concentric semicircles. If they are not concentric, suspect loss of parenchyma, with the calix extending closer to the outer margin of the kidney (try this in Fig. 5.10 c to help answer the quiz). In this way one can also see how much parenchyma is medial to the most medial calix of the superior pole. This polar region is a common site of parenchymal loss in reflux nephropathy. Similarly, the distance from the lower calices to the spine should be checked for parenchymal loss. There may be a vascular impression on either the fornix, calix, or renal pelvis. On multiple views these can be identified as vascular changes by their tubular contour.

Next, inspect the renal pelvis and ureters. The renal pelvis may be intrarenal or extrarenal (inside or outside the renal contour). If the pelvis is extrarenal, it tends to be larger and more easily distensible with osmotic loads. However, even in these instances the calices remain normal. The renal pelvis tapers at the ureteropelvic junction into the proximal ureter. As the ureters descend to the pelvis, they generally overlie the transverse processes of the spine. If they do not, a medial mass (enlarged lymph nodes, etc.) should be suspected. Oblique and lateral views are helpful in this situation. Once again, we are looking at size, contour, and position when we view the ureters. Frequently as the bladder fills, the upper tracts become dilated.

Delayed Films

► *Reed's Rule No. 11:* During intravenous urography, continue to take films as long as they provide needed information.

When there are abnormalities of the urinary system, delayed visualization of the kidney's collecting system is not uncommon. In instances of urinary tract obstruction, hypotension, or abnormal handling of the contrast, 12-, 24-, and 48-h films are helpful. Normally, 50% of the contrast is excreted in 2 h, and all is gone within 24 h. When taking delayed films, supine, prone, and lateral views may be requested selectively until the entire system is visualized. The value of the prone film is that the more anterior structures – renal pelvis and ureter – may be aided by gravity and fill to better advantage.

When a kidney is obstructed, the collecting system distends at the expense of the parenchyma. The more chronic the obstruction, the greater the distention. The parenchyma is compressed, with the tubules assuming a more nearly horizontal orientation. Thus, during the early phase the urine-filled calices are lucent, and the tubules form a parenchymal rim (do you see an example of this in the quiz Fig. 5.10?). As the delayed films are obtained, the collecting system slowly fills.

Contrast accumulates along the outer portion of the fluid-filled calix, forming a calyceal crescent. Prone films are very helpful.

What abnormalities can be detected on the different IVUs in Fig. 5.10?

Evaluation of the neonatal urinary system is somewhat more difficult. In the first week or two of life the neonate's renal blood flow, glomerular filtration rate, and renal tubule concentrating ability are decreased

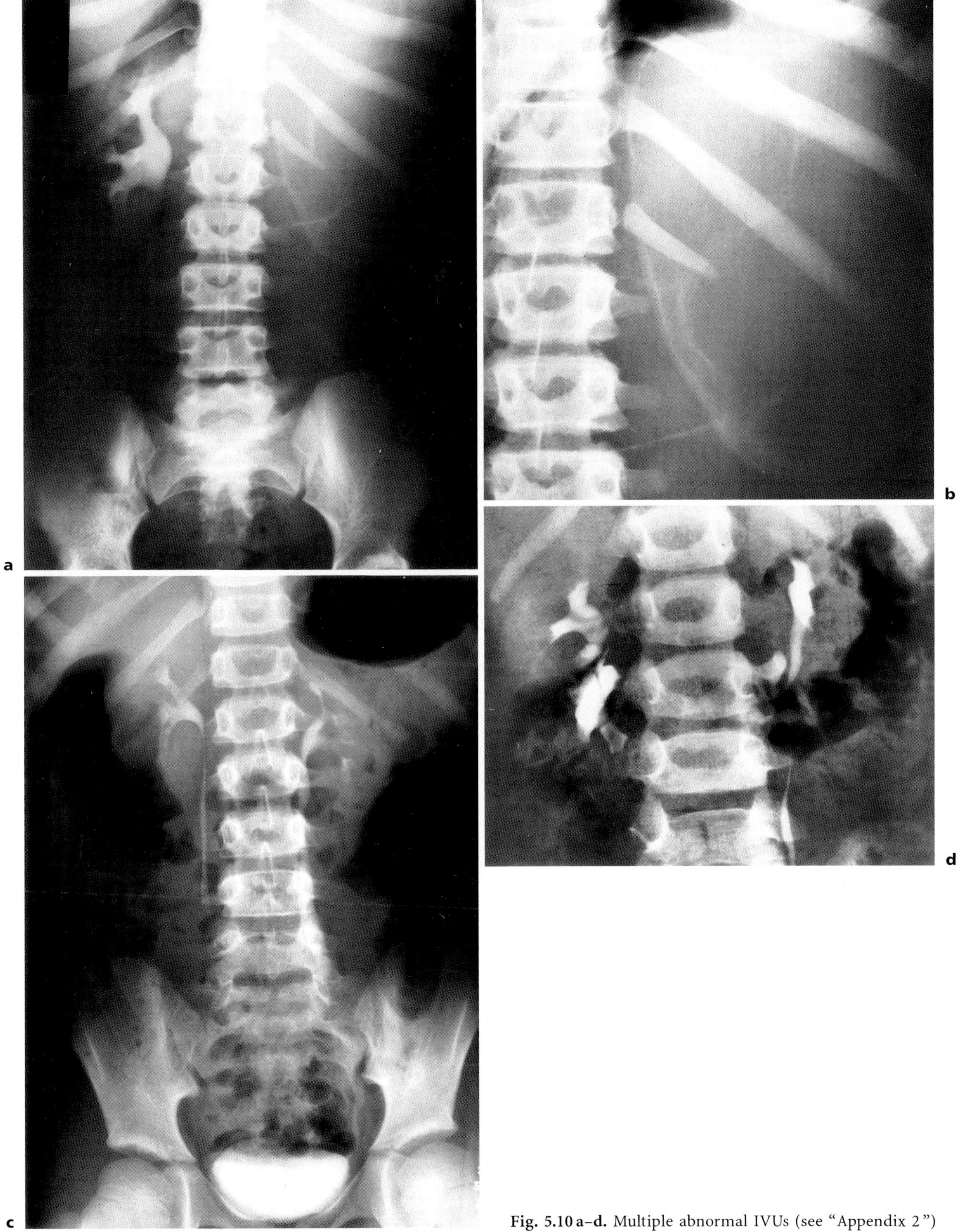

Fig. 5.10 a–d. Multiple abnormal IVUs (see "Appendix 2")

compared to that of older infants. For these reasons other imaging modalities, such as ultrasound or radionuclide imaging, are frequently utilized. Nonetheless, it is possible to obtain an adequate IVU of the neonate if the following modifications are made. The study must be prolonged; that is, the ability to see the kidneys in the nephrogram phase and collecting systems must be delayed so that a good nephrogram may be seen at 5–10 min. Films over 30–90 min may be necessary for optimal visualization of the renal pelvis and ureters. In addition, it may be crucial to order tomograms and/or a lateral film because renal outlines may be obscured by gas on the frontal projection.

The neonate is a prime example of the need to tailor the urogram specifically. Another example is the neurologically impaired child with abundant fecal material in the colon; this patient is uncooperative and may need a specific bowel preparation. Under some of these circumstances oblique projections, tomographic studies, or delayed films are mandatory.

The ureters are usually seen but not necessarily throughout their entire length on any one film. For more optimal visualization of the ureters a prone or upright film can be obtained utilizing the effects of gravity. In pediatric radiology compression devices are seldom necessary. The paths of the ureters course over the transverse processes of the vertebral bodies as seen on the frontal film. Although the medial position of the ureters is variable, the lateral position should not be lateral to the transverse processes.

Computed Tomography

CT is a tomographic modality in which axial cross-sections of the urinary tract are most easily obtained (Fig. 5.11). CT images are routinely performed at 10-mm intervals and thicknesses (contiguous 10-mm sections), although for specific regions 1.5- to 5-mm sections can be made. It is possible to make direct images in the coronal and sagittal planes, but these views are more difficult. The best reconstructions result when the initial data are derived from the thinnest possible sections, i.e., 1.5–3 mm. Patient preparation is similar to that with the excretory urogram except that oral contrast is given to opacify the bowel and allow definite identification of retroperitoneal spaces and intraperitoneal structures. The ability to define the entire retroperitoneum is a huge advantage for CT. The three components of the retroperitoneum are: (a) the anterior pararenal space, (b) the perirenal space, and (c) the posterior pararenal space (Fig. 5.12). The anterior pararenal space extends from the posterior peritoneum to the anterior renal fascia of Gerota. It contains the extraperitoneal portions of the gastrointestinal tract including the ascending and descending colon, the duodenal loop, and the pancreas. Because it contains the pancreas, it crosses the midline, and it is laterally confined by the lateroconal fascia. The perirenal space defined by the anterior and posterior layers of Gerota's fascia contains the adrenal gland and the kidney with its surrounding fat. These two fascial layers fuse laterally to form the lateroconal fascia and help form the paracolic gutters. The posterior pararenal compartment extends from the posterior renal fascia to the transversalis fascia and contains no viscera. This space continues laterally as the properitoneal fat of the abdominal wall.

CT of the kidneys without contrast allows the radiologist to detect calcifications, define the exact levels of interest, and appraise the tissue characteristics of a lesion (fat versus fluid, for example). Contrast is then given as a bolus in a dose of 2 ml/kg (our maximum is 150 ml). After one-third to one-half of the contrast medium is injected, images may be obtained to allow visualization of the vascular phase of the nephrogram. At this point the contrast medium fills the aorta, vena cava, and cortex of the kidney (primarily the glomeruli and tubules). The medulla is not yet opacified, and the pyramids are quite stark in their lack of contrast. Within 1–2 min the nephrogram phase begins as the contrast equilibrates between the medulla and the cortex. As with the excretory urogram, a differential diagnosis of a nonuniform or prolonged nephrogram can be made. At 3–4 min the pyelogram phase begins as contrast enters the calyces, renal pelvis, and ureters. The scan can be carried out dynamically, allowing ei-

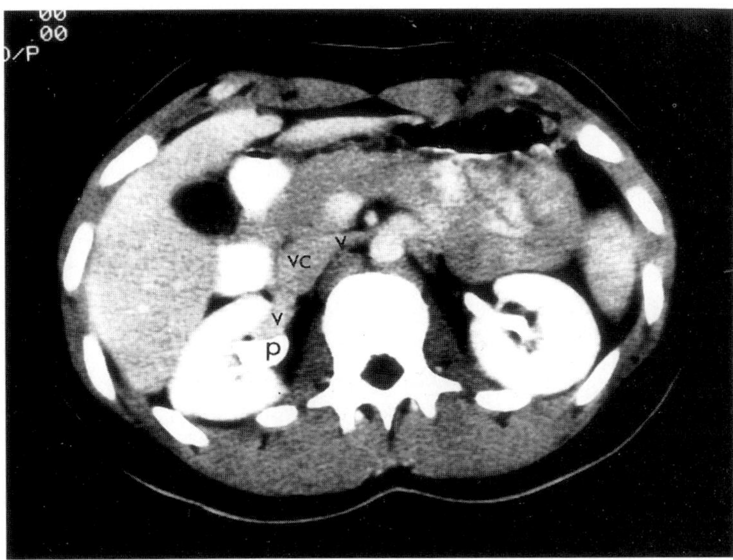

Fig. 5.11. CT of the kidney. Axial section, the mid-kidney shows the right and left renal veins (*v*) entering the vena cava (*vc*), renal pelvis (*p*), and kidney, liver, and aorta

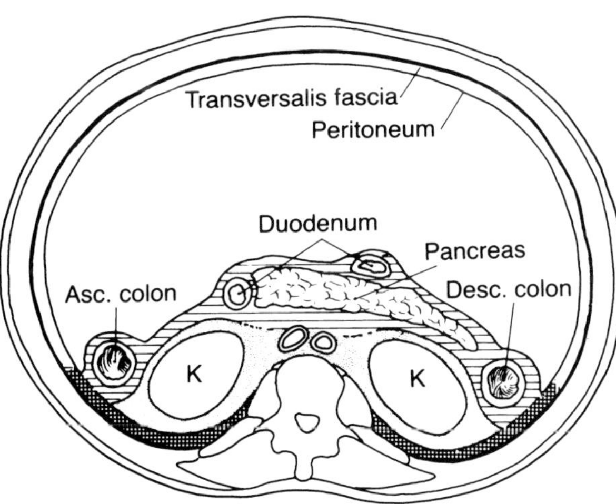

Fig. 5.12. The retroperitoneal spaces as described by Meyer [2]. *Striped area*, anterior pararenal space; *white areas around kidneys*, perirenal space; *cross-hatched areas*, posterior pararenal space

ther repetitive images of the same area as time passes or rapid sequential images.

Magnetic Resonance of the Kidneys

MR has not been used extensively in children for renal evaluation. With MR imaging there is no radiation, and there are no known biological hazards in the diagnostic range. Multiple planes of view can be obtained, but the patient must be still for an extended period of time. The ability of MR imaging to differentiate tissue characteristics (except calcium) is much greater than that of CT, and all of the planes are of the same image resolution, unlike the reconstructed planes of CT (Fig. 5.13). Cortical-medullary relationships are superbly analyzed; attenuations of cortical-medullary relationships are sensitive but nonspecific indicators of renal disease in adults. With MR imaging, as with ultrasound and nonenhanced CT, normally sized ureters are not seen. Contrast (gadolinium) may be necessary to detect tumors.

Angiography

Angiography is the most invasive way to study the kidneys. This topic is covered in Chap. 9.

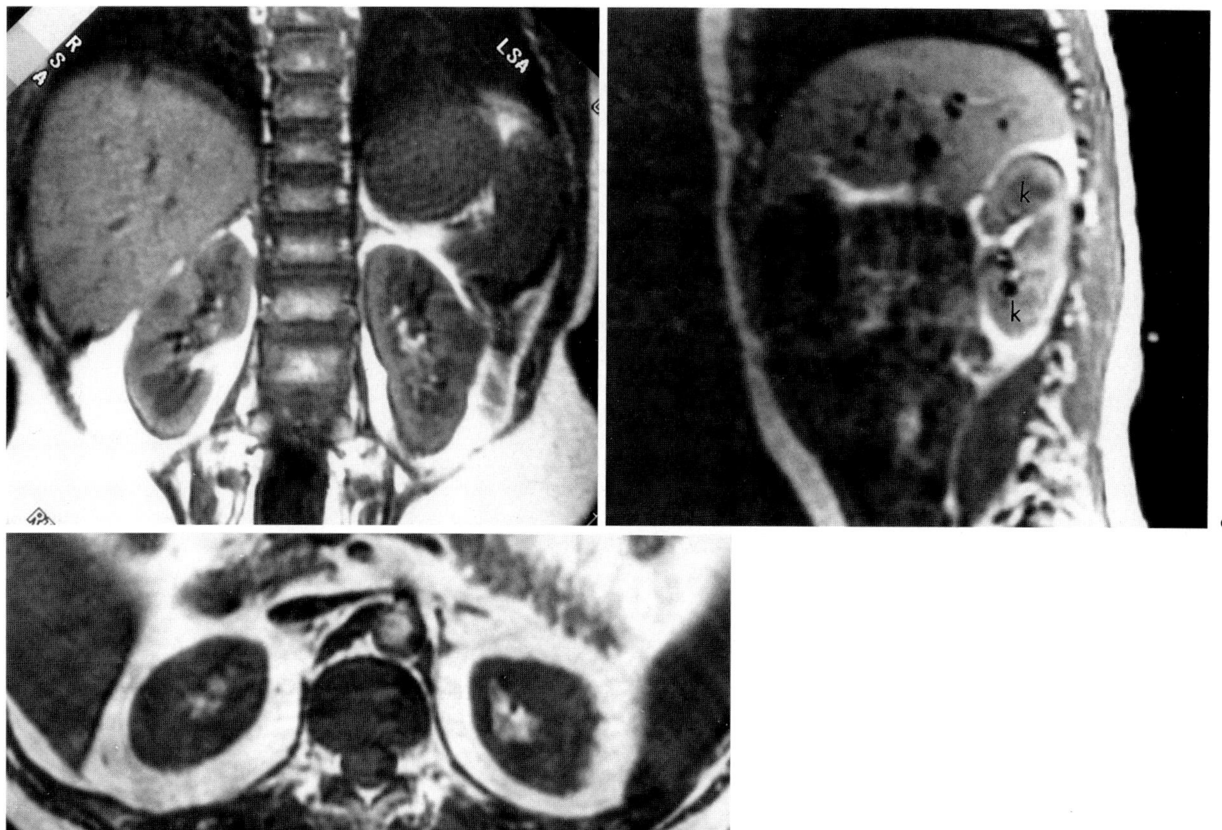

Fig. 5.13 a–c. MR imaging of kidney. **a** T1 spin-echo coronal view allows for definition of all adjacent organs. The cortex has higher signal than the medulla. **b** T1 spin-echo axial view has all the advantages of CT. This patient has abundant fat (*white-high signal*) around the kidneys. **c** T1 spin-echo sagittal image. Multiplanar imaging is the big advantage of MR. *k*, Kidney

Fig. 5.14 a, b. Nuclear studies of acute pyelonephritis. **a** Posterior scan with ^{99m}Tc-GH shows large photon deficient areas in both kidneys corresponding to areas of infection in this 2-year-old girl. **b** Posterior scan of the right kidney in another child shows photon deficient areas most prominent in the upper and lower poles. The left kidney is normal. This child complained of right flank pain and was febrile ▶

Integration of the Imaging Modalities

The basic questions to ask before ordering an imaging modality of the urinary tract are:

- Why am I doing this study?
- What do I hope to learn?
- Do I want an anatomical evaluation (i.e., tumor, anomaly, or obstruction) or a functional evaluation (i.e., decreased renal function)?

An appropriate imaging modality can be selected only after the goals are clear in your mind. Table 5.1 summarizes these modalities. The decision as to which imaging modality one selects is really a tradeoff. In screening or looking for a low-yield abnormality, the appropriate procedure is the one that can provide the answer with the least radiation and least danger. It is for this reason that ultrasound is frequently selected as the first imaging modality. On the other hand, in evaluating a tumor of the abdomen or the kidney, the most precise information is crucial; therefore, CT studies are frequently utilized. The four imaging modalities discussed in this chapter may be complementary. For example, an anechoic lesion on ultrasound may be a renal cyst, hydronephrosis, or a duplicated kidney. Only by correlating this finding with IVU results can the correct diagnosis be made.

Table 5.1. Imaging modalities

	Urography	Ultrasound	Nuclear medicine	Computed tomography	Magnetic resonance
Anatomy	++	++	+	+++	+++
Function	+	–	+++	+	+
Radiation	Low	None	Low	Highest of group	None
Injection of contrast/radio-nuclide	Yes	No	Yes	Yes	Sometimes
Patient preparation	Yes	No	No	Yes	No
Sedation under age 5	No	No	Probably	Probably	Yes

Common Clinical Situations

Urinary Tract Infection

Upper urinary tract infection must be documented before radiographic studies are requested. Although the presence of bacteria on Gram stains of a fresh, unspun, clean-catch specimen is very suggestive of a urinary tract infection, this must be confirmed with a quantitative urine culture. A colony count of 100 000 per millimeter of midstream voided specimen is considered a positive urine culture. Imaging should be used in the evaluation because: (a) This is the first *diagnosed* urinary tract infection, not necessarily the first *actual* infection. Urinary tract infection may be missed for some time, and kidney damage may well be present. (b) The imaging of urinary tract infection is controversial. There is general agreement that the younger the child is the greater the risk of kidney damage from infection, and that pyelonephritis must be present to lead to scarred kidney and renal damage.

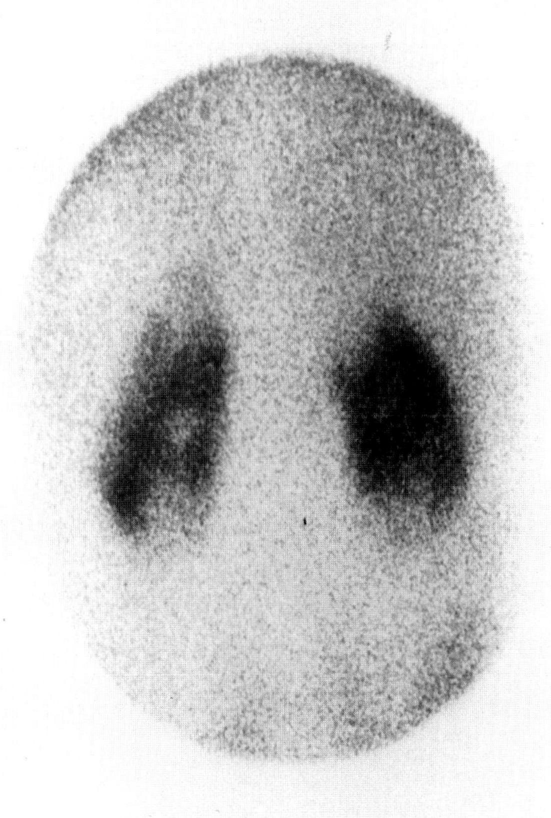

a

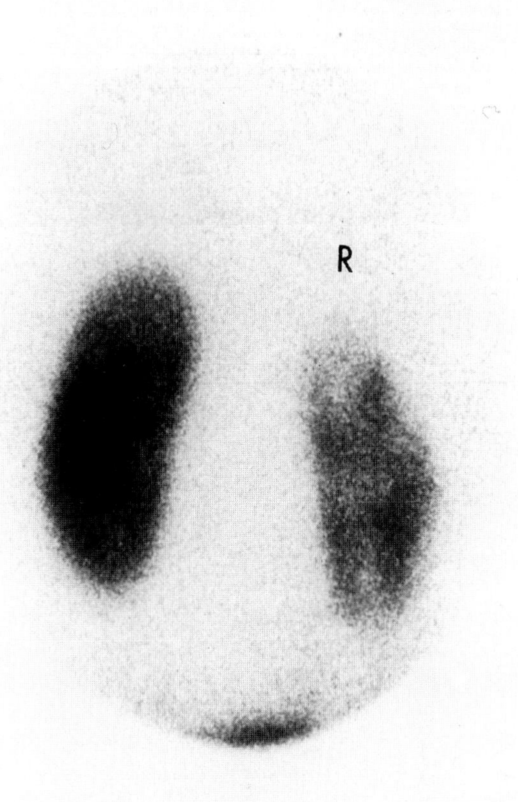

b

In the past it was thought that ureterovesical reflux is the major risk factor for pyelonephritis. However, 50% of children with sequelae of pyelonephritis never have documented reflux. Therefore it appears that imaging the kidney for pyelonephritis is the most appropriate first step in the high-risk groups (neonate to 5 years). This should be conducted with ^{99m}Tc-DMSA or ^{99m}Tc-GH (Fig. 5.14). If positive, ultrasound and voiding studies are usually carried out.

In low-risk groups (age under 5 years), a DMSA scan might be all that is necessary. Remember: reflux decreases with age.

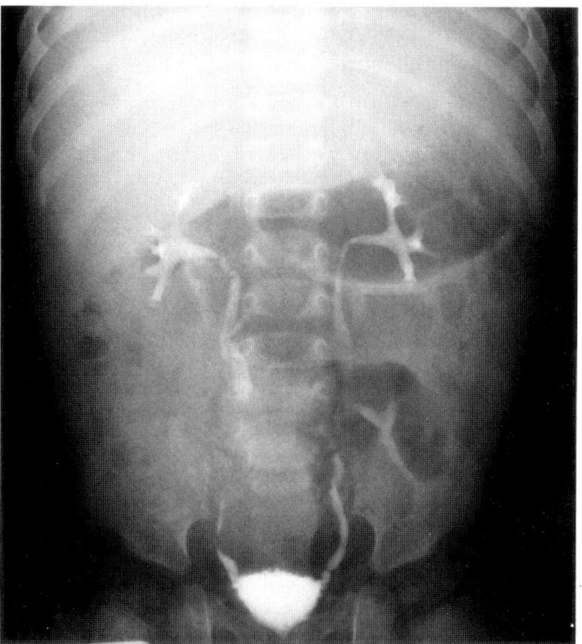

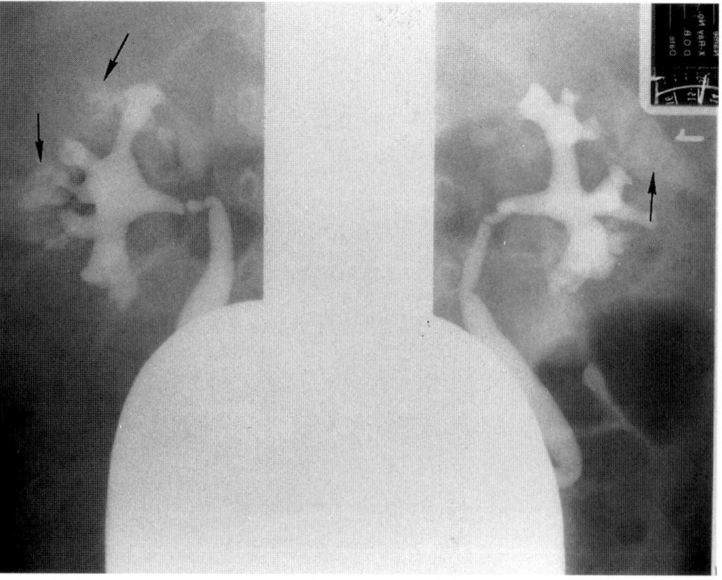

Fig. 5.15 a, b. Reflux. **a** This infant demonstrates bilateral grade II reflux (contrast refluxes to calyces without distention). **b** Bilateral grade IV reflux is seen (moderate distention of calyces). There is also bilateral intrarenal reflux (into the parenchyma) an ominous sign (*arrow*)

Enuresis

Most nocturnal bedwetters do not require any imaging studies. Careful history, centering on the symptoms of urinary tract infection, neurogenic bladder, and persistent versus intermittent wetting, should clarify the problem. If an imaging work-up is pursued, an ultrasound to rule out anomalies and a VCU to detect a neurogenic bladder or abnormalities such as an ectopic ureteral insertion are performed.

Abdominal Mass

This clinical phenomenon is discussed fully in Chap. 6.

Hematuria

Blunt abdominal trauma is a common cause of renal injury. When the trauma involves the upper abdomen, CT may be performed for the gross evaluation of renal function and the precise evaluation of anatomical detail. CT studies provide the best detail of the kidneys and adjacent visceral injury and in some circumstances may be the initial procedure. When there is injury to the lower abdomen and pelvis, a VCU is obtained (remember: the anterior urethra may need to be studied). At the same time, precise detail of the surrounding tissues and upper tracts can be obtained with CT and contrast enhancement. The latter may be preferable because it avoids instrumentation of the urethra in an acutely injured patient.

In nontraumatic hematuria, the need for an imaging modality reflects the clinical diagnosis. Acute β-streptococcal glomerulonephritis and Henoch-Schönlein purpura are not indications for an intravenous pyelogram or CT. However, since tumors çan present with hematuria, a precise anatomical evaluation is appropriate if the diagnosis is uncertain. Because of the lower radiation dose and, in many instances, the ease of obtaining the examination, an ultrasound scan is usually performed first.

Dilated Collecting System Seen on Antenatal Ultrasound Examination

Because of ever increasing use of prenatal sonographic screening, pediatricians are confronted with a relatively new problem: the neonate who is found on prenatal ultrasound to have "fullness" or dilated collecting system. The postnatal follow-up, however, is relatively simple. The infant will need a follow-up (preferably after the first few days of life) and voiding study to rule out reflux (Fig. 5.15). When there is no reflux, but there is a dilated renal pelvis, a radionuclide scan (^{99m}Tc-DTPA) to rule out obstruction is in order. This should be performed with Lasix to determine the exact degree of obstruction (Fig. 5.16).

References

1. Slovis TL, Sty JR, Haller JO (1989) Imaging of the pediatric urinary tract. Saunders, Philadelphia
2. Meyer MA (1982) Dynamic radiology of the abdomen, 2nd edn. Springer, Berlin Heidelberg, New York
3. National Council on Radiation Protection and Measurements (1981) Radiation protection in pediatric radiology. NCRP report 68. Bethesda, National Council on Radiation Protection and Measurements

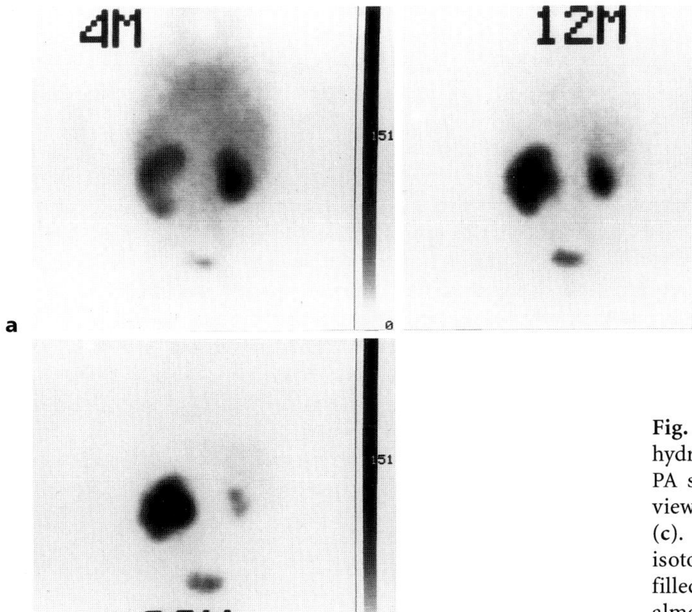

Fig. 5.16 a–c. Neonatal hydronephrosis. This neonate had left hydronephrosis on prenatal ultrasound. Posterior ^{99m}Tc-DTPA scan was performed; remember: the patient's left is the viewer's *left*. The scans at 4 min (**a**), 12 min (**b**), and 28 min (**c**). At 4 min the left kidney is bigger, and there is lack of isotope in the renal pelvis. By 12 min the renal pelvis has filled. Lasix was given, and at 28 min the right kidney is almost empty, but the large dilated left renal pelvis remains. This was a ureteral pelvic junction obstruction

6 Abdominal and Pelvic Masses

The pediatrician frequently asks the pediatric radiologist to verify the existence of an abdominal or pelvic mass and to suggest possible diagnoses. The imaging approach to such problems varies, but these basic principles must be followed:

- The initial procedure should be a three-view abdominal series (Chap. 4).
- When there is only a *question* of a mass, the least invasive procedure should be done first.
- Once a mass has been established, the work-up is guided by the patient's age, the location of the mass, and the symptoms (Table 6.1).
- The following priorities should be kept in mind: (a) Since barium interferes with ultrasound, radionuclide imaging, CT, and excretory urogram, any barium examination should follow these studies. (b) If both a barium enema and an upper GI series are necessary, the barium enema should be performed first because barium is more readily cleared from the colon.
- The pediatric radiologist is the best source of information as to how the imaging work-up should proceed.

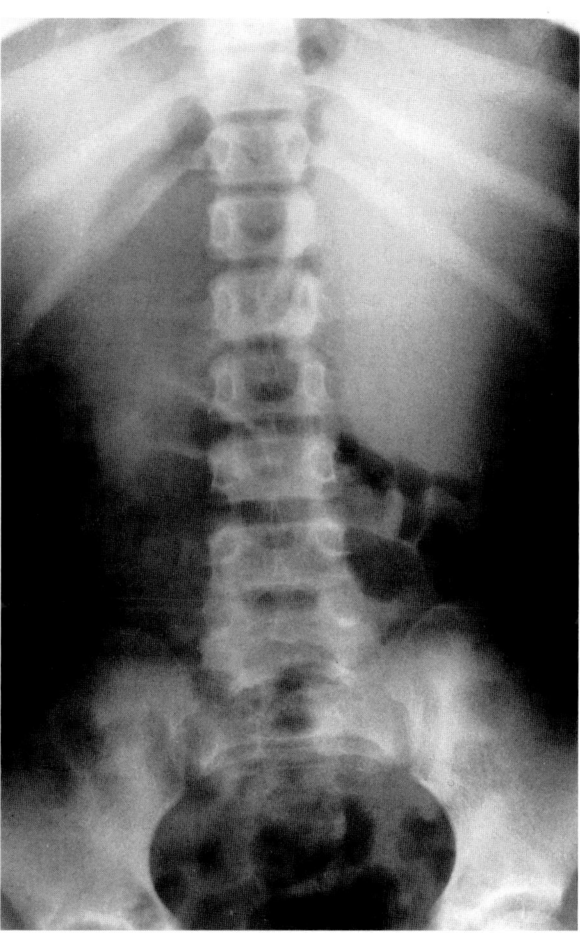

Fig. 6.1. Mass (*left upper quadrant*) – an enlarged spleen and effects. The gas-filled gastrointestinal tract is displaced inferiorly and to the right. The differential diagnosis of anatomical origin for the mass includes muscle, peritoneum, stomach, kidney, spleen, and adrenal gland. These are structures that are found "skin to skin." This child had isolated splenomegaly due to portal hypertension

Begin the Work-Up with an Abdominal Series

Almost every child who presents with an abdominal mass should have abdominal films as an initial screening procedure (except for girls over 9 years of age, who may be pregnant). Plain film findings and abdominal series are discussed in Chaps. 4 and 5. Specifically, one should look for a mass, the effects of the mass, and calcifications.

Mass effect (see Fig. 6.1) is the effect of the mass on contiguous structures, such as bowel or viscera. Divide the abdomen into quadrants and apply your knowledge of anatomical structures in this quadrant.

► *Reed's Rule No. 12:* Try to find the effects of the mass on adjacent organs on each abdominal film. Draw the mass, if necessary.

Table 6.1. Most frequent abdominal and pelvic masses by age (modified from 4–6)

Age and type of mass	Incidence (%)	
Neonate		
Renal	55	70%
Hydronephrosis		
Multicystic kidney		
Ureteropelvic junction obstruction,		
Ureteral vesical junction obstruction,		
Reflux (includes valves)		
Genital	15	
Hydrometrocolpos		
Ovarian		
Gastrointestinal	15	
Duplications		
Volvulus		
Nonrenal retroperitoneal	10	
Adrenal hemorrhage		
Neuroblastoma		
Teratoma		
Hepatosplenobiliary	5	
1 Month–2 years		
Renal	55	78%
Wilms' tumor		
Hydronephrosis		
Nonrenal retroperitoneal	23	
Neuroblastoma		
Teratoma		
Gastrointestinal (including biliary masses and appendiceal abscess) and intussusception	18	
Genital, miscellaneous	4	
Older than 2 years [a]		
Visceromegaly secondary to infection leukemia, lymphoma, splenomegaly secondary to portal hypertension	Frequent	
Wilms' tumor and neuroblastoma	Frequent to age 5; decreases thereafter	
Appendiceal abscess	Frequent over age 5	
Intussusception	Most frequent at age 2; decreases thereafter	
Pregnancy	Most common pelvic mass in females over age[a]	

[a] It is difficult to obtain precise numbers for this age group.

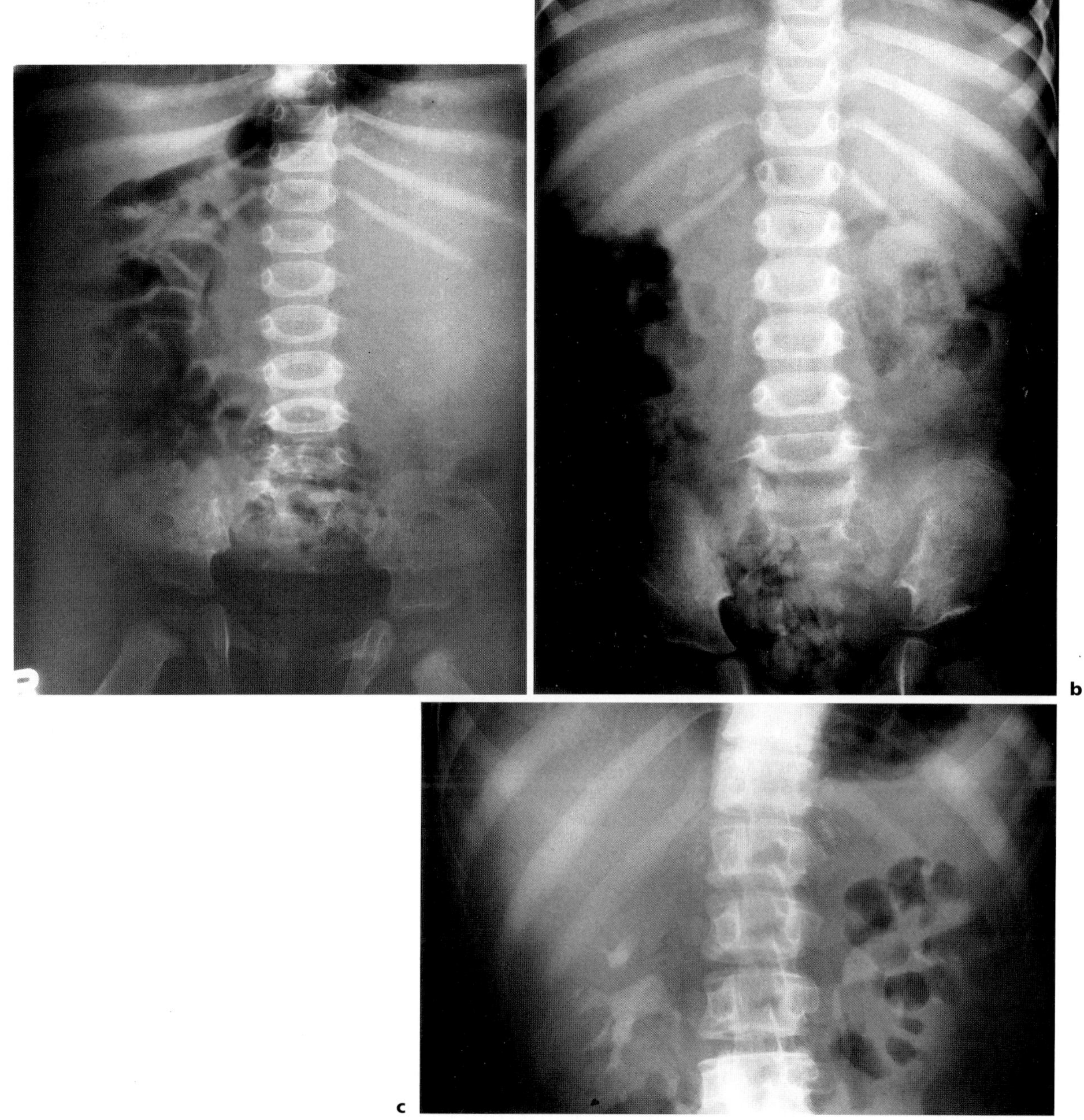

Fig. 6.2 a–c. Calcification on the plain film. a A 1-year-old with left-sided abdominal mass. There are diffuse, fine calcifications within the mass. b An 18-month-old with right upper quadrant mass. There is fine stippled calcification between T11 and T12. c A 16-year-old with coarse calcification in the region of the adrenals as seen on this excretory urogram. a, b Neuroblastomas. c An old adrenal hemorrhage

Calcifications (see Fig. 6.2) are an important clue to the type of mass present. Fine, punctate calcifications next to the upper pole of the kidney may well represent an adrenal neuroblastoma, while large, coarse calcifications may merely mean the presence of calcified adrenal hemorrhage. It is common for the neuroblastoma to calcify, while it is distinctly less common for a Wilms' tumor to calcify. An appendicolith is ordinarily round, solitary, and laminated, while a calcification in a dermoid or teratoma may have a structure similar to

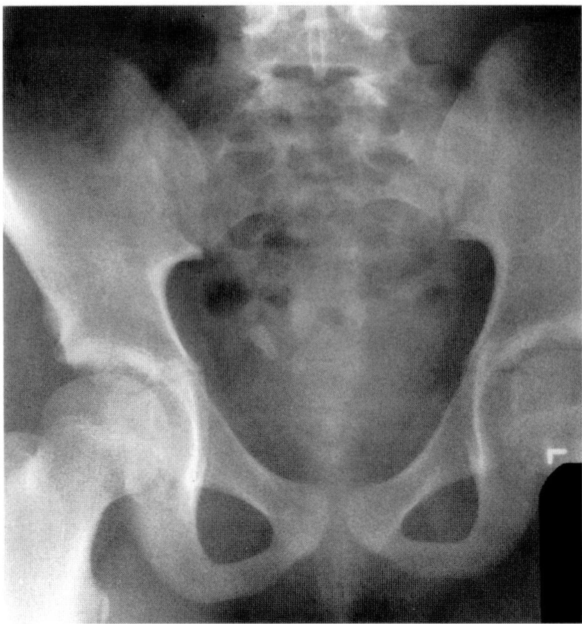

Fig. 6.3. Dermoid. An 8-year-old girl with pelvic mass. The plain film revealed a calcified lesion resembling a tooth

a tooth within it (Fig. 6.3). It must then be determined where the mass originated, and whether it is neoplastic, inflammatory, etc.

► *Reed's Rule No. 13:* After the mass has been defined, find the center of the lesion. Then consider all the structures, gross and microscopic, near the center of the lesion as possible sources of the mass. Think skin to skin.

Remember: an abdominal mass may be an enlarged organ, such as the liver, spleen, or kidney. Frequently, children with leukemia have visceromegaly. Isolated splenomegaly is found in portal hypertension (Fig. 6.1).

Begin with the Least Invasive Study When There is a Questionable Mass

Frequently the clinician is not sure whether there is a mass. In a constipated child fecal masses in the colon are easily palpated and may be mistaken for a lesion. Other putative masses include the distended urinary bladder and the abdominal aorta in a particularly thin child. Therefore, evacuation of both bowel and bladder contents should precede any work-up to obviate the majority of "pseudomasses."

In girls over the age of 9 years any pelvic mass should be considered an intrauterine pregnancy until proved otherwise. For this reason, ultrasound is initially utilized because it is the least invasive modality without ionizing radiation (Fig. 6.4).

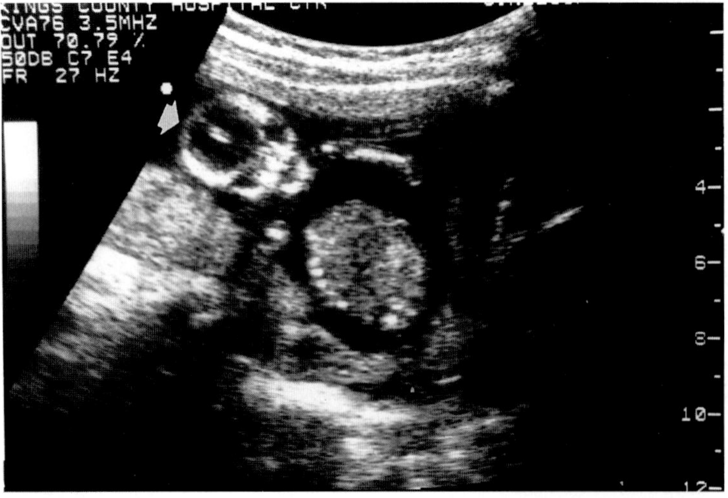

Fig. 6.4. Intrauterine pregnancy. This 11-year-old girl presented with a pelvic mass. Ultrasound revealed an intrauterine fetus. *Arrow*, fetal head. The face is looking at you. Yes! Those are the orbits and the mouth

Let the Patient's Age, Symptoms, and Location of the Mass Direct the Work-Up

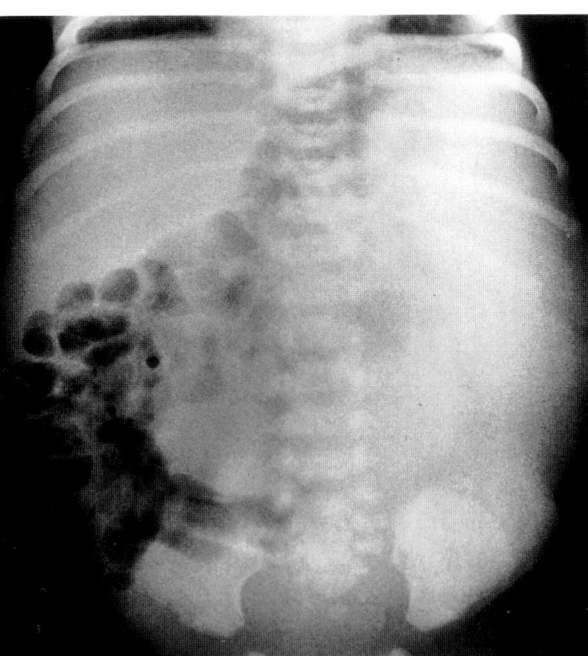

Newborn. Seventy percent of abdominal and pelvic masses in neonates originate in the genitourinary tract. Hydronephrosis (ureteropelvic junction obstruction, ureterovesical junction obstruction, and reflux) and multicystic kidneys account for the majority of urinary masses (Table 6.1; Fig. 6.5), while the most common genital masses are hydrometrocolpos and ovarian cysts (Fig. 6.6). Malignant abdominal masses are uncommon in this age group (although neuroblastoma occurs rarely), but pelvic masses with malignant potential (e.g., sacrococcygeal teratoma) do occur.

One Month to 2 Years of Age. Once again, the urinary masses predominate, with Wilms' tumor and hy-

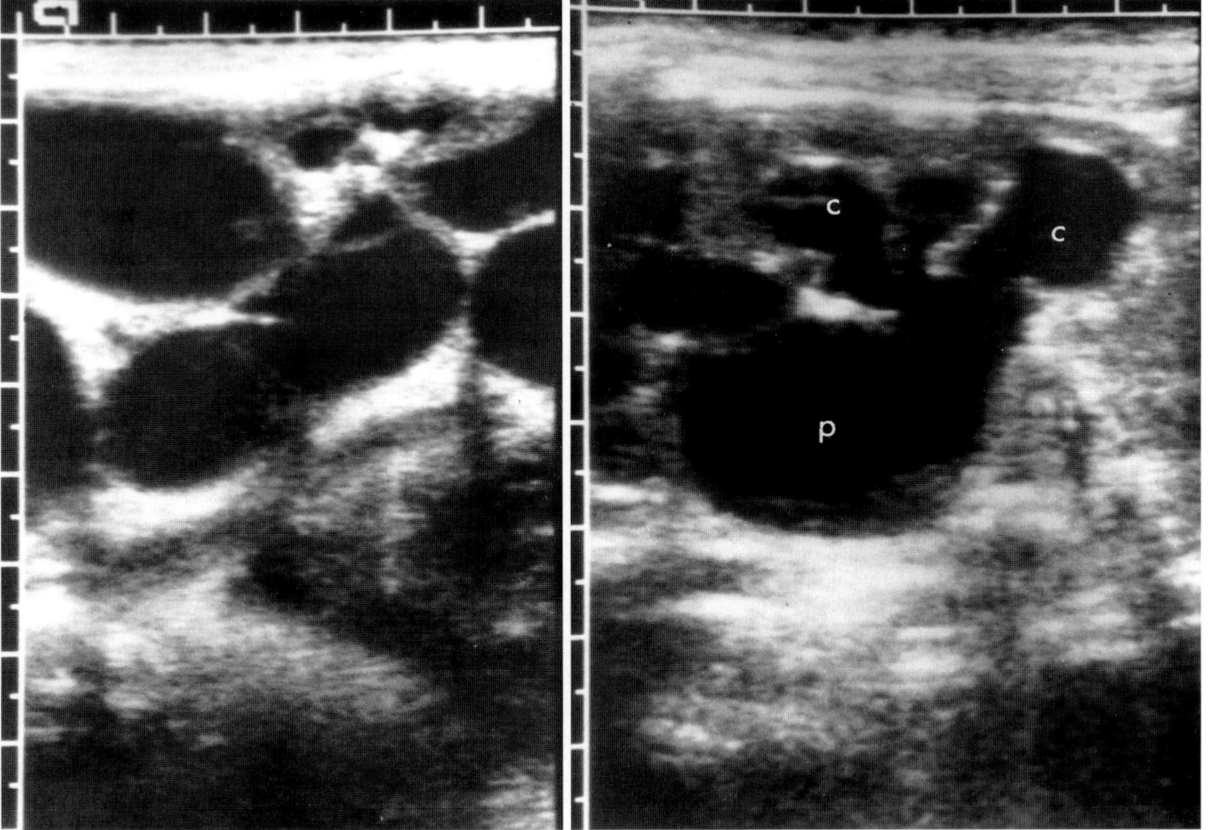

Fig. 6.5 a–c. Newborn abnormalities. **a** Plain film shows left flank mass. **b** Ultrasound reveals a multicystic kidney. There are septa between cysts and no renal parenchyma. **c** Another child with hydronephrosis and dilated renal pelvis (*p*) and calyces (*c*)

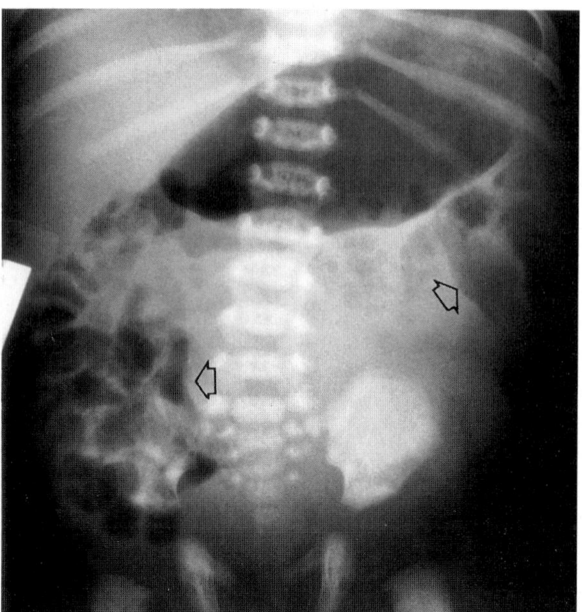

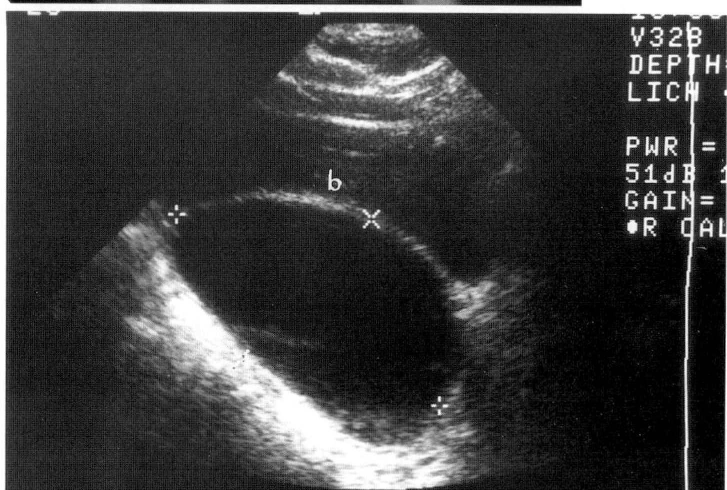

Fig. 6.6 a, b. Ovarian cyst. **a** This 6-month-old girl presented with a central lower abdominal mass. The plain film of the abdomen reveals bowel displaced away from this mass (*arrows*). Pelvic masses, when they enlarge, leave the true pelvis and are found in the infraumbilical region. **b** Ultrasound shows a cystic (*all black*) mass (*x*) behind the bladder (*b*)

dronephrosis occurring with equal frequency. Nonrenal retroperitoneal masses such as neuroblastoma now become more common (Fig. 6.7). The gastrointestinal mass of most concern now becomes the intussusception (Chap. 4).

Older than 2 Years. Once a child reaches 2 years of age, the incidence of genitourinary system masses declines, and the differential diagnoses broaden. Traumatic lesions, inflammatory processes (e.g., from a perforated appendix; see Chap. 4), and the more unusual hepatic lesions are now considered. However, Wilms' tumor and neuroblastoma remain high in the differential diagnoses. The lymphomatous masses in the abdomen become a strong consideration in the older age group (Fig. 6.8).

Location of the Mass. After age, the location of the mass is the next important consideration. If a neonate has a flank mass, the chances are great that it will be a hydronephrotic or multicystic kidney. A less likely right upper quadrant mass is a hepatoblastoma. In a 2-year-old a right upper quadrant mass suggests a neuroblastoma or Wilms' tumor. A good trick is to put your finger where you think the center of the mass is and then consider all the normal viscera under your

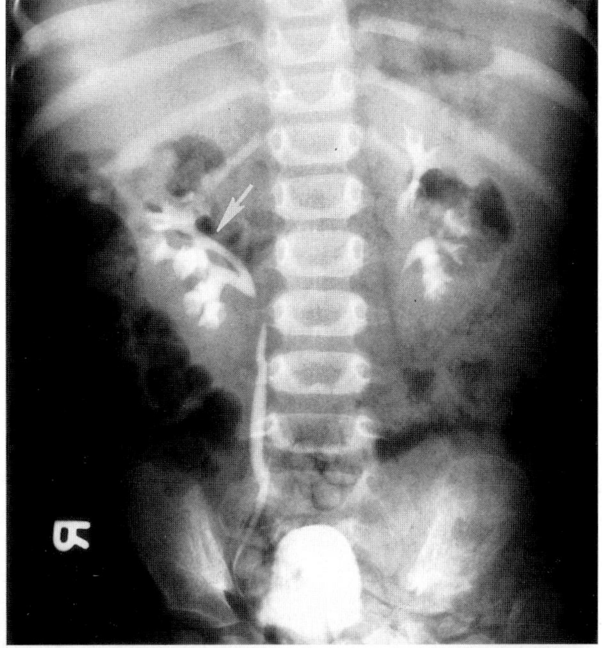

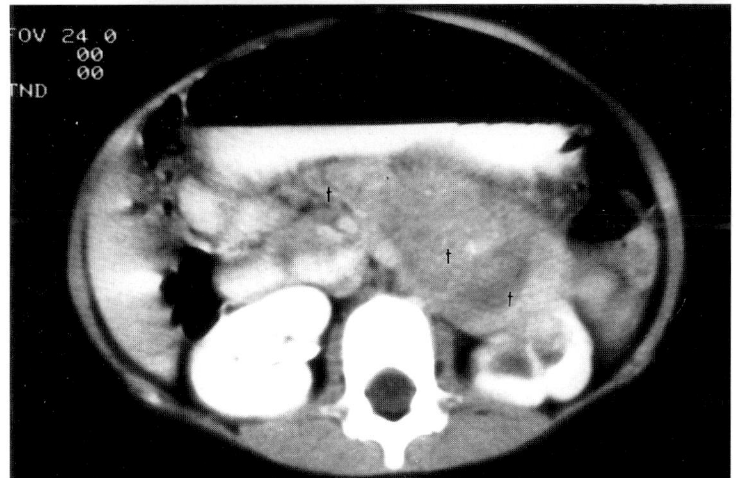

Fig. 6.7 a, b. Neuroblastoma. **a** Excretory urogram on same patient as in Fig. 6.2b. A 5-min film shows the right collecting system displaced inferiorly and laterally (*arrow*). The renal axis is wrong with the upper pole more lateral than the lower pole. Note that the calyces are not distorted but displaced. This is a typical finding in neuroblastoma. **b** CT on another child reveals encasement of vessels and amorphous margins of the tumor. The tumor (*t*) extends across the midline. The top of the left kidney is flattened

finger from skin to skin. Then think of common pathology affecting those viscera. This helps form the differential diagnosis.

Symptoms. In many instances when a mass is palpated, either by the parents or a physician, the child experiences no symptoms. However, symptoms or signs such as jaundice or profuse diarrhea provide clues. A jaundiced patient with a right upper quadrant mass may have a choledochal cyst, while one with a flank mass and profuse secretory diarrhea may have a catecholamine-secreting neuroblastoma. Specific attention should be paid to symptoms in children with pelvic masses. Because of the relationship of the pelvic mass to the bladder, bowel, and sacral nerve complex these children may present with dysfunction of one or more of these systems (Fig. 6.9). Since masses (other than those associated with the ovaries and uterus) occur in the pelvis nearly as frequently as they do in the upper abdominal retroperitoneal areas, any child with bladder, bowel, or neurological symptoms should be suspected of having a pelvic mass. In addition, the diagnostic work-up – appropriate history, physical examination and imaging procedures (Table 6.2, Fig. 6.10) – should proceed accordingly.

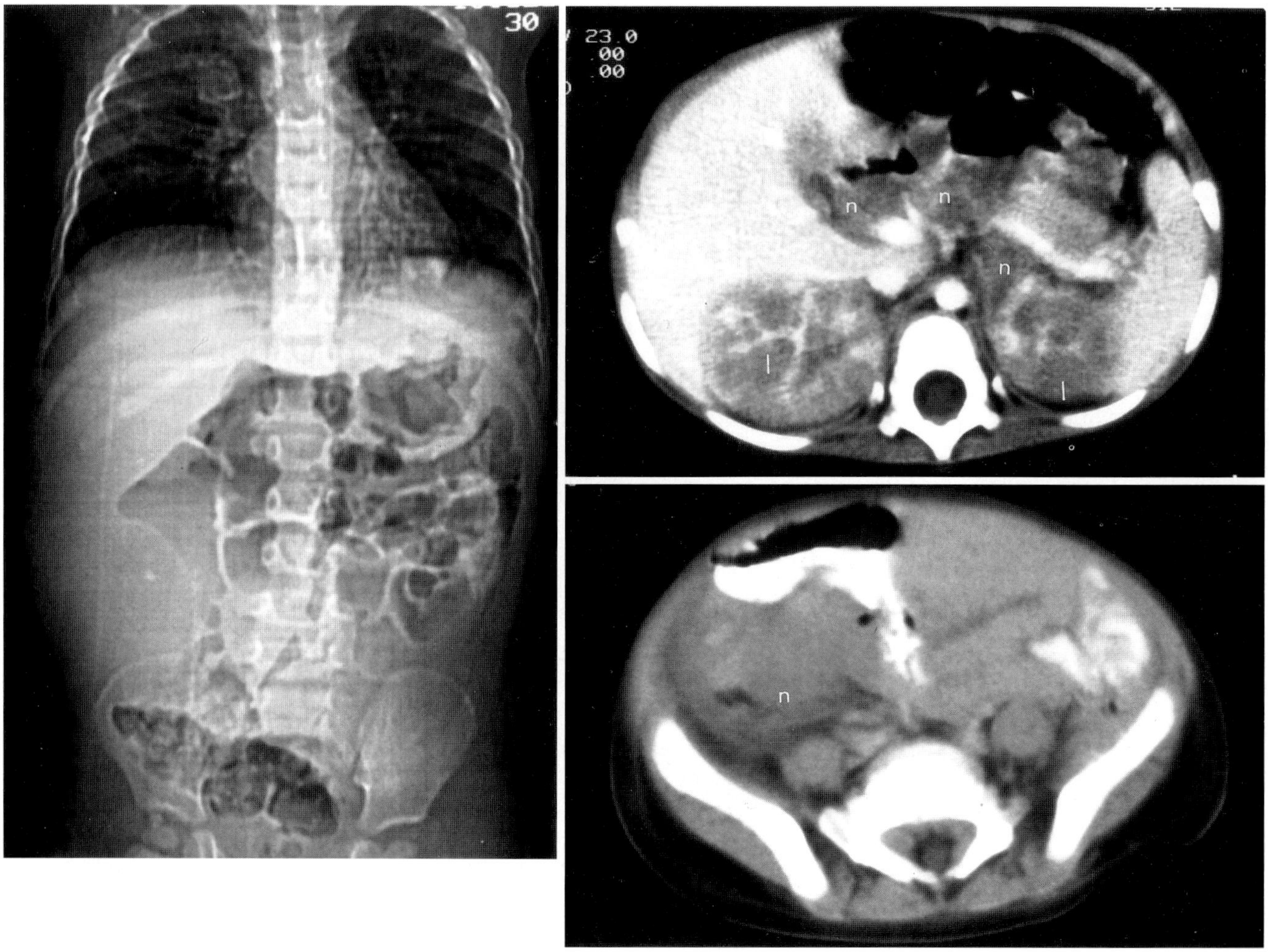

a

b

c

Table 6.2. Imaging procedures by signs and symptoms in children with an abdominal-pelvic mass

	First	Later	
Hypertension	US with Doppler	MRI	Renal or suprarenal tumor, renal vascular lesion
Jaundice	US	NM	Obstruction of biliary system, choledochal cyst
Fever, right lower quadrant mass	US	CT or BE	Appendicitis or appendiceal abscess[a]
Colicky abdominal pain, bloody diarrhea	Enema (barium or air)		Intussusception
Projectile vomiting, nonbilious	UGI or US		Pyloric stenosis[b]
Hepatic mass	US w/Doppler	NM, CT, MRI, angiography	Hepatoblastoma, vascular tumor, resectability
Splenomegaly	US with Doppler		Patency of portal vein, liver pathology, portal hypertension, masses of spleen

BE, Barium enema; CT, computed tomography; MRI, magnetic resonance imaging; NM, nuclear medicine; US, ultrasound; UGI, upper gastrointestinal examination.

[a] If diagnosis of acute appendicitis is made clinically, no imaging procedure is necessary; if chronic or atypical, may do US to show mass effect.

[b] When pyloric tumor ("olive") is felt, no imaging procedure is needed.

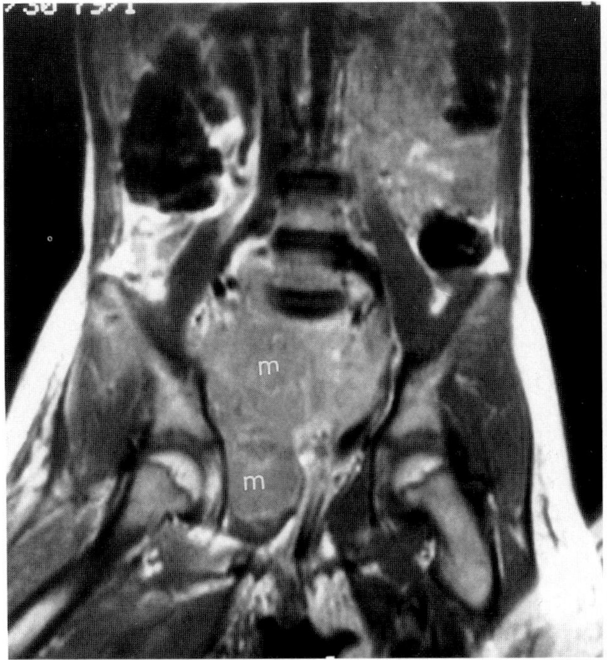

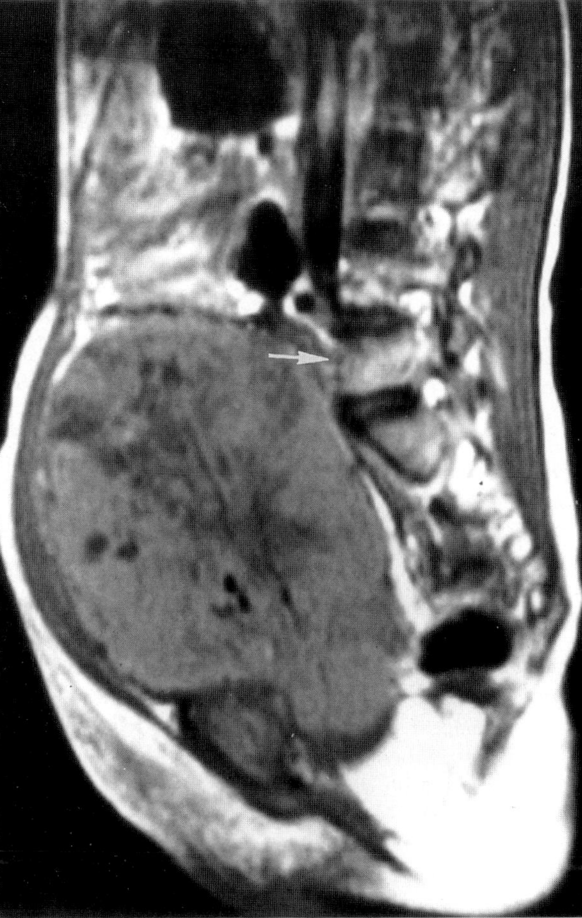

◀ **Fig. 6.8 a–c.** Lymphoma. **a** A 3-year-old girl with right flank mass. **b** Contrast-enhanced CT shows low-density renal lesions (*l*) bilaterally and retroperitoneal and para-aortic adenopathy (*n*) surrounding the abdominal midline vessels. **c** The mass of nodes extended down the right flank into the pelvis

▲ **Fig. 6.9 a, b.** Pelvic mass. A 6-year-old girl with recent onset of gait disturbance and bowel dysfunction. Coronal MR reveals a large soft tissue mass encasing the sacrum and extending into the right groin (*m*). **b** Lateral views shows vertebral body involvement (*arrow*) and compression of rectum and bladder. This was a soft tissue Ewing's sarcoma

Fig. 6.10. Imaging work-up of a child with an abdominal mass. *NM*, Nuclear medicine; *US*, ultrasound; *EU*, excretory urogram; *VCUG*, voided cystourethrogram; *MRI*, magnetic resonance imaging; *UGI*, upper gastrointestinal examination. *Asterisk*, confirms changing size. (Modified from [1])
▼

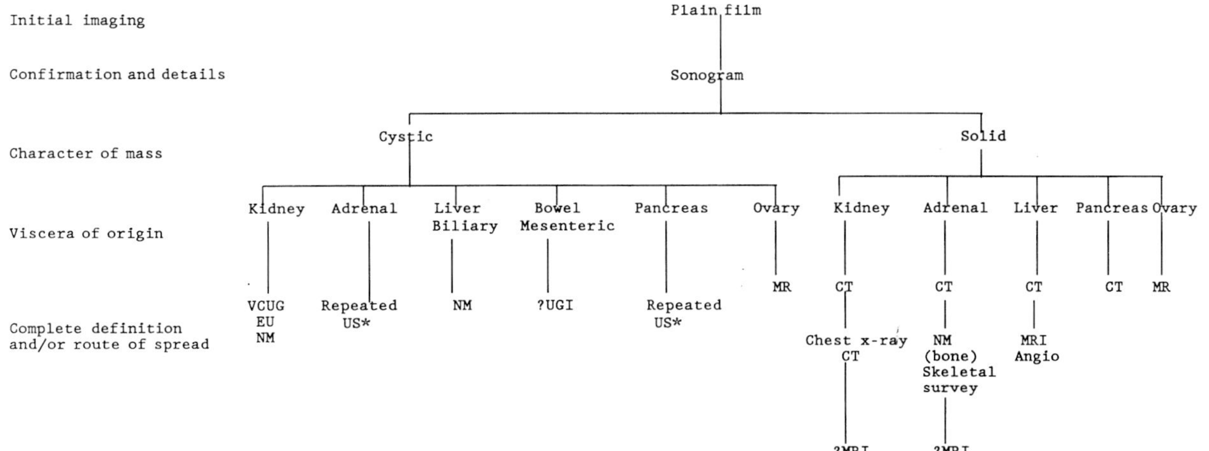

Imaging Principles

Many of these principles are discussed in previous chapters. For newborns, after initial plain abdominal films, ultrasound is generally the first test because most masses are of genitourinary origin (hydronephrosis, multicystic kidney), and most of them are cystic with characteristic ultrasonic appearance.

Once the presence of a mass is firmly established and its site determined, the extent of the lesion should be defined. CT and MR imaging are the most precise imaging methods to define the intra-abdominal and pelvic extent of a tumor.

Specific Lesions

The most common abdominal or pelvic tumors of childhood are Wilms' tumor and neuroblastoma. The following are helpful clues for identifying the abdominal mass on CT and ultrasound:

- Tumor motion: helps separate tumor from organs not invaded by the tumor (e.g., liver, kidney)
- Fat displacement: helps to distinguish visceral (renal) from extravisceral (nonrenal) tumors
- Compressed rim of liver tissue: when present, suggests extravisceral as opposed to intravisceral tumor
- Caval thrombus: Wilms' tumor, hepatoblastoma
- Calcium: more common in neuroblastoma
- Spinal involvement: most often neuroblastoma
- Nodal encasement: more common in neuroblastoma
- Portal vein displacement: suggests extrahepatic origin as opposed to hepatic invasion

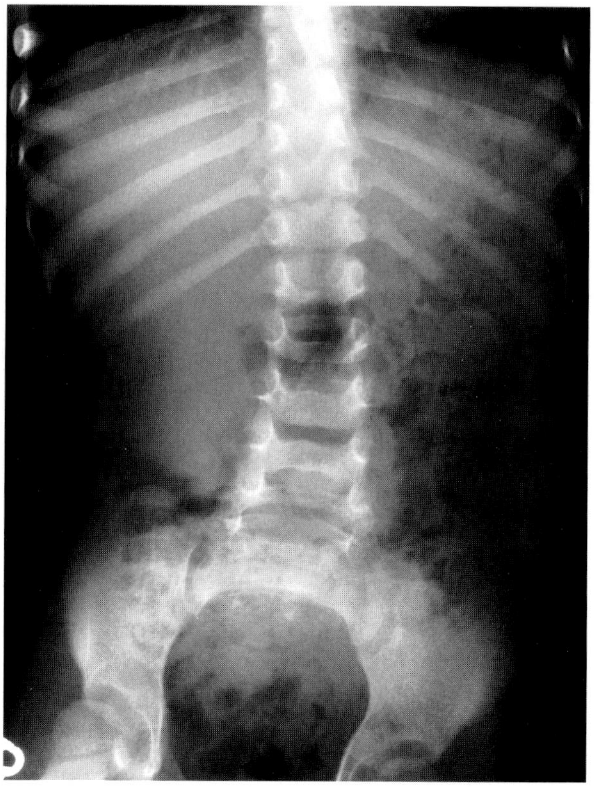

a

Fig 6.11 a–c. Wilms' tumor. **a** A 3-year-old girl presented with a right flank mass. There was no calcification. **b** CT reveals the mass to be within the right kidney, causing hydronephrosis. The mass (*m*) is well defined, does not cross the midline or encase the great vessels. The opposite kidney is normal. **c** In another child with Wilms' tumor, there are multiple chest metastases

Wilms' Tumor

Wilms' tumor is an intrarenal tumor (Fig. 6.11) with peak incidence between 2 and 5 years of age. Although the presenting symptom is frequently an abdominal flank mass, the tumor is associated with hematuria in 20% of patients. It is commonly asymptomatic, but occasionally fever and pain are symptoms. Hypertension may be present. The radiographic findings are those of distortion of the internal renal architecture. Infrequently, the tumor is large enough to completely obstruct the kidney. It is uncommon to see calcification. In general, the prognosis is good, but it depends almost entirely on the histological type (favorable versus unfavorable) and staging of the lesion. For the work-up of a child with an abdominal mass, see Table 6.2 and Fig. 6.10. However, once the primary diagnosis is made, the extent of the tumor should be evaluated on the basis of biological behavior of tumor spread and sites of common metastases. Its routes of spread may be:

- Local
  - Renal vein
  - Inferior vena cava
  - Perihilar lymph nodes
  - Contiguous invasion of the liver
- Remote
  - Lungs: "cannonball" metastases
- Rare
  - Hematogenous to the liver
  - Bone

With Wilms' tumor, it is crucial that the inferior vena cava and renal veins be evaluated, as the tumor often

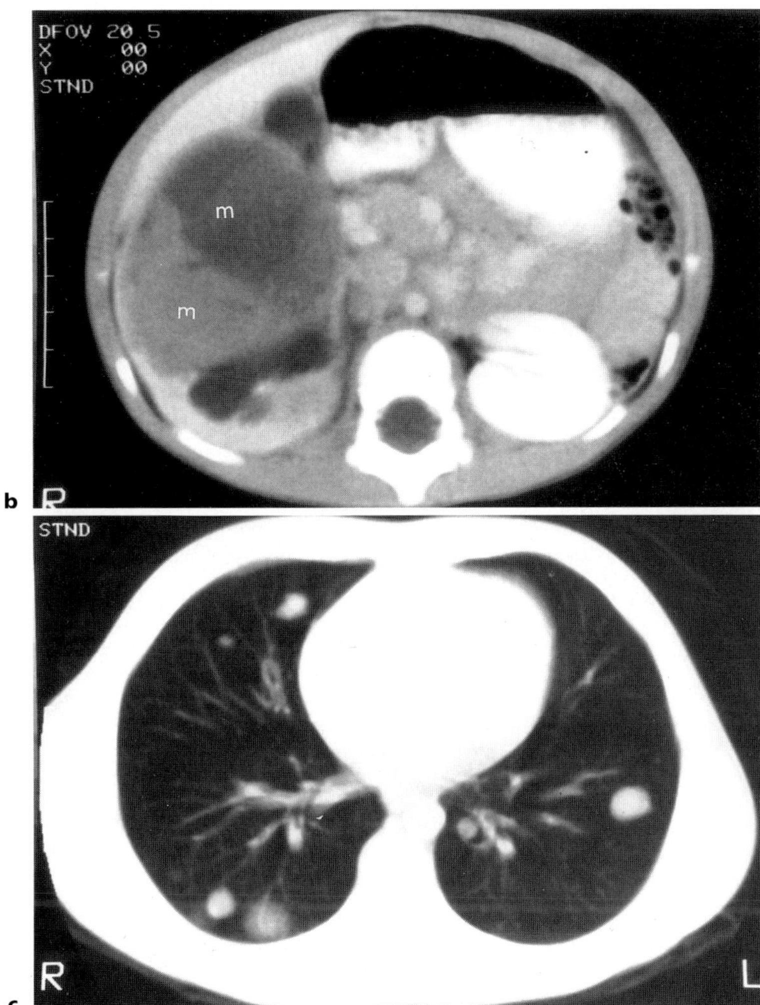

b

c

grows directly into the renal veins, the inferior vena cava, and occasionally the heart. Detection of tumor in this region determines whether thoracoabdominal exploration is necessary. The vena cava is best and least invasively evaluated by real-time ultrasound or MR imaging. The other kidney must also be examined to rule out bilateral Wilms' tumor and/or the presence of nephroblastomatosis (primitive rests of cells with tumor potential), a precursor of Wilms' tumor.

Evaluation of the chest, liver and lymph nodes – common sites of tumor metastases – is best done by CT (see Fig. 6.11).

Neuroblastoma

Neuroblastoma is a lesion of the sympathetic nerve chain and may arise anywhere along the axis of these sympathetic nerves (see Fig. 6.7). About 66% of these tumors arise in the abdomen and appear most frequently in the adrenal gland – the suprarenal region. The possible routes of spread are:

- Local
  - Lymph nodes and extensive nodal masses
  - Invades neural foramina causing deviation of dural sac
  - Encases great vessels
- Remote (hematogenous)
  - Bone
  - Central nervous system: extradural space and orbits

The majority of neuroblastomas occur in children aged 6 months to 5 years. Unlike the asymptomatic presentation of a child with Wilms' tumor, many children with neuroblastoma present with weight loss, irritability, fever, and anemia. A few show excessive catecholamine production and have such symptoms as skin flushing, perspiration, diarrhea, and/or headaches. On physical examination, there may well be hypertension and tachypnea.

The plain film findings frequently show stippled calcification, with lateral and downward displacement of the kidney (Figs. 6.2, 6.7). Neuroblastoma has a rather poor prognosis if the child is over 1 year of age. By the time it is diagnosed, it has frequently metastasized to the skeleton, as well as to the bone marrow and the liver.

After the primary neuroblastoma is discovered, evaluation of the bones and the liver is necessary. Liver metastases can be shown by CT and radionuclide studies, while radiographs and/or radionuclide studies are best for bone lesions.

Because of the high frequency of intraspinal involvement with neuroblastoma, MR imaging is essential to the work-up (see Chap. 8).

Hepatic Tumors

These lesions are certainly less common than either Wilms' tumor or neuroblastoma. They are presented here because their imaging evaluation is complex and demands the use of multiple procedures. The two malignant liver tumors seen most frequently are hepatoblastoma and hepatocellular carcinoma. The more common benign hepatic lesions are vascular, such as the hemangioendothelioma. Children with these tumors come to the physician with complaints either of a mass in the upper abdomen or enlargement of the abdomen. Liver dysfunction with jaundice and ascites is seen less frequently.

The initial imaging procedure, after the plain film, is an ultrasound of the right upper quadrant. Doppler is used with ultrasound to diagnosis arteriovenous malformations, hemangiomas, and portal vein patency. Because in most instances the surgeon would like to know about the resectability of the lesion, the studies that best demonstrate anatomical detail are performed next. These include CT and/or MRI–MRA. The latter is the preferred imaging modality in preoperative staging of liver tumors because it gives excellent soft tissue contrast while allowing visualization of hepatic vascular structures to rule out possible tumor invasion. This, then, is quite different from the evaluation for Wilms' tumor or neuroblastoma. Knowledge of the natural history of the disease, as well as the necessity for precise anatomical detail for surgical resection, demands an extensive multimodality preoperative work-up.

Lymphoma

Hodgkin's and non-Hodgkin's lymphomas (Fig. 6.8) are frequent malignancies of childhood. Although most children do not present with an abdominal mass, occasionally a palpable abdominal mass is the initial presenting sign. The reason for including lymphomas in this discussion is to remind one that lymphomatous infiltration (as well as leukemic infiltration) of the kidneys, liver, and spleen does occur. When evaluating the abdomen for visceromegaly or mass, these diseases should be considered.

Rhabdomyosarcoma

Rhabdomyosarcoma is the most common of the soft tissue sarcomas. In 16% of cases the tumor originates in the genitourinary system. The vagina, bladder, testicular or paratesticular region, or prostate may be the primary site. It originates from the same embryonic mesenchyme that gives rise to skeletal muscle and is a major diagnostic consideration when facing a solid pelvic mass. It occurs in any age group, with 10% appearing in the first year of life; these young infants have an especially poor prognosis. The tumor metastasizes via the lymph and the bloodstream; no specific organ system predominates in metastatic spread. Therefore, the radiographic work-up would include evaluation of bone, chest, lymph nodes, etc.

Pregnancy: The Most Common Pelvic Mass in Girls

Evaluation of pelvic masses begins, for girls over 9 years of age, with a pregnancy test or an ultrasound study (see Fig. 6.4). Careful longitudinal and transverse scans are done to rule out the easily diagnosable intrauterine pregnancy. The pelvic mass is defined, and the diagnostic possibilities may be limited to a select few. After pregnancy, ovarian lesions are the next most common mass. The lesion may be benign or malignant and may be predominantly cystic or solid.

References

1. Slovis TL, Sty JR, Haller JO (1989) Imaging of the pediatric urinary tract. Saunders, Philadelphia
2. Silverman FN (1993) Caffey's pediatric X-ray diagnosis, 9th edn. Mosby, St. Louis
3. Cohen MD (1992) Imaging of children with cancer. Mosby, St. Louis
4. Griscom NT (1965) The roentgenology of neonatal abdominal masses. AJR Am J Roetgenol 93:447
5. Kasper TE et al (1967) Urological abdominal masses in infants and children. J Urol 116:629
6. Melicow MD, Uson AC (1959) Palpable abdominal masses in infants and children: a report based on review of 653 cases. J Urol 81:705

7 Skeleton

The second most frequent radiographic study, after the chest film, is that of the pediatric skeleton. The most common indication for such studies is of course trauma. In order to understand the disease processes that occur in the pediatric age group one must first know the skeletal anatomy. The skull and spine are covered in Chap. 8.

Anatomy

Long Bones

The two physiological mechanisms of bone production and development are endochondral (long bones) and intramembranous ossification (flat bones). The long bone of a child is divided into four areas (Fig. 7.1):

- diaphysis: the shaft of the long bone
- metaphysis: the area of cartilaginous calcification and ossification where the bone flares
- physis: the lucent line where growth takes place prior to calcification of the cartilage
- epiphysis, or secondary ossification center: a portion of which interfaces with the joint as the articular cartilage and allows movement within the joint

The center of the long bone is the medullary cavity, while the outer bone is called the cortex. Some long bones (e.g., the femur) have a nonarticulating *apophysis* (see Fig. 7.1), which is similar to the epiphysis but does not contribute to the length of the bone (e.g., the greater trochanter). In the growing child's skeleton blood supply is primarily to the metaphysis, and many of the disease processes and roentgen findings are seen in this region. For example, hematogenous osteomyelitis is visible most often in the metaphysis; similarly, metastases travel hematogenously to the metaphysis.

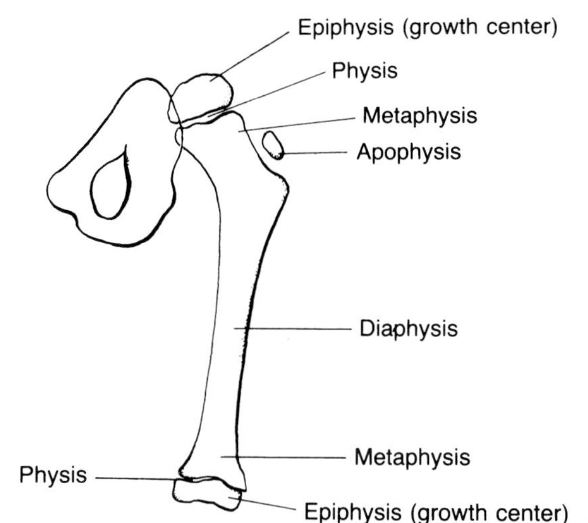

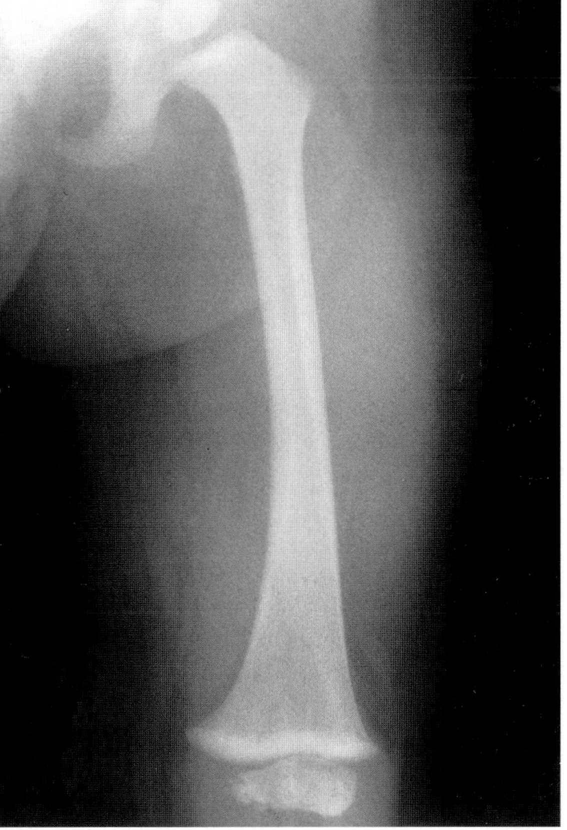

Fig. 7.1 a, b. The normal femur. **a** Schematic drawing of a normal femur. **b** Radiograph of a normal femur (apophysis not present yet)

Flat Bones

In the flat or membranous bones there is no diaphysis, metaphysis, or physis but rather a mesenchymal network or membrane attracts osteoblasts, which form osteoid. Membranous bones include the mandible, pelvis, scapula, base of the skull, the clavicles, and the sternum. There are equivalent diaphyseal, metaphyseal, and epiphyseal areas, however, which behave very similarly to their counterparts in the appendicular skeleton.

Unique Features

The skeleton of children is quite different from that of adults. The child's bones are obviously still growing, developing, and modeling; therefore many ossification centers are constantly appearing and fusing with the main skeleton (Fig. 7.2). Because these ossification centers may appear fragmented and may ossify in a multicentric fashion, they can easily simulate chip fractures. One should therefore obtain comparison views if there is any question.

Injuries to the metaphyseal region, physis, and epiphysis are much more damaging in children than in adults because the growth plate is disturbed. These are called Salter-Harris fractures and carry a prognostic rating according to the severity of the growth plate injury (I–V, with V being the worst; Fig. 7.3). Severe length discrepancies and other growth disturbances can occur from fractures in these regions.

Another unique difference between the child's and the adult's skeleton is the low incidence of dislocations (complete disruption of the joints with loss of contact between articulating surfaces) of otherwise normal joints. Because children's capsular and ligamentous structures are two to five times stronger than the weakest part of the growth plate, the growth plate fractures first, and dislocation occurs less frequently.

The growing bones of children are also unique in that they are more "plastic" and more likely to bend before they fracture (Fig. 7.4). Because of this resiliency children are more likely to have "incomplete fractures," two of which have characteristic names – the *greenstick* fracture and the *torus* fracture. The greenstick fracture is characterized by a bowed long bone

Fig. 7.2 A–C. The normal elbow at different stages of development. Note the appearance of the various ossification centers as the child matures

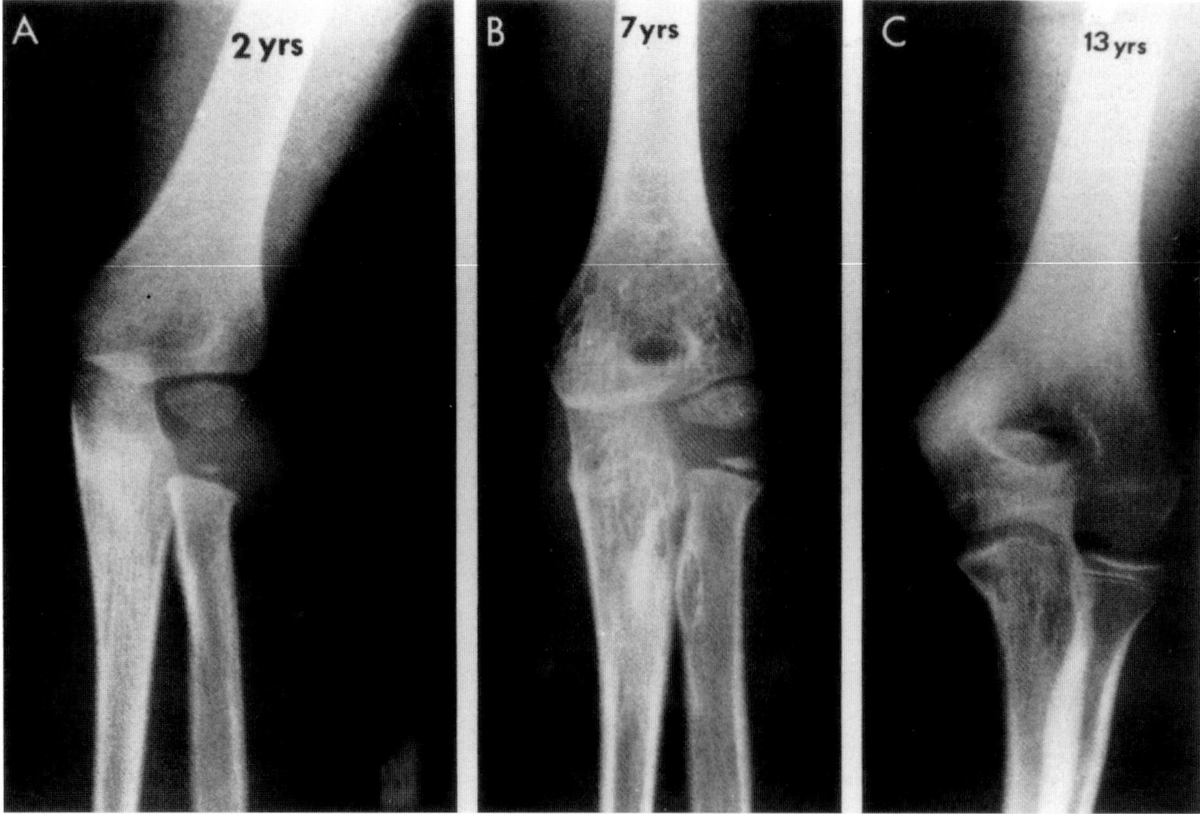

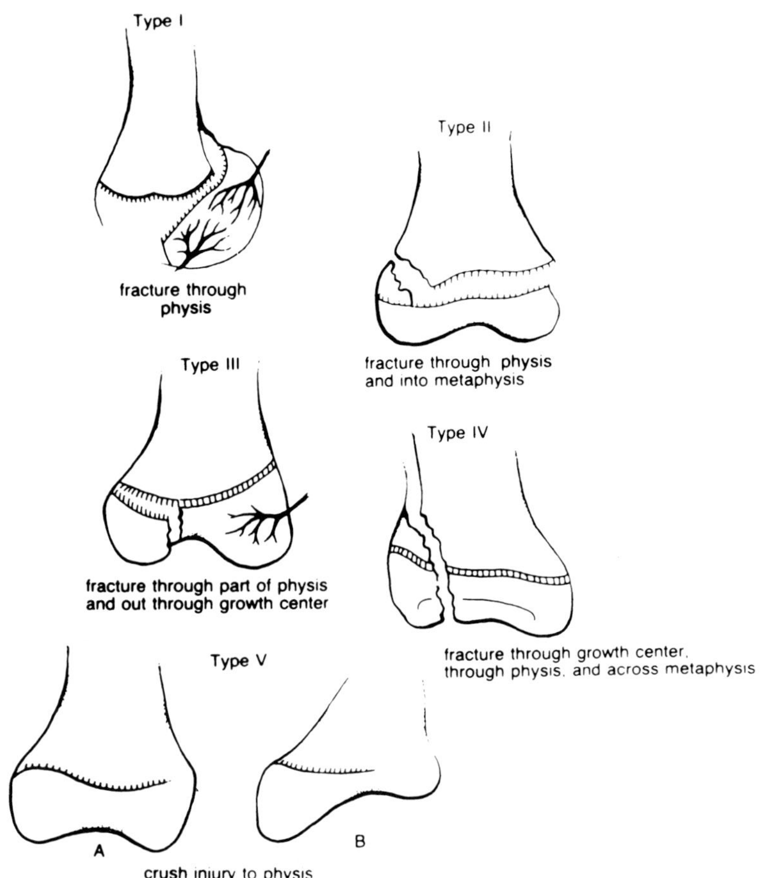

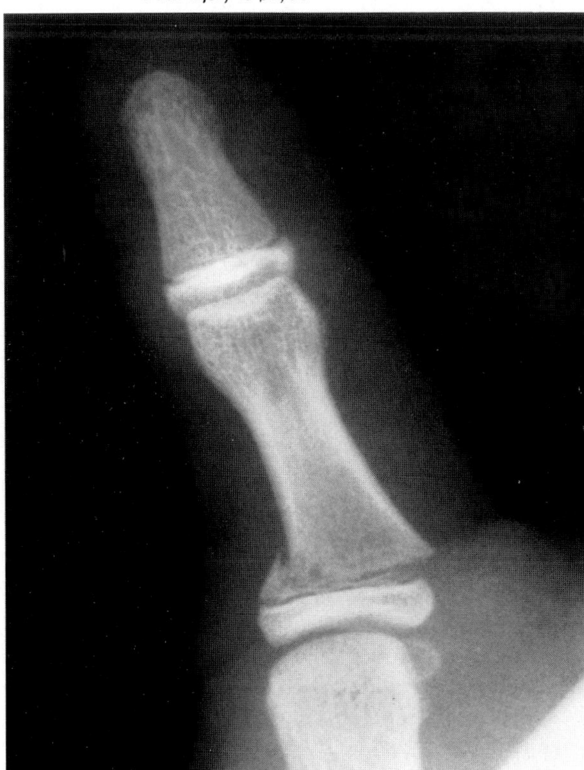

Fig. 7.3. a Salter-Harris classification of fractures involving the growth plate. Prognosis depends on integrity of the blood supply and fracture type. Salter IV and V have a worse prognosis than I, II, and III. **b** Salter II fracture of the proximal phalanx of the thumb. The fracture involves the metaphysis and physis

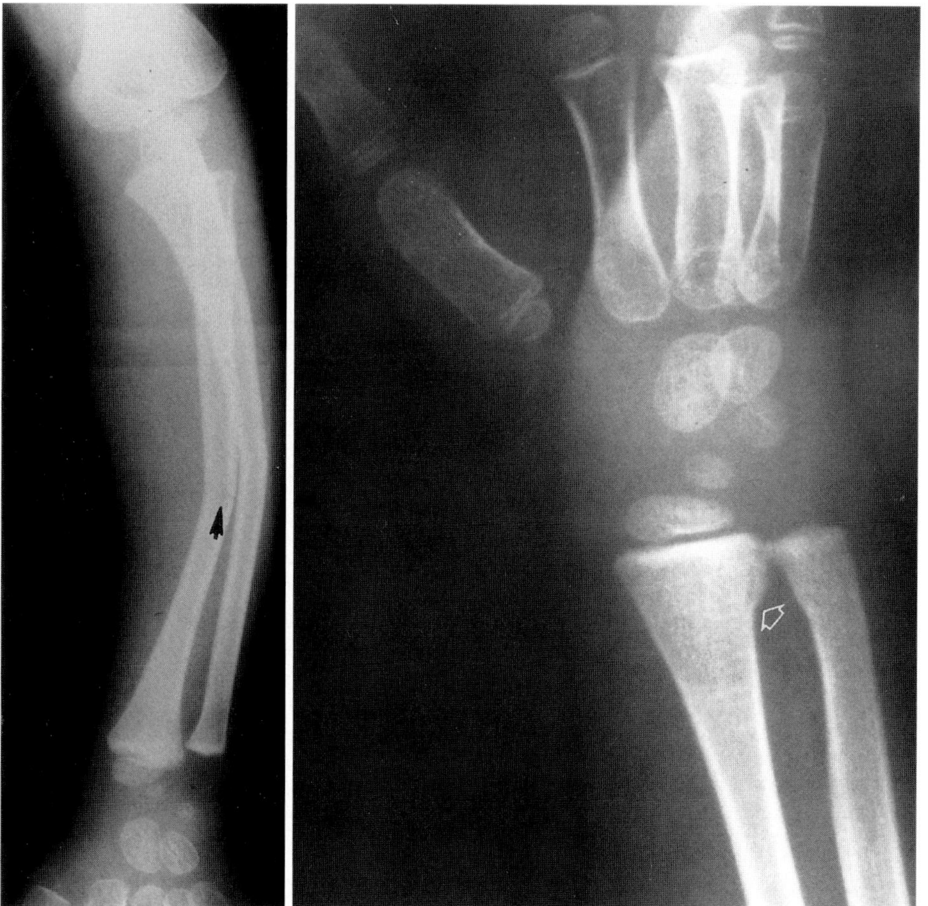

Fig. 7.4. a Greenstick fracture. The fracture appears to extend halfway through the diaphysis (*arrow*). **b** Torus fracture. Note the buckling at the medial aspect of the distal radius (*arrow*)

with a break on the convex surface but apparent cortical continuity on the concave surface. In the torus fracture there is buckling on one side of the cortex (see Fig. 7.4). In both of these fractures, however, microscopic examination shows nondisplaced fractures of osteoid across the bone.

In children the periosteum is constantly growing. Therefore it is less firmly attached to the diaphysis, or shaft, of the long bone and is more likely to tear and thus be elevated by trauma and hematoma formation. The periosteum reacts by laying down a thick layer of new bone. In contrast, the periosteum at the ends of the long bones is not loosely attached but rather firmly adherent to the metaphyseal regions. Twisting injuries here cause avulsion of a piece of bone from the metaphysis. This type of "bucket-handle" injury or avulsion "corner fracture" is commonly found in cases of child abuse (Fig. 7.5; discussed below).

Another difference between the adult and child is the ability to estimate bone maturation in those in the pediatric age range. This is done by comparing radiographs of the wrists and hands with those in an atlas by Greulich and Pyle [1].

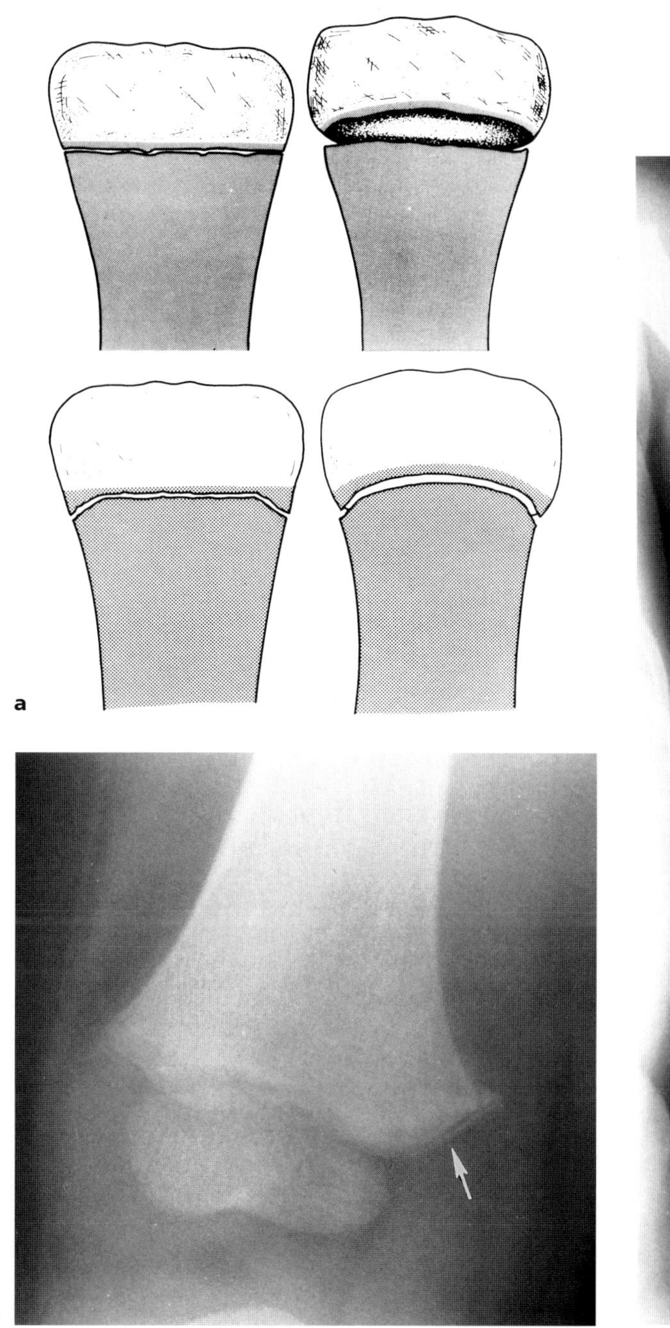

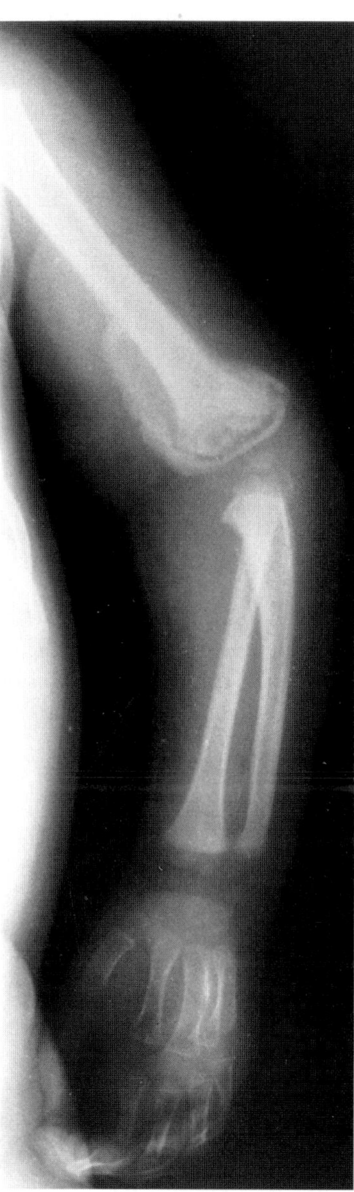

Fig. 7.5 a–c. Bucket handle fractures. **a** Drawings of a metaphyseal fracture as it appears with various radiographic projections and distractions. **b** Bucket-handle fracture of distal femur. A thin avulsion of bone at the femoral metaphysis (*arrow*) resembles the resting handle of a bucket. This fracture is commonly seen in the battered child syndrome. **c** Another child with profuse periosteal reaction about distal left humerus. This defines the "bucket-handle" lesion. Note bucket-handle fracture of olecranon

The General Approach to the Skeletal Plain Film

Before diagnosing specific bony abnormalities it is important to evaluate the film as a whole. Is the film overexposed? This can be judged by looking at the soft tissues and seeing whether they are "burnt out" or clearly visible. If they are not clearly visible, the film is overexposed. If the bones are so light that the trabecular pattern is indistinct or invisible, the film is underexposed. The overexposed film can sometimes be salvaged by viewing it in front of a high-intensity illuminator. The underexposed film is ideal for examining soft tissues but not for much else.

It is also important to look at any bony abnormality in two or more views. Fractures are easily missed if one relies on only a single view of the area. Comparison views are frequently necessary.

We use the ABCS system [2] to evaluate the bones: A = alignment, B = bone size, shape, texture, mineralization, and maturation, C = cartilage and joint space, S = soft tissue. Below we discuss the components of this system in reverse order.

Soft Tissues (Including "Fat Pads"). As in other areas of the body, the soft tissues give clues to the site and kind of injury (Table 7.1, Fig. 7.6). See the section on imaging the soft tissues and cartilage, below.

Cartilage and Joint Space. Remember, one does not see the joint space alone on plain films – rather the noncalcified articular cartilage and joint space (Fig. 7.7). Since only a small portion of this region is joint space, any narrowing may well be significant. The "joint space" should be symmetric and smooth without any calcifications or disruptions (see Fig. 7.7). The cartilage and joint space are superbly visualized by MR (see below).

Bone Size, Shape, Texture, Mineralization, and Maturation. The configuration of the bone and its special relationship helps determine the presence of fractures, dislocations, or congenital anomalies. Many normal and abnormal findings can be detected by looking at the bone surface – the cortex. Periosteal reaction, with the exception of so-called physiological appositional new bone found symmetrically in infants 2–6 months of age (see below), should be regarded as abnormal. Remember, periosteum is *normally not visible*. It is seen only when it has been stimulated to lay down new bone, or the bone beneath it has been resorbed. With an osteomyelitic process one can see cortical destruction along with reparative periosteal new bone (Fig. 7.8).

▶ *Reed's Rule No. 14:* The periosteum is normally not seen.

Next we look at the texture of the bone with its normally uniform trabecular pattern and uniform mineralization. We diagnose metastatic disease and infection by the permeative destructive nature of bone involvement (Fig. 7.9). These lesions do not have well-defined margins. At this time we can also detect metabolic disorders such as rickets and scurvy (Fig. 7.10). The medullary cavity is another important component to evaluate. The major component of the medullary cavity – the bone marrow – is not seen on plain films but is seen extraordinarily well on MR (see below). Bone maturation (see above) becomes important when suspecting certain diseases such as hypothyroidism, where the bone age is markedly decreased.

Table 7.1. Abnormalities of soft tissue (modified from [7])

What to look for	Disease
Soft tissue swelling	Most likely site of bone abnormality, hemorrhage, traumatic edema, inflammation, neoplastic abnormality
"Fat-pad" elevation	Fluid within a joint displacing the periarticular fat
Muscle wasting	Disuse, neuromuscular abnormality, chronic disease of any etiology requiring lots of bed rest
Calcifications	Old trauma; hemangiomas; metabolic, parasitic, or connective tissue disorders (dermatomyositis, scleroderma)
Opaque foreign bodies	Glass (even nonleaded glass) is often visible on a radiograph
Gas in tissue planes	Penetrating trauma, infection by gas-forming bacteria
Adjacent surprises	Unsuspected renal or appendiceal calculi, especially on lumbar spine films

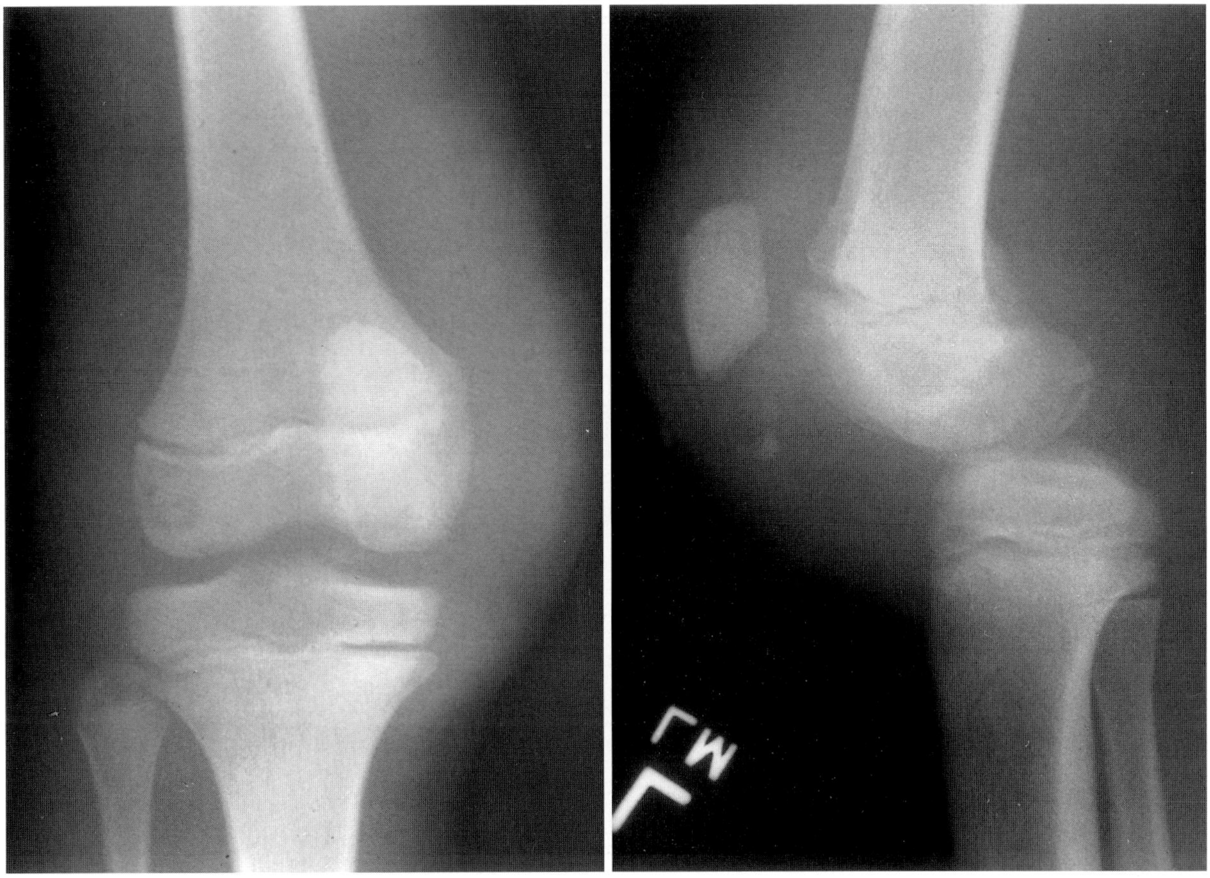

Fig. 7.6 a, b. Soft tissue swelling and fracture. **a** Frontal radiograph of the knee shows the soft tissue swelling of the knee. **b** Lateral radiograph shows fragmentation of the patella and fracture of the epiphysis. This child has insensitivity to pain and ambulated on this fractured distal femur and patella

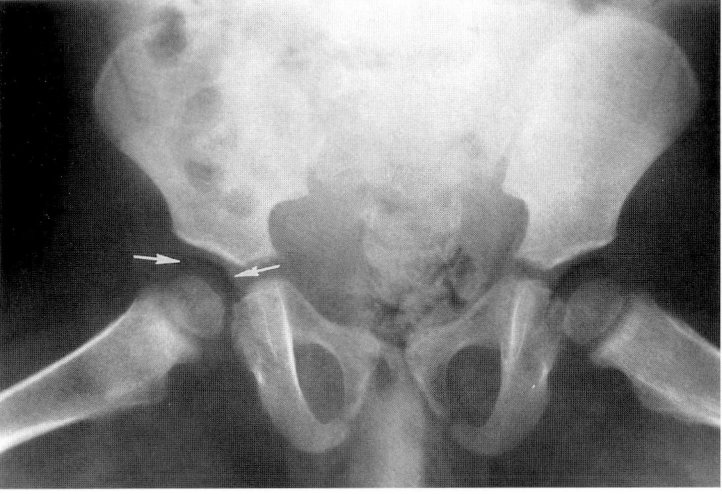

Fig. 7.7. Vacuum phenomenon. A lucent (*black*) line outlines the cartilaginous head of the femur (*arrows*). This lucency, often seen in the large joints of children, is caused by pulling, resulting in a vacuum in the joint that allows nitrogen to enter and outline the articular cartilage of the bone

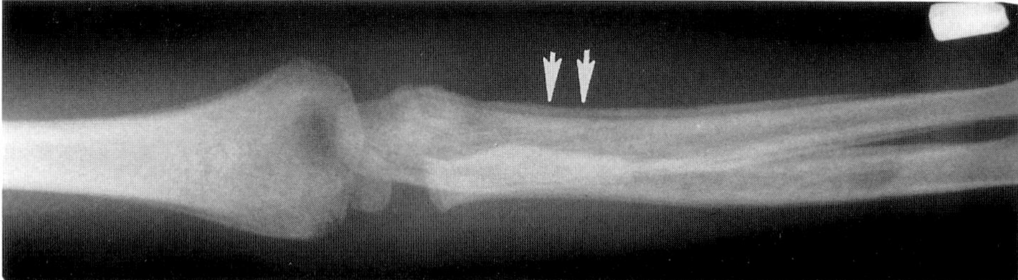

Fig. 7.8. Osteomyelitis. The ulna, radius, and humerus all exhibit a smooth periosteal reaction (*arrows*). The radius has a lytic defect at its distal position. This child has sickle cell disease with multifocal osteomyelitis

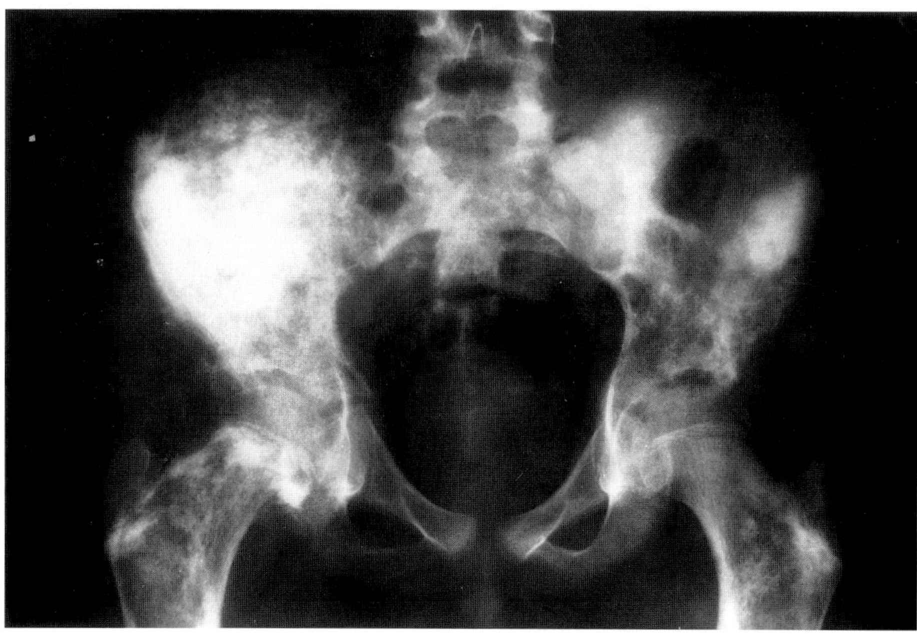

Fig. 7.9. Metastasis. Careful attention to the texture of the bone shows areas of lucency (*black*) and sclerosis (*white*). These correspond to lytic and blastic lesions caused by a medulloblastoma that metastasized to bone. While lytic metastases are commonly seen, blastic ones are quite infrequent

Alignment of Bones. Disruption of bone cortex and articular surfaces is easy to spot when you look for it!

▶ *Reed's Rule No. 15:* When viewing an extremity, try to imagine the appearance of the patient. An excellent example is bowed legs or knock knees.

In order to make an intelligent decision about the radiograph of a child's bones the radiologist must know a few important clinical facts, such as the patient's age, sex, race, prior treatment, and whether this is a generalized or local bone disturbance.

Age. As discussed in the work-up of a child with an abdominal mass, the occurrence of lesions at different ages helps to form the differential diagnosis. For example, a 6-year-old is more likely to have aseptic necrosis of the capital femoral epiphysis (Legg-Calvé-Perthe disease), while hip disease in a teenager is often a slipped capital femoral epiphysis.

Sex. Hemophilia affects males; therefore it follows that arthropathy and bone changes are found only in males.

Race. Sickle cell anemia, Gaucher's disease, and thalassemia are important considerations in different racial and ethnic backgrounds – sickle cell disease in blacks, Gaucher's disease in Jewish children, and thalassemia in children of Mediterranean ancestry.

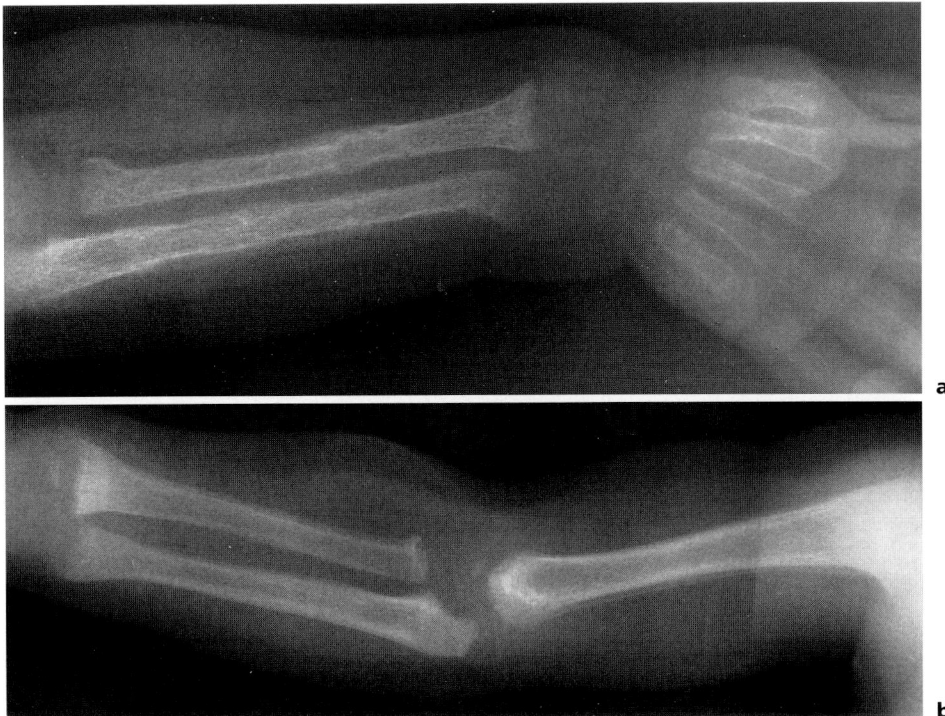

Fig. 7.10 a, b. Rickets. a In a young child the bones are demineralized and fractured. The distal radial-ulnar metaphysis are indistinct, frayed, and cupped. b In an older child, note how far the distal epiphysis is from the metaphysis

Prior Treatment. It is important for the radiologist to know whether the lesion has already been partially treated since it may display a much different roentgenographic appearance in the treated state. For example, a healing or treated bone cyst appears much different than the untreated variety.

Generalized or Local Disease. Finally, the radiologist must know whether this is the only bone involved, or whether the disease affects multiple bones. Histiocytosis, fibrous dysplasia, and metastases are systemic bone diseases, while simple bone cysts and Brodie's abscess are most commonly isolated focal disorders (see Fig. 7.9). Therefore, a skeletal survey or bone scan frequently is helpful. After plain films of the bones, CT and MR are often necessary. CT is excellent for bone alignment after trauma because it allows for visualization in the axial or coronal plane and detects bone or calcium in joint spaces. However, cartilage is imaged poorly. MR, on the other hand, images cortical bone poorly but is superb for bone marrow, ligaments, tendons, cartilage, and muscles. MR is frequently used to evaluate sports injuries and is the procedure of choice prior to surgery.

Common Pediatric Problems

Trauma

Since trauma is the most frequent indication for skeletal examinations, it is important to know the normal variants that may appear (see Fig. 7.2). An excellent source of normal variants is found in the books of Keats [3] and Kohler [4]. It is important to compare both sides when one is in doubt about the presence of a fracture (Fig. 7.11).

Let us start by looking at the fetus, which is rarely traumatized because it is in a protected environment – an amniotic fluid "water bath." Fractures, however, may occur in congenital diseases such as osteogenesis imperfecta. This disease is characterized by multiple partial and complete fractures in many bones (Fig. 7.12).

During difficult deliveries, such as breech presentations, fractures may be sustained; the most common ones involve the clavicles and skull. Since the infant is not very mobile during the first year of life, most injuries and fractures are secondary to various kinds of accidents. Particular findings, however, lead the radiologist to suspect child abuse – the battered child syndrome. These include multiple fractures in different stages of healing (indicating multiple episodes of inflicted injury), metaphyseal corner ("bucket-handle")

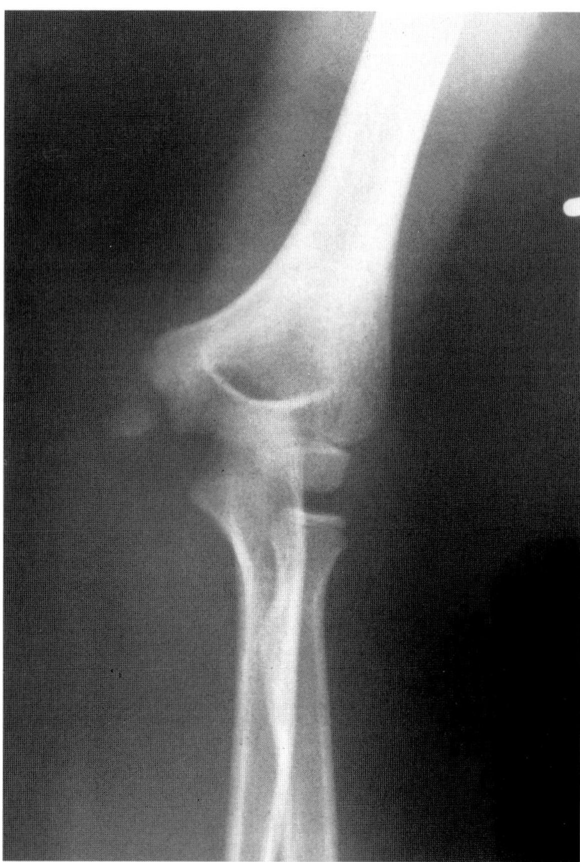

Fig. 7.11. Do you see the abnormality? (See "Appendix 2") Compare this elbow with those in Fig. 7.2

Fig. 7.12. Osteogenesis imperfecta. This newborn (the umbilical clamp is still in place) shows bowed and fractured lower extremities. Note the "crinkling" of the left femur. These fractures occurred in utero and resulted from unusually fragile bones due to a congenital defect in collagen architecture ▼

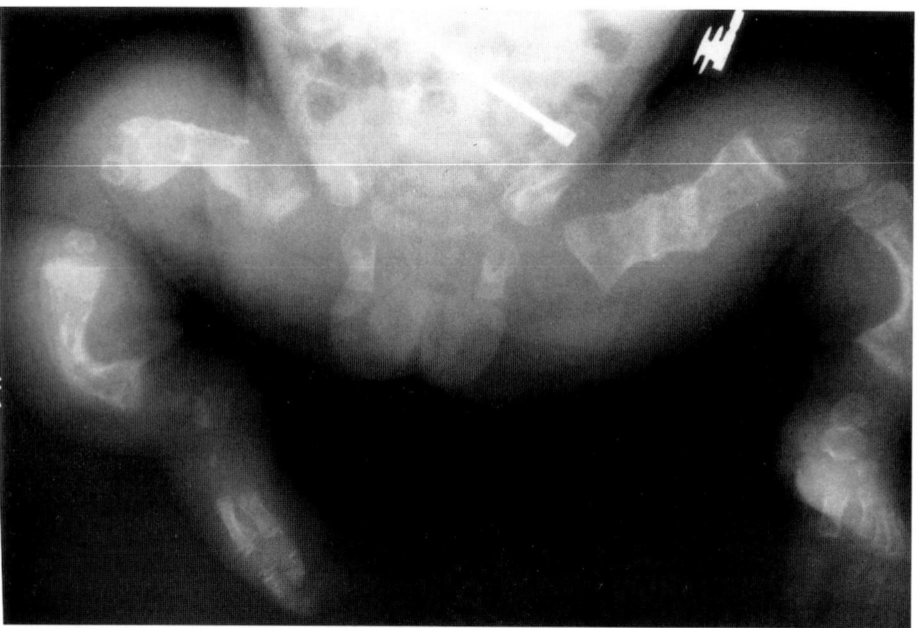

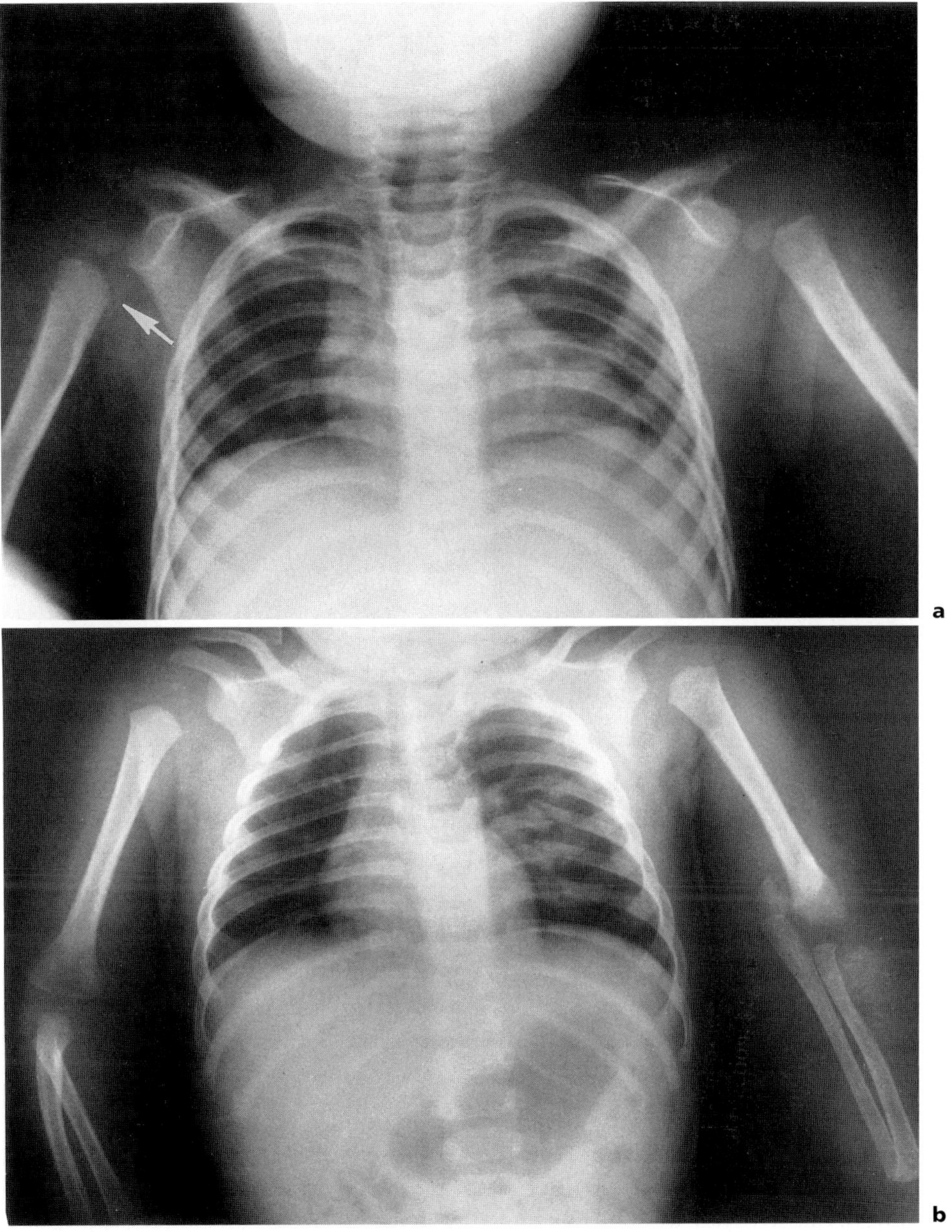

Fig. 7.13. **a** A bucket-handle fracture of the proximal right humerus (see Fig. 7.5). **b** Can you find all the abnormalities in this battered child? (see "Appendix 2")

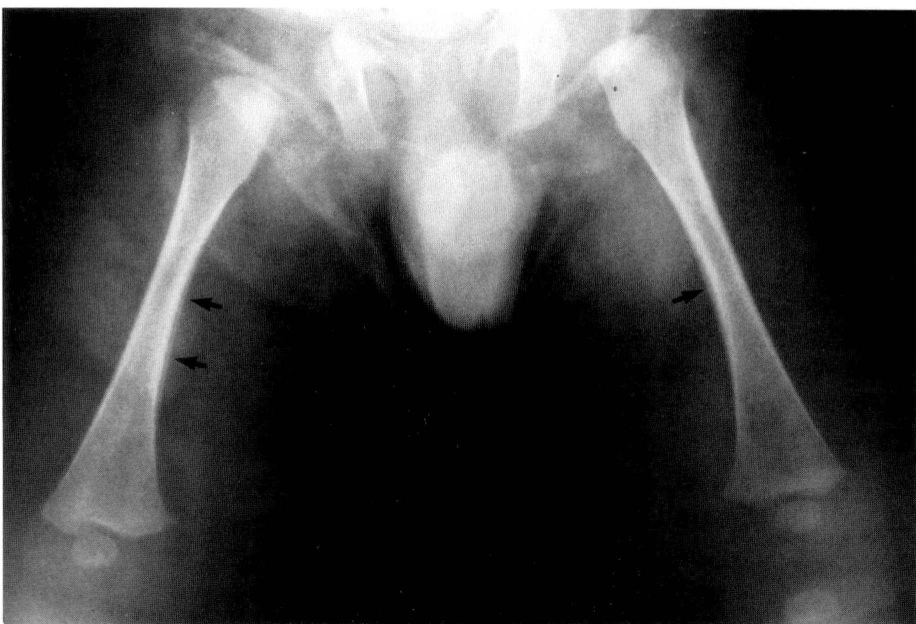

Fig. 7.14. Appositional new bone formation. This frontal view of a 2-month-old child shows what could be mistaken for pathological periosteal reaction on medial aspects of both the femurs (*arrows*). This normal variant can be present up to 6 months of age and reflects rapid bone growth rather than a disease state

Fig. 7.15 a–d. "Nursemaid" or "supermarket" elbow. **a, b** ▶ Frontal and lateral elbow films with a line drawn through the shaft of the radius on the lateral shows that the radius does not articulate with the capitelum (*arrowhead*). This dislocation is caused by a sharp pulling motion, caused in the old days by a nursemaid and in more modern times by a parent or guardian pulling a child. It often occurs in the supermarket, hence the name. **c, d** Normal realignment

fractures (Figs. 7.5, 7.13) and, particularly, posterior rib fractures (Fig. 7.13).

One must not, however, confuse the normal appositional new bone formation in infants from 2 to 6 months of age with pathological periosteal elevation. Rather, this is, as previously stated, normal periosteal bone deposition. It is bilaterally symmetric and found in the humeri, femora, and tibiae and extends to the metaphysis but no further. These are not fractures, nor do they denote any trauma (Fig. 7.14).

When it is necessary to determine the age of a fracture, remember: the younger the child, the faster the healing. In all children, however, the initial reparative process, periosteal reaction, begins 7–14 days after the original injury.

During the reading of children's radiographs we have found it useful to keep in mind the following "trauma tips" - factors unique to pediatrics:

- The clavicle is prone to greenstick fractures, which may be hard to visualize. One must take films in at least three views to make sure the child does not have a fracture.
- The elbow has so many secondary ossification centers that it is frequently necessary to view the opposite elbow for comparison.
- The *supermarket elbow* usually results from a sudden pull on a child's arm, as a parent is rushing through his/her shopping. If the radius is dislocated, the child will not move the arm (Fig. 7.15). The radius must be in direct relationship to the capitelum, regardless of the position of the elbow. The fat-pad sign is an especially valuable clue in trauma (Fig. 7.16).
- Stress fractures, although unusual, may occur in the proximal tibia, usually following extreme exercise (Fig. 7.17).
- A toddler's fracture, seen in children between the ages of 9 months and 3 years, is an oblique, nondisplaced fracture of the distal tibial shaft (Fig. 7.18).
- The slipped capital femoral epiphysis is a Salter I fracture of the femoral head (Fig. 7.19). This injury is found in adolescents, and there is a significant incidence of bilaterality.
- Metaphyseal corner fractures, multiple injuries, and, particularly, posterior rib fractures, are clues to child abuse (see Fig. 7.13).

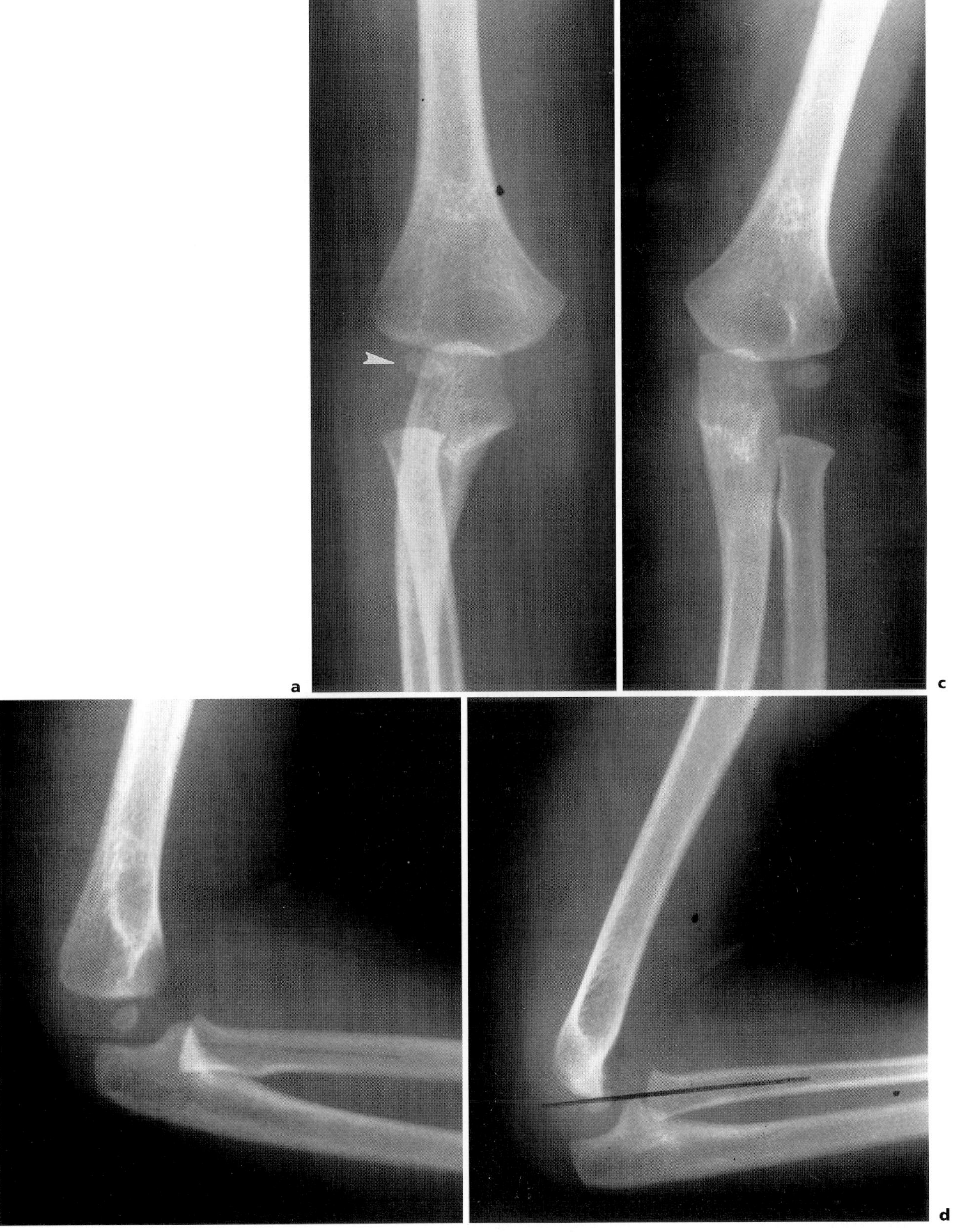
a
c
b
d

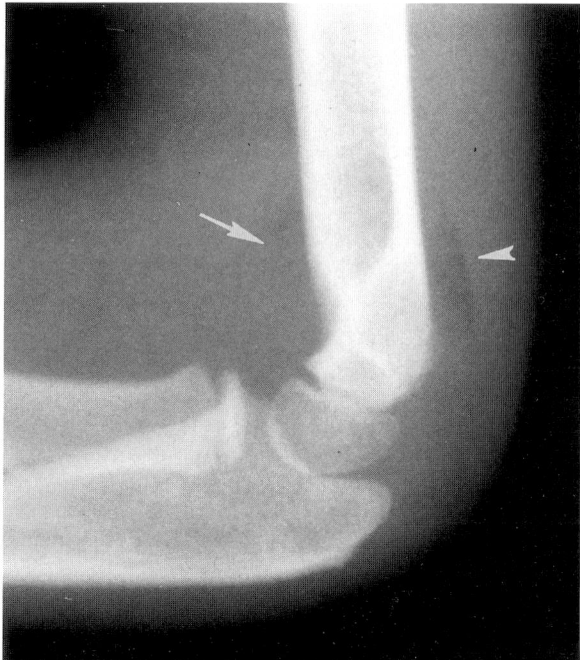

Fig. 7.16

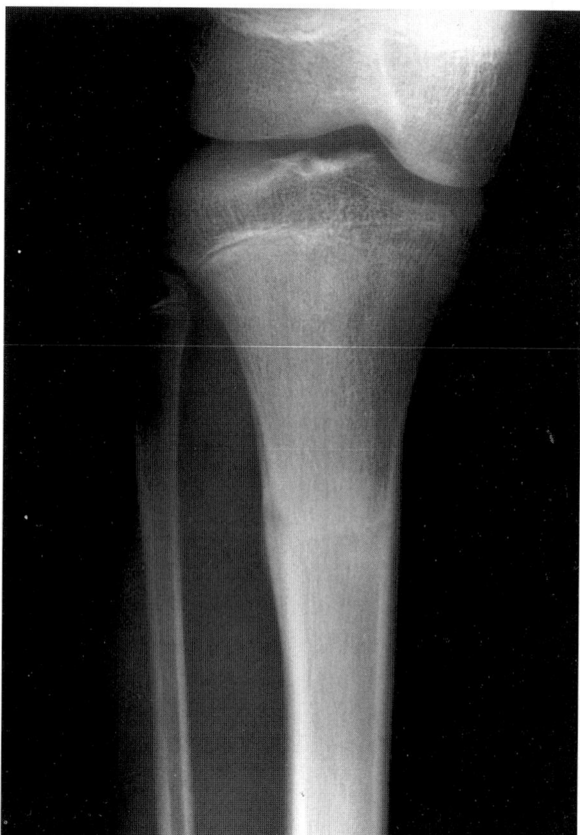

Fig. 7.17

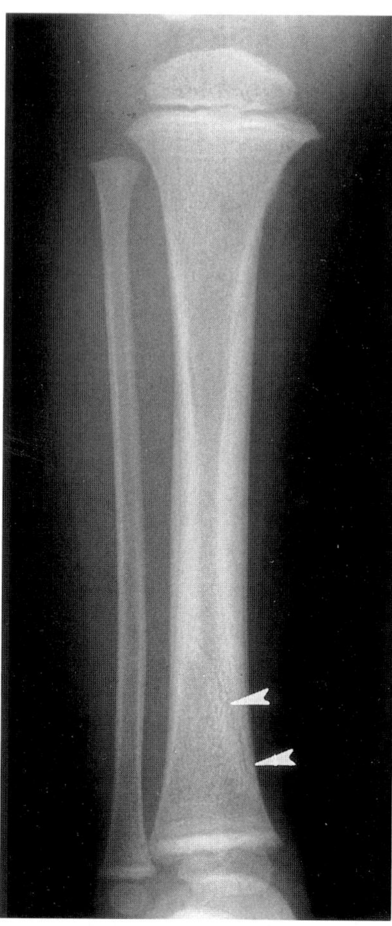

Fig. 7.18

Fig. 7.16. Positive fat pad sign. While the fracture is not visible, the posterior fat pad is displaced so that it is now visible (*arrowhead*). This is an indirect sign of trauma and reflects joint effusion. There is also a large anterior fat pad sign (*arrow*). This is less specific for a fracture

Fig. 7.17. Stress fracture. Frontal radiograph of the tibia shows a zone of sclerosis along the midshaft. There is also periosteal reaction

Fig. 7.18. Toddler's fracture. 18-month-old girl with a limp. The tibia shows a subtle oblique fracture (*arrowheads*)

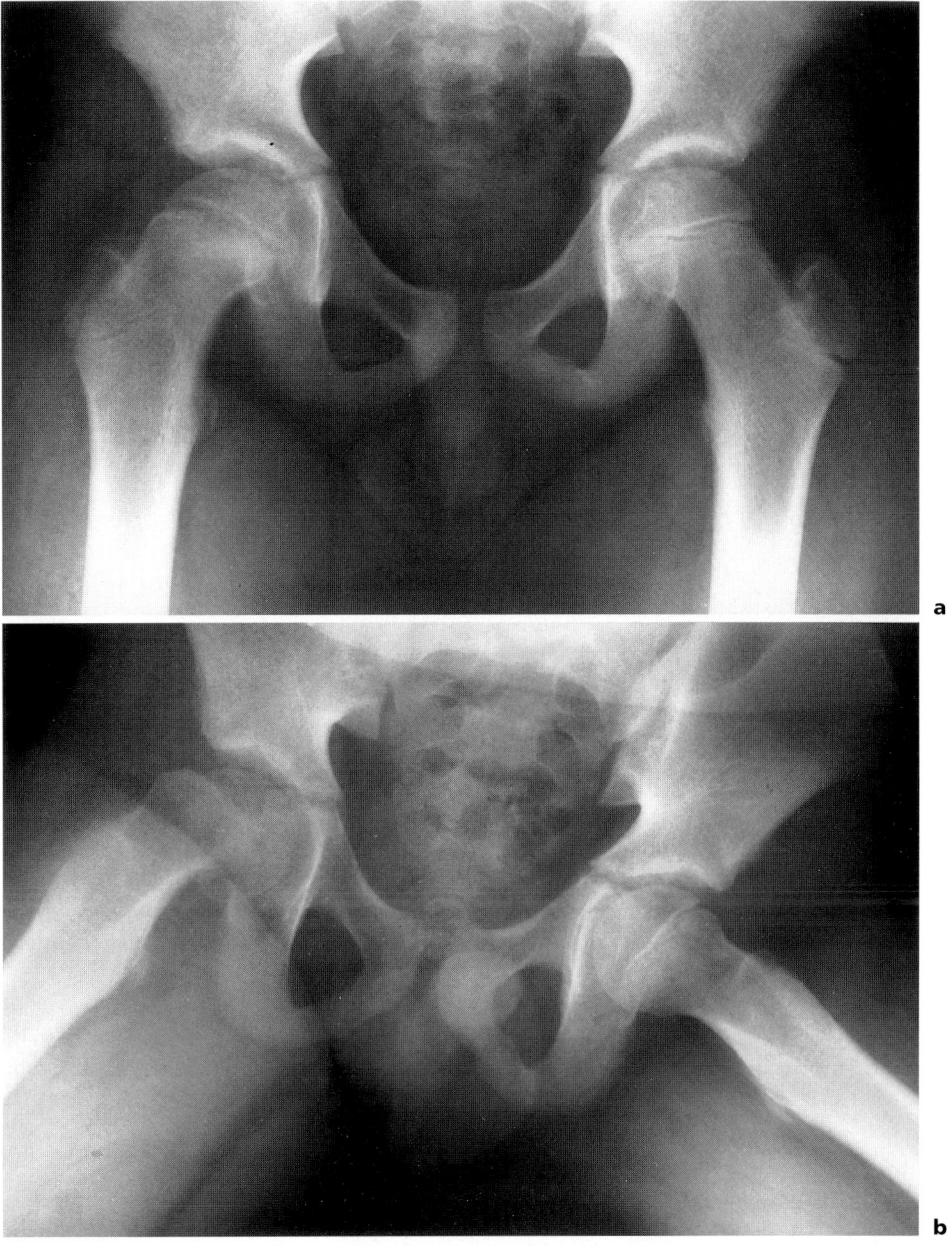

Fig. 7.19 a, b. Slipped capital femoral epiphysis. **a** This film of the hip was taken in neutral position and shows asymmetry of the physis. The right physis appears wider, and the femoral head appears medially displaced. In all suspected cases of slipped capital femoral epiphyses, a frog-leg lateral film is taken. **b** Frog-leg lateral film shows complete separation of the right femoral head. This requires surgery – hip pinning

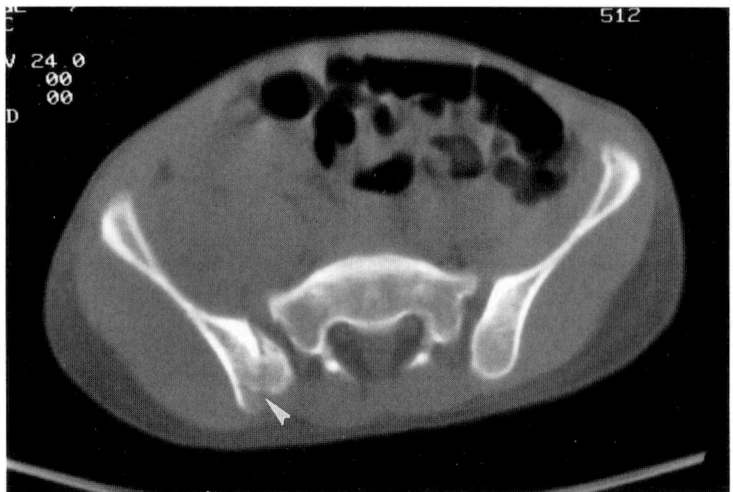

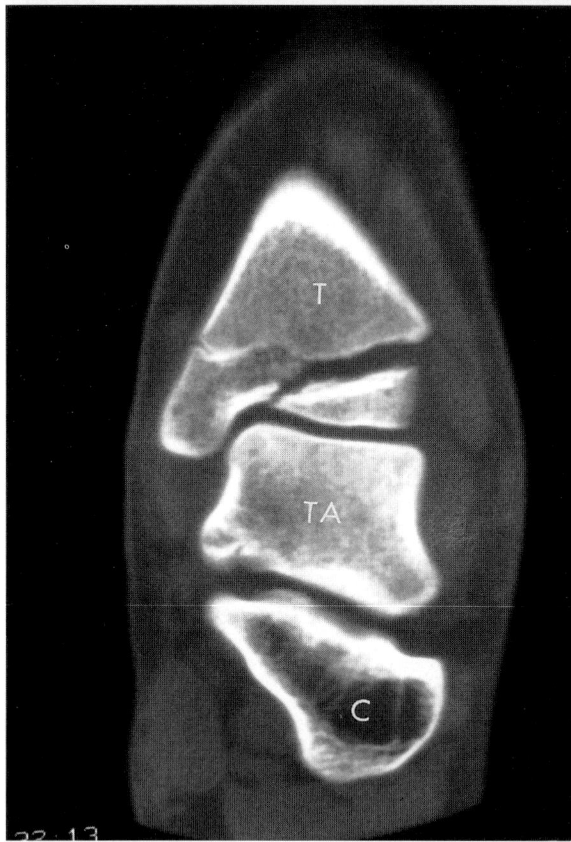

Fig. 7.20 a, b. Fracture on CT. **a** A 7-year-old with back pain and negative plain films. Axial CT section with bone windows revealed a subtle fracture of the right ileum (*arrowhead*). **b** Coronal view of an ankle fracture in another child shows the epiphyseal fragment and distortion of the ankle mortis. *T*, tibia; *TA*, talus; *C*, calcaneus

Cross-Sectional Imaging of Trauma

Suspicion of fracture on the plain film can be further investigated with CT. Certain fracture dislocations are best evaluated with CT. This is true in areas difficult to "see" with routine radiographs. These include the sacrum, pelvis, hips, and ankle. Because CT affords us cross-sectional imaging, the exact location and orientation of fractures are best imaged with this modality (Fig. 7.20).

Where does MR fit in in the work-up of skeletal trauma? MR is superb when one is interested in detecting injury to the growth plate or the formation of a cartilaginous bar crossing the growth plate (a bar may subsequently develop secondary to trauma and prevent further growth in that region; the entire bone can be deformed). MR is also indicated for osteochondritis dessicans, internal derangement of joints, and ligament and tendinous injury. This is especially true of knee injuries, where MR has revolutionized the work-up of trauma (Fig. 7.21). It is not unusual to find a low-signal lesion in the proximal tibia or distal femur which was not seen on plain film. This represents a bruise (or contusion) of bone and often can explain the patient's symptoms.

Even ultrasound has a place in the work-up of trauma. Radiopaque foreign bodies such as metal or glass are easily demonstrated by plain films. Sonography is excellent in finding and guiding the removal of nonopaque soft tissue foreign bodies. CT may also be good in this regard, although sonography is easier, quicker, has no radiation, and is less costly.

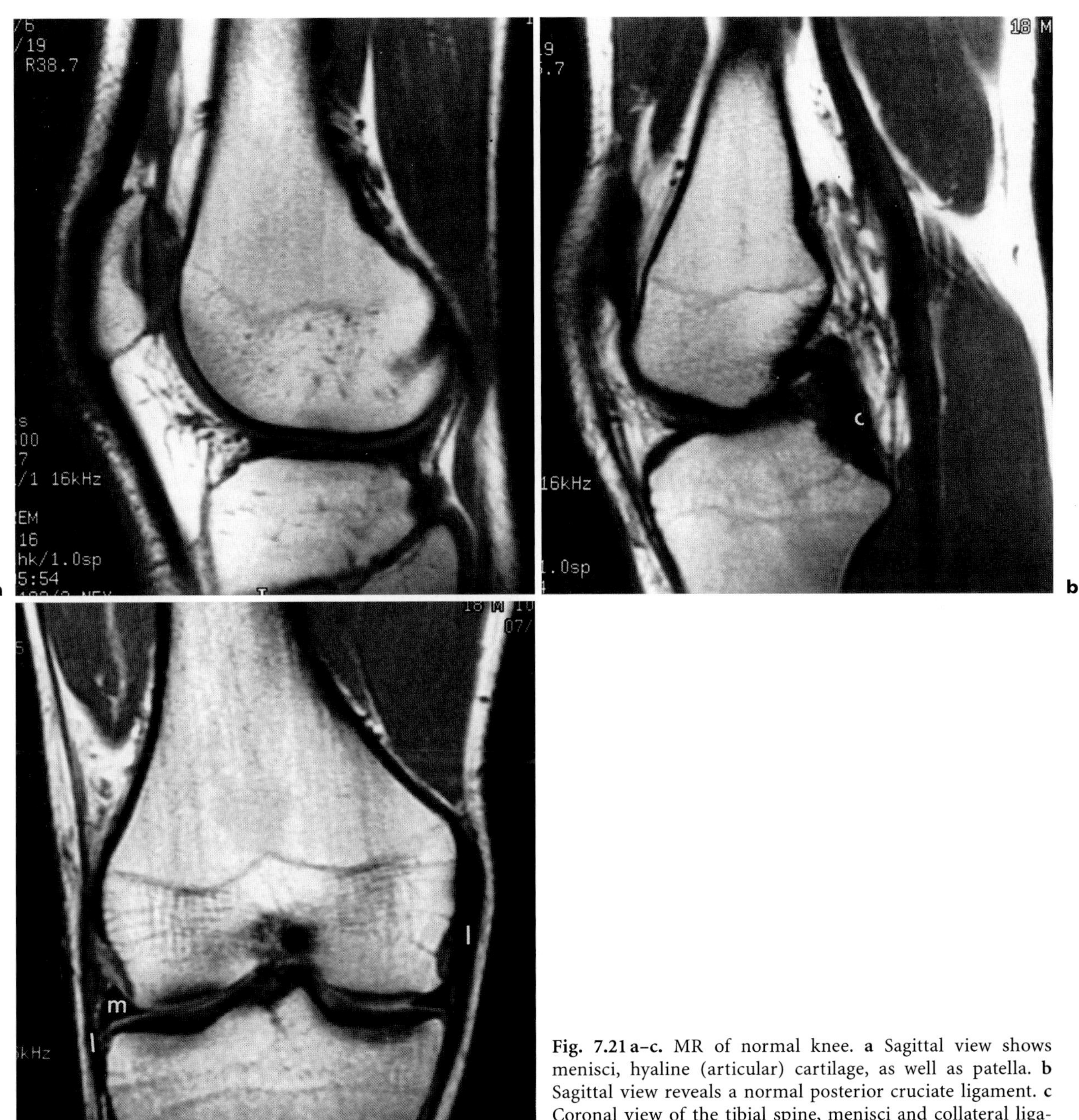

Fig. 7.21 a–c. MR of normal knee. **a** Sagittal view shows menisci, hyaline (articular) cartilage, as well as patella. **b** Sagittal view reveals a normal posterior cruciate ligament. **c** Coronal view of the tibial spine, menisci and collateral ligaments. *m*, Meniscus; *c*, cruciate ligament; *l*, collateral ligaments

Congenital Dislocation of the Hip (Developmental Dysplasia of the Hip)

Congenital dislocation of the hip (CDH) occurs in about 1 in every 1000 neonates. Girls are more prone to this disorder than boys, with the left hip involved more frequently than the right. For years, radiographic screening has been the best that we could do; instability is not diagnosed, but the persistently dislocated hip is readily seen. The hip is displaced laterally and posteriorly. On plain films lateral displacement of the femoral neck implies that the femoral head (not visible in young infants) is not covered by the acetabulum (Fig. 7.22). Currently, hip sonography is used to diagnose the unstable hip. The hip may be scanned in neutral, flexed, adducted, and abducted positions with and without stress, and pre- and posttreatment evaluations can be made. Ultrasound and at times CT may be used for evaluating the hip in plaster.

Osteomyelitis

Osteomyelitis is usually acquired via hematogenous spread of organisms to the bone. Since the greatest blood supply is in the metaphysis, this region has a predilection for osteomyelitis. A small focus of these purulent organisms causes abscess formation in the marrow with an increase in local pressure, followed by local deossification and destruction of the cortex (Fig. 7.23). The epiphysis is usually spared because of the tight adherence of the periosteum to the metaphysis. However, the shaft of the bone is readily permeable to infection as the periosteum is loosely adherent, and organisms may ascend the shaft of the bone or the medullary cavity.

Deep puncture wounds may also cause osteomyelitis in children. One of the more common organisms introduced via a puncture wound is *Pseudomonas*, while staphylococcal osteomyelitis is most common in hematogenously spread disease (see Fig. 7.8). Patients with sickle cell disease are susceptible to *Salmonella* osteomyelitis.

The clinical symptoms precede the radiographic findings by 7–14 days. For this reason a radioisotope

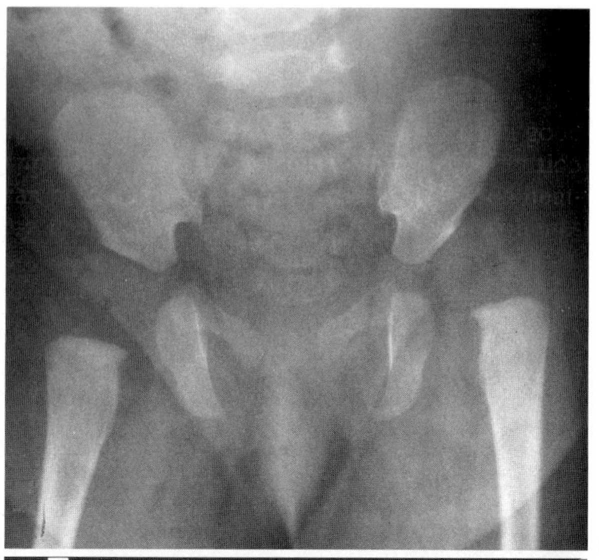

a

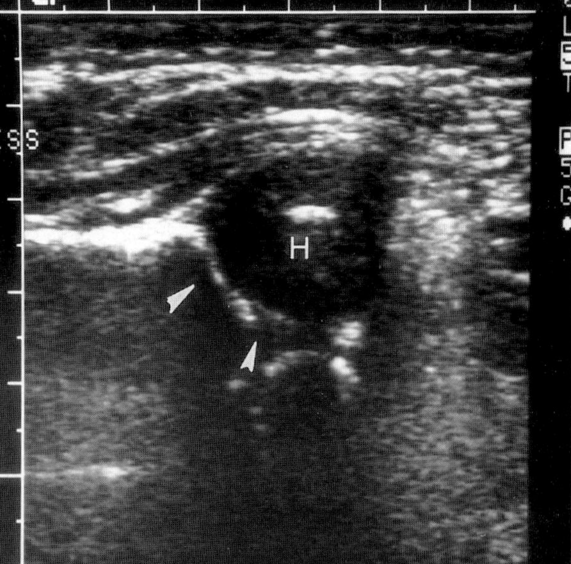

b

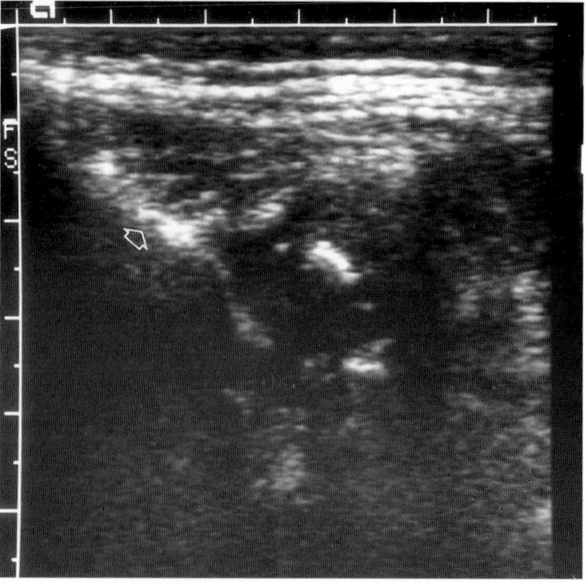

c

Fig. 7.22 a–c. Dislocated hip. **a** A 10-week-old infant with a left dislocated hip. **b** Another child with dislocation was studied with ultrasound while in a corrective harness. On the longitudinal view the partially ossified right femoral head (*H*) is seen in the acetabulum (*arrowheads*). **c** The same hip out of harness. Note that the ileum is not horizontal (*open arrow*) as in **b** and the lateral acetabulum is not seen. The hip is now dislocated

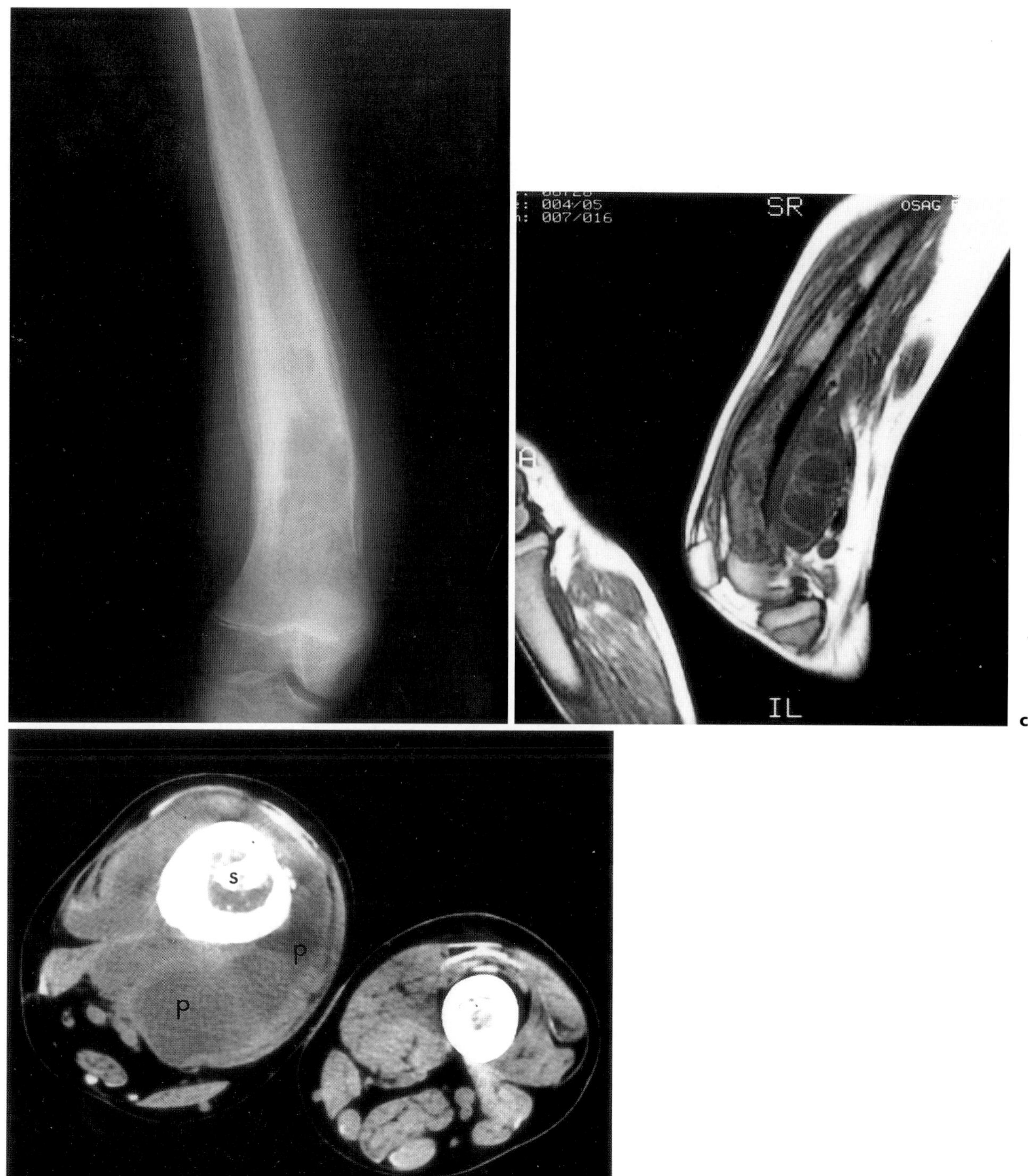

Fig. 7.23 a–c. Osteomyelitis. **a** Lateral view of the distal femur shows periosteal reaction and sclerosis (*white area*) in the diametaphysis. **b** CT of the same femur taken 1 month later. The osteomyelitis continued and now we see a sequestrum (*s*) in the center of the femur and pus (*p*) surrounding the cortex. **c** MR shows the marrow involvement and soft tissue abnormalities in exquisite detail

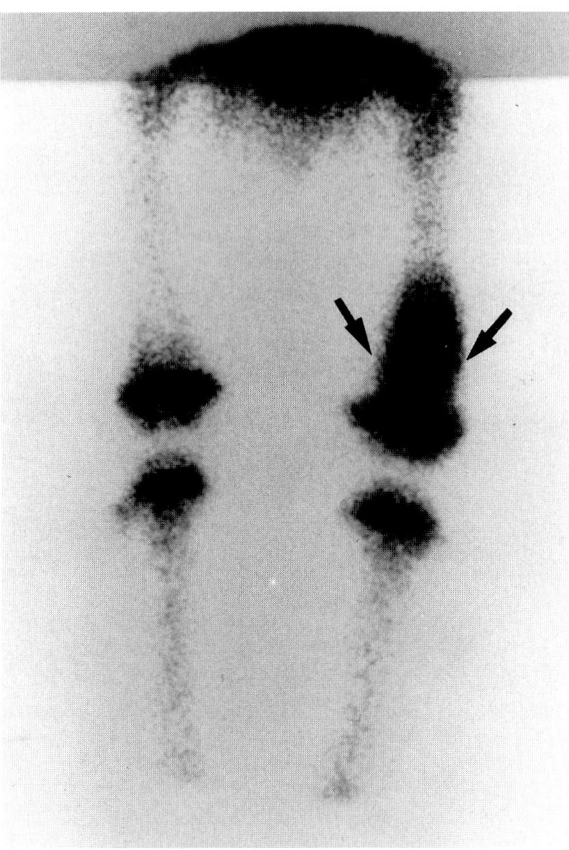

Fig. 7.24. Osteomyelitis on bone scan. Anterior view of the femurs on 2-h delayed images of a ^{99m}Tc-labeled diphosphonate bone scan reveals increased uptake in the distal left femur (*arrows*)

study is frequently more helpful in the early diagnosis of acute osteomyelitis. The proper study is a "three-phase" bone scan with ^{99m}Tc-labeled diphosphonate. The initial phase is the blood pool and the second phase is soft tissue segment. These are obtained immediately after injection. Positive results mean increased blood flow and soft tissue infection (cellulitis). The delayed scan is the third phase, and is positive in osteomyelitis and septic arthritis (Fig. 7.24).

If the diagnosis is made promptly and treatment is successful, healing usually occurs without significant growth disturbance. However, prolonged infection prior to the diagnosis or severe involvement of a joint – septic arthritis – can have long-term sequelae.

The radiographic findings of acute, healing, and chronic osteomyelitis are summarized below:

- Acute osteomyelitis (0–2 weeks)
  - Soft tissue swelling initially
  - Loss of cortical margin
  - Focal demineralization of bone
  - Faint periosteal new bone formation (7–14 days after onset)
- Healing phase (2–4 weeks)
  - Destroyed bone with irregular areas of sclerosis and lysis
  - Sequestrum – dense devascularized bone fragment within an area of pus and granulation tissue
  - Involucrum: peripheral shell of supporting bone laid down by the periosteum around the old disease
- Chronic osteomyelitis (either unusual localized osteomyelitis or improperly treated)
  - Diffuse bone production with little or no destruction
  - Occasional draining sinus or lucent area in the midst of the sclerotic bone

CT and MR have a definite role in the work-up of osteomyelitis, especially in the chronic and indolent form (Fig. 7.23). MR is especially useful in septic arthritis as it can demonstrate cartilage loss, joint effusion, synovial hypertrophy, and bone destruction. When the radiographic or scintigraphic findings are equivocal or hard to evaluate, MR is also useful. This is especially true when dealing with certain "flat" bones that are hard to visualize on plain radiographs such as the sternum, scapula, and pelvis (Fig. 7.25).

Certain children, however, are at high risk for osteomyelitis and its complications. These include neonates who have a high incidence of both β-streptococcal osteomyelitis and septic arthritis. In neonates osteomyelitis is frequently multifocal. Patients with sickle cell disease have a high incidence of *Salmonella*

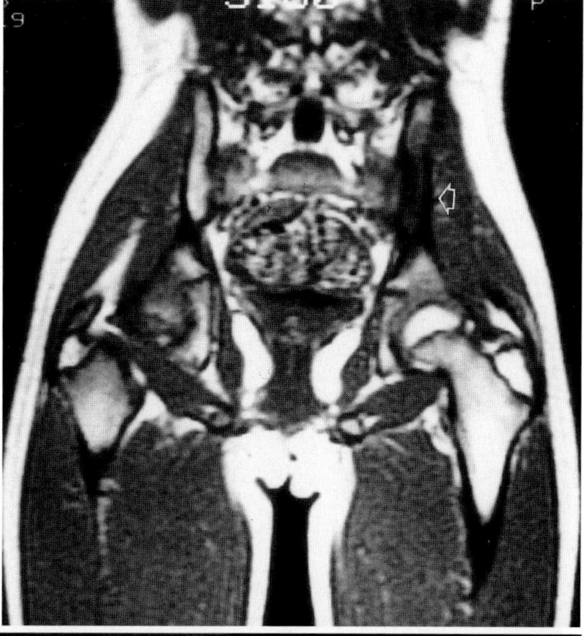

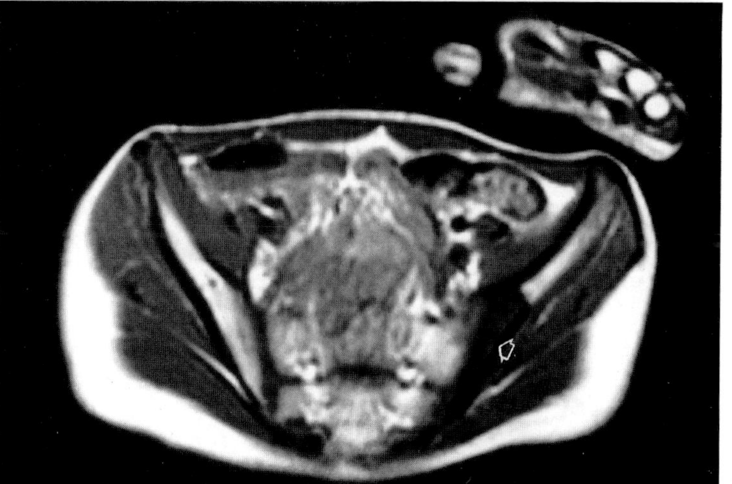

Fig. 7.25 a, b. MR of osteomyelitis. **a** Coronal T1 scan shows diminished signal in the left iliac bone (*arrow*). **b** This is confirmed in axial T1 images

osteomyelitis, which is also frequently multifocal, but the most common organism in bone infection of patients with sickle cell disease is *Staphylococcus*. Children with immune deficiencies such as chronic granulomatous disease and agammaglobulinemia are prone to multifocal osteomyelitis or osteomyelitis in unusual areas such as the iliac bones; this is frequently due to unusual organisms (Fig. 7.25).

Bone infarcts are seen in a number of disorders, including sickle cell anemia, pancreatitis, Gaucher's disease, and steroid therapy. When it is idiopathic and affects the femoral head, it is called Legg-Calvé-Perthe disease (Fig. 7.26). Plain films have never been able to differentiate infection from infarction in sickle cell disease, but in other disorders dense bone that eventually fragments is typical for infarction. MR is especially well suited for the diagnosis of infarction since it is a marrow disorder.

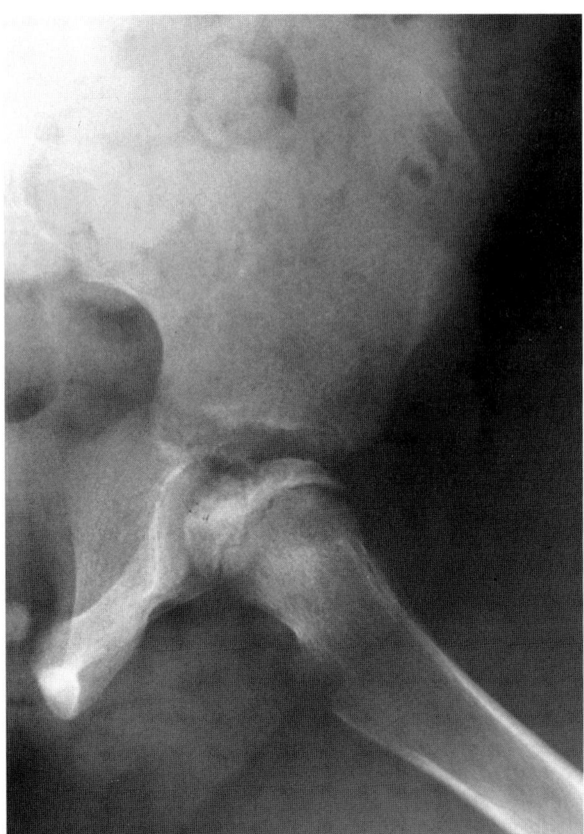

a

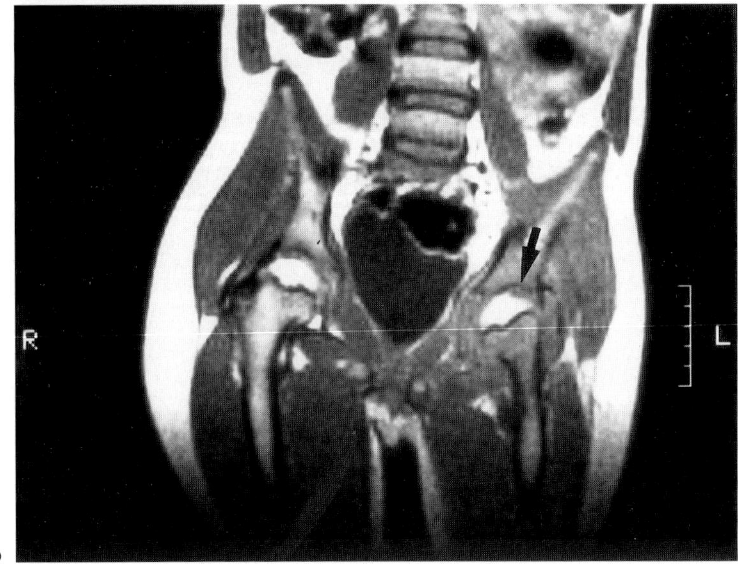

b

Fig. 7.26 a, b. Legg-Calvé-Perthe disease. **a** Frog leg view of the left hip reveals fragmentation of the capital femoral epiphysis. **b** Coronal MR shows the white (fat-filled) epiphysis except laterally where there is diminished signal (*arrow*)

Metabolic Disorders

The growing skeleton is susceptible to many nutritional deficiencies and reflects the adequacy of the homeostatic mechanisms (gastrointestinal tract, liver, kidneys) for handling calcium. Two of the more common disturbances in this category are rickets and hyperparathyroidism, which is usually secondary to chronic renal disease.

Rickets. In rickets there is a deficiency of vitamin D and, therefore, poorly mineralized osteoid tissue. The trabeculae are fuzzy and irregular and certainly not as distinct as those in normal bone. The metaphyseal regions are irregular, with cupped and frayed metaphyses (Fig. 7.10). The apparent space between the metaphysis and the ossification center is greater than normal, as there is an abundance of uncalcified cartilage. Despite all our advances, the most common cause of rickets in the world today is still nutritional vitamin D deficiency. However, in most medical centers the most common cause of "rickets" is chronic renal disease. Children with liver disease also may manifest rachitic changes.

Hyperparathyroidism. In this disorder bone resorption far exceeds bone proliferation (osteoclasis far exceeds osteoblastic activity), and as a result the bone is resorbed. Radiographically one sees subperiosteal bone resorption most often along the diaphyses of the phalanges, at the distal clavicles, and along the lamina dura of the teeth. Diffuse demineralization and focal lucent lesions (brown tumors) are other signs of this disorder (Fig. 7.27). In chronic renal disease, calcium loss through the urinary system is usually so great that the parathyroids must draw calcium into the blood system from the existing stores in bones to maintain a normal calcium-phosphorous ratio.

Lead Intoxication. Heavy metals such as lead or bismuth stimulate increased calcification of cartilage which causes increased density in the metaphyseal regions. The density is found in both large, weight-bearing bones as well as smaller ones (e.g., tibia and fibula) and in other areas where longitudinal bone growth is occurring most rapidly (Fig. 7.28). Remember: the ulna and fibula are the key bones for determining lead intoxication. The femur, humerus, and radius often have dense metaphyseal bands normally but never the ulna and fibula. The finding of "lead lines" correlates with chronicity of exposure and not with blood lead levels or acute symptoms.

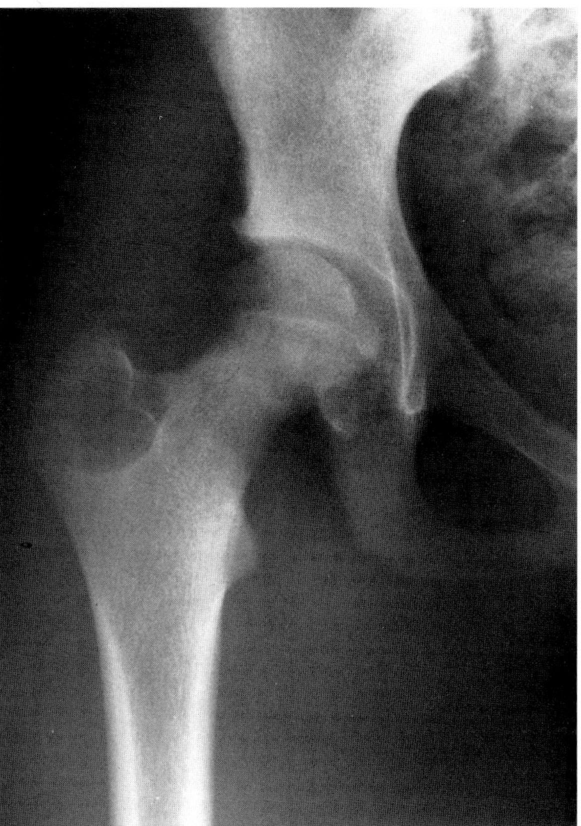

Fig. 7.27. Hyperparathyroidism. The cortical margins of the neck (both medial and lateral) of the femur are not visible due to bone resorption. (Compare to neck of femur in Fig. 7.1.) Also note the lytic lesion in the greater trochanter. This brown tumor is the result of accumulation of fibrous tissue and giant cells and has all the characteristics of a benign bone lesion. A sclerotic border and the clear zone of demarcation are evidence of its benignity

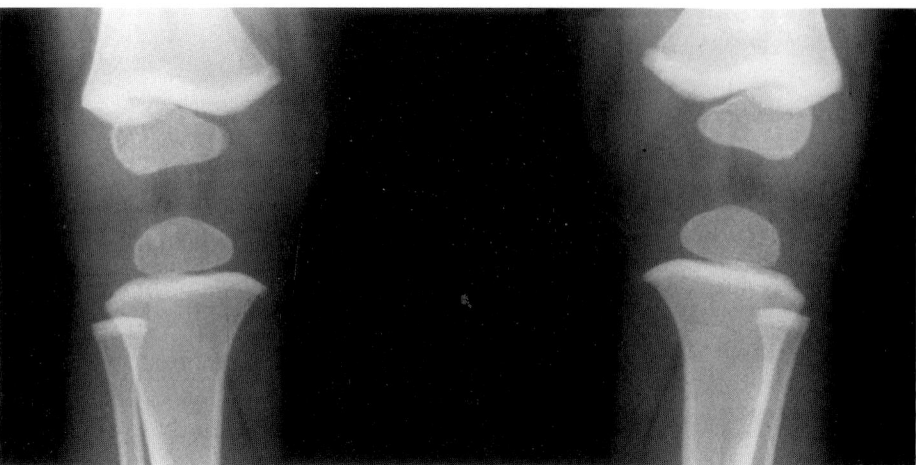

Fig. 7.28. Chronic lead intoxication. The metaphyses of all the bones, especially the fibula, are sclerotic. This is typical of heavy-metal ingestion. While the femur, tibia, and humerus often have equivocal density in the metaphyses, the ulna and fibula should not be dense at all. Consequently, any metaphyseal density noted in the latter two bones should raise the suspicion of heavy-metal intoxication

Bone Tumors

Malignant bone tumors are not common in children, but benign bone lesions are frequently seen. Some of the common benign and malignant lesions are described below.

Benign Lesions

Simple bone cyst is a lucent defect at the end of the long bone near but not touching the epiphyseal line; it is most often found in the humerus, femur, or tibia (Fig. 7.29). *Fibrous cortical defect* is a well-circumscribed, elliptical lucent lesion in the cortex at the end of a long bone, particularly the femur or tibia; the larger ones are called *nonossifying fibromas. Osteochondroma* is a protuberant growth of bone from the diaphysis that has contiguous cortical margins. *Enchondroma* is a cartilaginous, cystlike lesion often seen in the phalanges and ribs. *Osteoid osteoma* is a sclerotic lesion with a central lucent nidus. It occurs in many places, including the long bones and spine.

Malignant Lesions

Osteogenic sarcoma occurs mostly during adolescence, frequently in the long bones; this is the most common primary malignant tumor in the pediatric age group, and it is metaphyseal and bone-producing. *Ewing's sarcoma* is the second most common tumor in the pediatric age group; it is more common than osteogenic sarcoma in those under 10 years of age (Fig. 7.30). This lesion may occur in any bone in the middiaphyseal region and is permeative. There is a large, soft tissue component. It is frequently found in

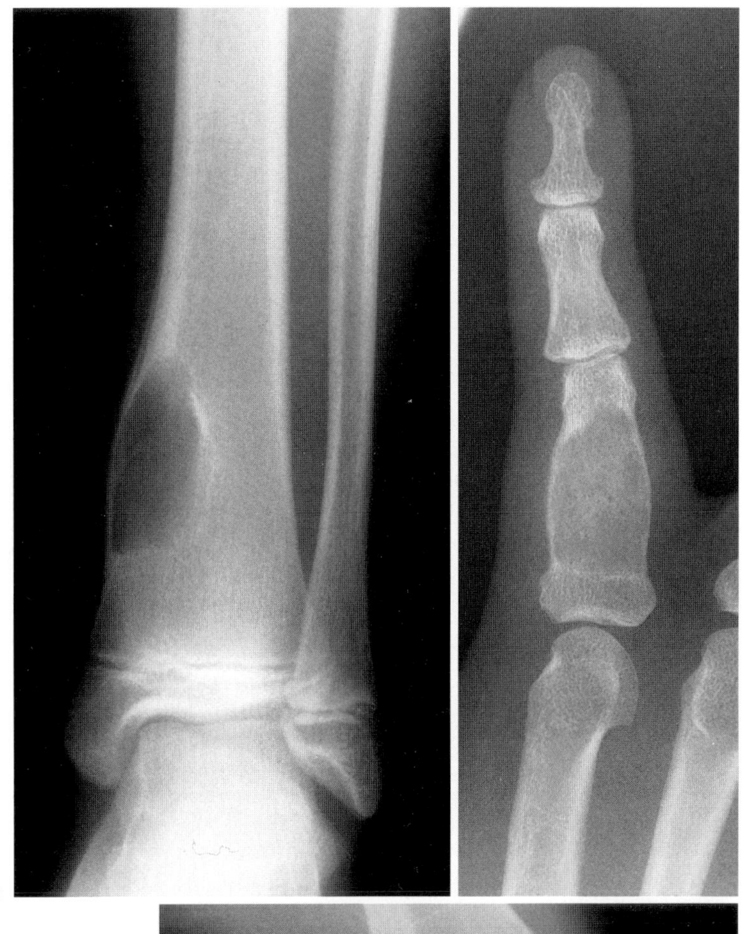

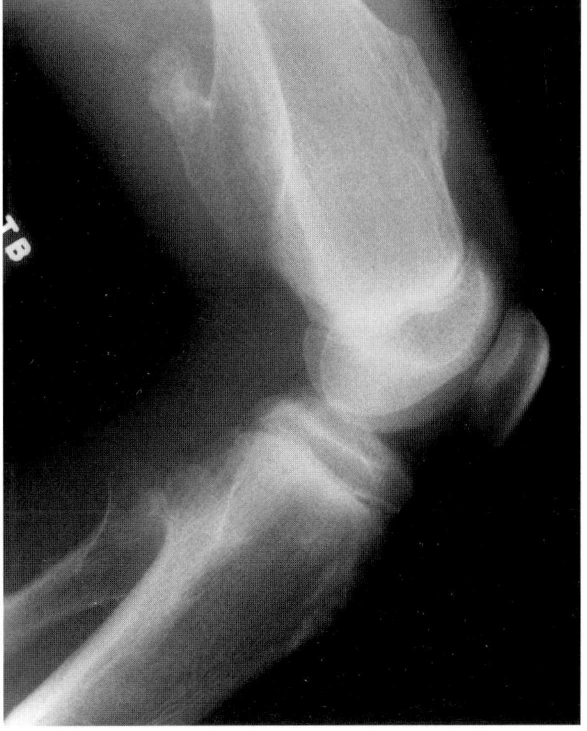

Fig. 7.29 a–c. Benign bone lesions. **a** Simple bone cyst. The distal tibial lesion is well demarcated and is of lower density. It has no septations. The lesion bows the medial cortex – somewhat unusual for a simple bone cyst and suggests that an aneurysmal bone cyst should be in the differential. **b** Multiple osteochondroma are present in the distal femur and proximal tibia and fibula. There is continuity of cortex and the lesions point away from the joint. **c** Enchondroma: A well-defined cystic lesion with very fine punctate calcifications is often found in the finger

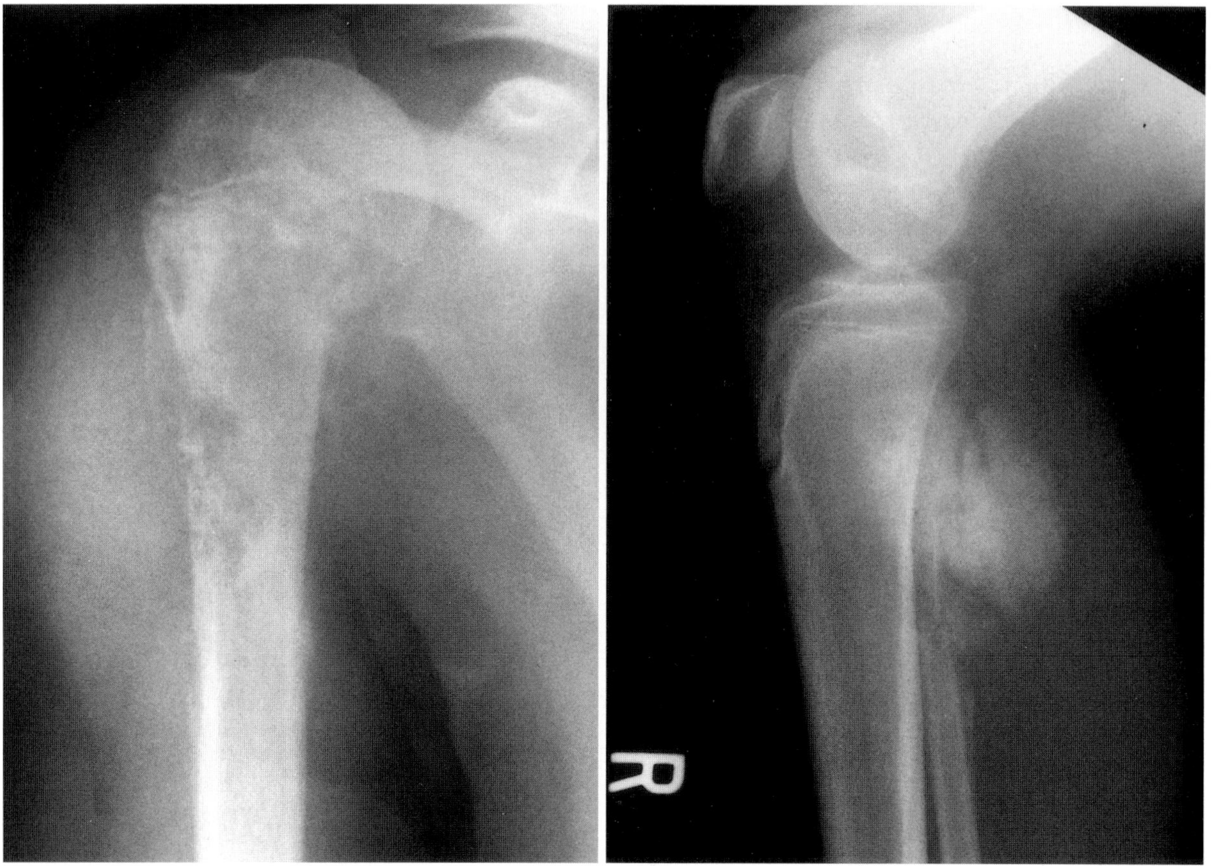

Fig. 7.30 a–e. Malignant lesions. **a** Ewing's sarcoma. This radiograph displays many of the findings of a malignant bone lesion. The disordered periosteal reaction both medially and laterally and the extensive bone destruction without a clear zone of demarcation between normal and abnormal suggest malignancy. **b** Osteogenic sarcoma. Lateral film of the proximal fibula shows dense prolific periosteal reaction and irregularity of the bony cortex. **c** Axial T2 MR of the same patient reveals the amount of soft tissue involvement (*bright signal – gray to white*) surrounding the bony cortex [*dark (black) circle*]. **d** Osteogenic sarcoma in another patient. Radiograph of the femur shows the bone formation in the soft tissues and sclerosis of the diaphysis of the femur. The cortex is indistinct. **e** Coronal T1 MR demonstrates the extent of marrow involvement (compare to other side) as well as the soft tissue component of the tumor

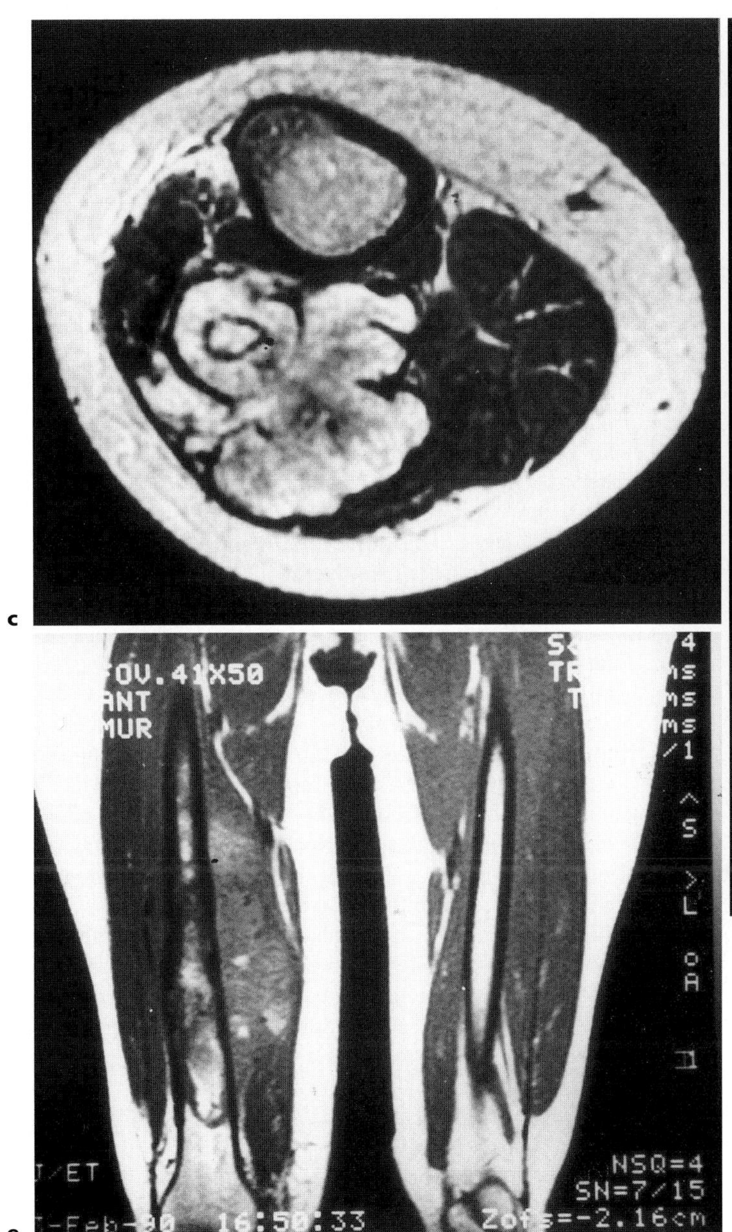

c

e

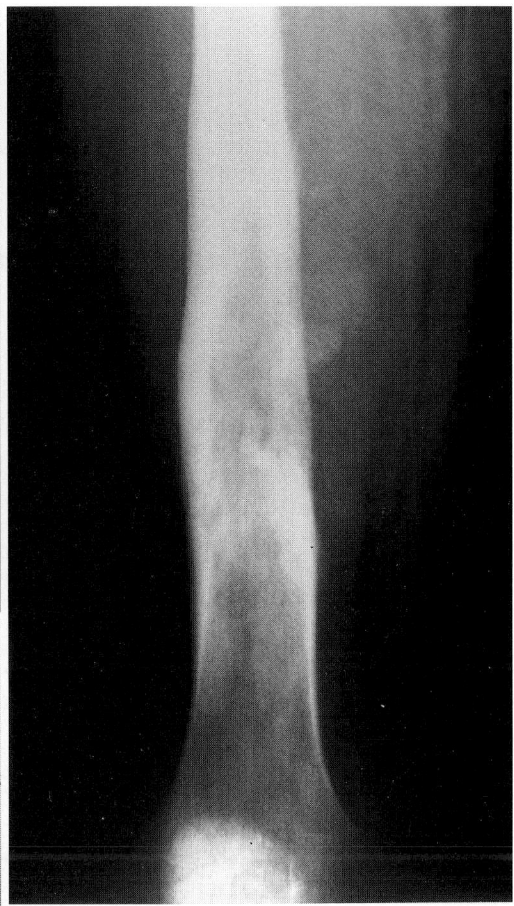

d

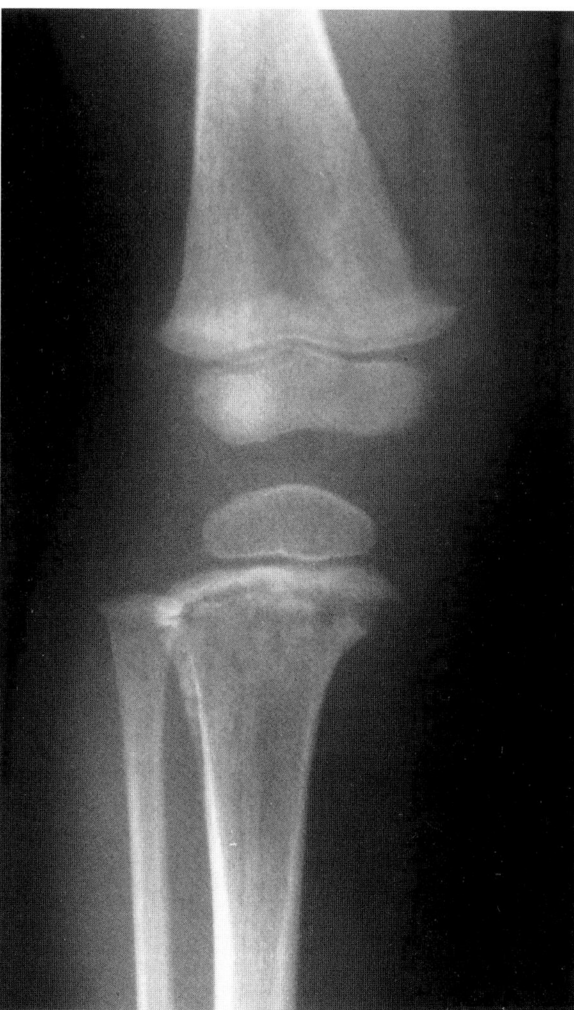

Fig. 7.31. Metastatic bone disease. Neuroblastoma has permeated the proximal tibia and to a lesser extent the distal femur. Not the similarity to Fig. 7.30

flat bones, such as those of the pelvis. Systemic malignancies of bone – leukemia, neuroblastoma (metastatic), retinoblastoma (metastatic), hepatoblastoma (metastatic) are important in the differential of permeative lesions. The appearances of these four diseases plus Ewing's sarcoma and osteomyelitis are all similar and cannot be *specifically* diagnosed by X-ray (Fig. 7.31).

The radiologist must decide whether the lesion is benign or malignant. Clear signs of a benign lesion include sharp demarcation between the lesion and the normal bone, a sclerotic margin around the lesion, and a nonaggressive pattern of growth. The characteristics most often associated with a malignancy include an accompanying soft tissue mass, an indistinct zone between the normal and abnormal bone – an indistinct zone of demarcation – and permeative, destructive changes in the bone (see Figs. 7.30, 7.31). Plain film radiography is usually adequate to diagnose most benign tumors. Sometimes CT can add diagnostic information that can be helpful, such as in osteoid osteoma, where location of the nidus is critical for operative management. While plain radiography is still quite reliable for predicting the histopathological nature of a specific lesion and in predicting its malignant characteristics, MR is the modality of choice once a malignant bone lesion has been diagnosed. The extent of the lesion including cortical and intramedullary invasion, or epiphyseal, joint space, ligamentous tendinous, and nerve bundle involvement are shown. MR evaluation aids in the decision to perform a limb salvage procedure or an amputation and is helpful in following response to chemotherapy. Remember, however, that histological diagnoses can only be suggested; only a biopsy can result in a firm diagnosis.

Soft Tissue Tumors

The first examination in evaluating any soft tissue mass is still the plain film. When the patient has a palpable lesion, plain films can rule out underlying skeletal deformity, such as exostosis or callus formation overlying a fracture. Calcium, in the form of phlebolith in hemangiomas or as periosteal reaction in myositis ossificans (calcifying hematoma and muscle damage after trauma), is an important clue. The plain film may be helpful in detecting periosteal reaction, destruction, and remodeling of underlying bone. When CT and MR were added to the diagnostic armamentarium, the work-up of patients with soft tissue tumors underwent a major change.

MR is superb for the diagnosis of soft tissue tumors because it can rule out masses in virtually 100% of cases. Benign soft tissue masses tend to be sharply

Fig. 7.32 a, b. Arthritides. **a** Hemophilia. Hemophilic arthropathy can be recognized by the squaring of the ends of the long bones (compare the distal femur to that in Fig. 7.1) and the erosive defects along the condyles (*arrows*). The joint space narrowing and erosions (the intracondylar notch is also eroded, *open arrowheads*) are typical of arthritis. **b** Juvenile rheumatoid arthritis. Note the joint space narrowing in both hip joints. Osteoporosis is the hallmark of this disease. The left hip is laterally displaced by the synovial proliferation

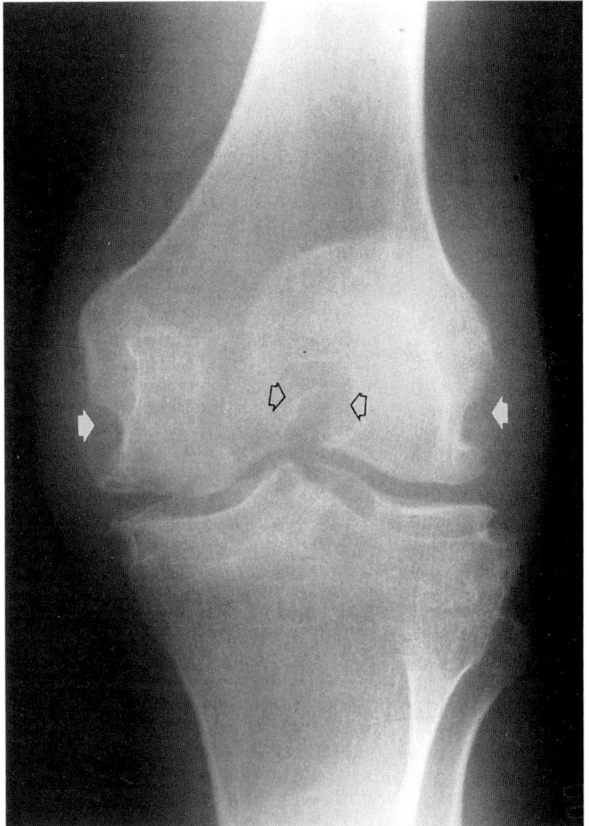
a

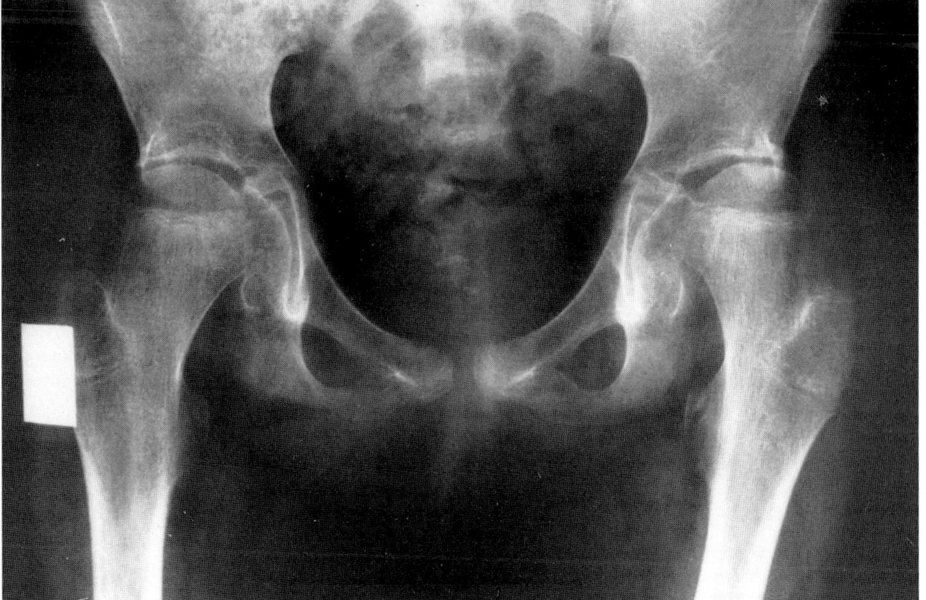
b

defined, encapsulated, and homogeneous with no peritumoral edema, while malignant masses tend to have indistinct margins, tend to be inhomogeneous, and have peritumoral edema in over 90% of cases. Specific diagnoses can be made for certain types of tumors if they contain fat or are vascular – lipoma, liposarcoma, hemangioma, arteriovenous malformation, pseudoaneurysm, ganglion cyst and hematomas. MR is also superb in detecting fluid levels inside certain lesions.

Marrow Disorders

MR has become the modality of choice in evaluating diseases of the bone marrow. Because MR can separate fat from other tissues, it is excellent in appreciating the normal patterns of bone marrow distribution and the response of the marrow to the stress of disease. The disorders in which MR imaging is superb are:

- Myeloid hyperplasia (anemia, cyanotic heart disease)
- Marrow replacement disorders (leukemia, Gaucher's diesease, neoplasms, lymphoma, metastases)
- Myeloid depletion (drugs, viral infections, radiation therapy toxins)
- Myelofibrosis (chemotherapy, radiation, infarction)

MR images the marrow by visualizing the fat content; fat-suppressing techniques aid in diagnosing infiltrative diseases. Marrow contains fat, and as the infant grows into adulthood, the amount of fat in the skeleton increases and the amount of cellular marrow (hematopoietic) decreases. The marrow changes in the appendicular skeleton first and gradually moves centrally towards the axillary skeleton. Since the fatty marrow is bright and the cellular marrow is darker, abnormalities are easily recognized (Fig. 7.25). For example, the epiphysis almost always contains fatty marrow. Thus, an infarct in the epiphysis is readily detected (it is black; Fig. 7.26).

Arthritides

The most common cause of joint-swelling in children is trauma. Usually the history is obtained, and the injury is short-lived. The second most common cause of "arthritis" is infectious – the septic joint. The common organisms in childhood are *Staphylococcus* and *Streptococcus,* but the ubiquitous gonococcus cannot be forgotten. Here again, radiographic signs of bone involvement may not be present, but there is joint effusion and swelling. Appropriate clinical maneuvers such as tapping the joint are diagnostic. Less commonly, hemophilic arthritis, rheumatoid arthritis, and arthritides of collagen disease are found (Fig. 7.32).

What abnormalities do you see in Fig. 7.33?

References

1. Greulich WW, Pyle SL (1970) Radiographic atlas of skeletal development of the hand and wrist, 2nd edn. Stanford University Press, Stanford
2. Forrester DM, Brown JC, Nesson JW (1987) Radiology of joint diseases, 3rd edn. Saunders, Philadelphia
3. Keats TE (1992) An atlas of normal roentgen variants, 5th edn. Year Book Medical, Chicago
4. Köhler A (1968) Borderlands of the normal and early pathologic in skeletal roentgenology, 11th edn., Grune and Stratton, London
5. Ozonoff MB (1992) Pediatric orthopaedic radiology, 2nd edn. Saunders, Philadelphia
6. Schultz RJ (1990) The language of fractures, 2nd edn., Williams and Wilkins, Baltimore
7. Troupin RH (1978) Diagnostic radiology in clinical medicine, 2nd edn., Year Book Medical, Chicago

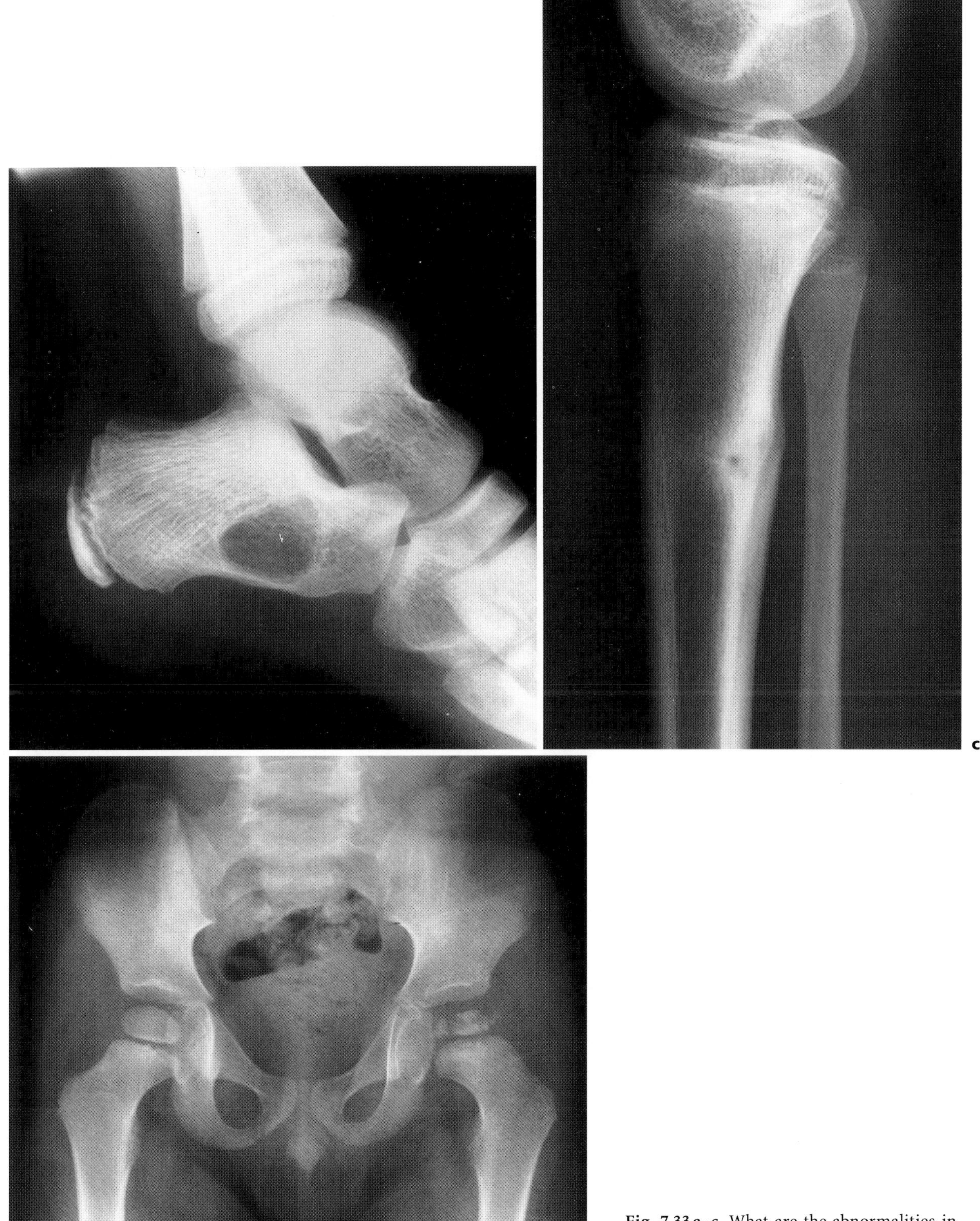

Fig. 7.33 a–c. What are the abnormalities in these three cases? Answers in "Appendix 2"

8 Central Nervous System

Cross-sectional imaging (ultrasound, CT, and MR) has completely revolutionized the way in which we look at the central nervous system. Once again, the ordering physician must ask, "What do I want to know?" If the concern is about the bony vault, a skull series may suffice, but if the real interest is diagnosing an intracranial lesion, one of these cross-sectional modalities should be used. We begin with the skull for anatomy of the cranial vault and then cover intracranial anatomy. Lastly, indications for imaging evaluation of the head, neck, and spine are discussed.

Skull

The cranial sutures and fontanelles divide the skull into its major bones (Fig. 8.1). A suture is a nonossified portion of the membranous bone. (Remember: most of the skull is derived from membranous tissue, while the base of the skull and long bones are derived from enchondral ossification.) The metopic and coronal sutures begin at the large, diamond-shaped anterior fontanelle. The midline sagittal suture separates the parietal bones. It extends from the anterior fontanelle to the posterior fontanelle at the posterior aspect of the parietal bones.

The complex occipital bone is composed of six individual bones: two interparietal, one supraoccipital, two extraoccipital, and one basioccipital bone. The temporal bone, located inferior to the parietal bone and anterior to the occipital bone, includes the mastoid process and structures of the internal ear. The temporal bone extends anteriorly to the sphenoid bone. The sphenoid bone is the dense structure at the base of the skull which includes the greater and lesser wings and the sella turcica. The largest bone of the face is the mandible. A routine skull examination should include the mandible, maxilla, orbital structures, and paranasal sinuses (maxillary, ethmoidal, and frontal).

The time of closure of various intracranial sutures and fontanelles and the appearance of the paranasal sinuses are summarized below:

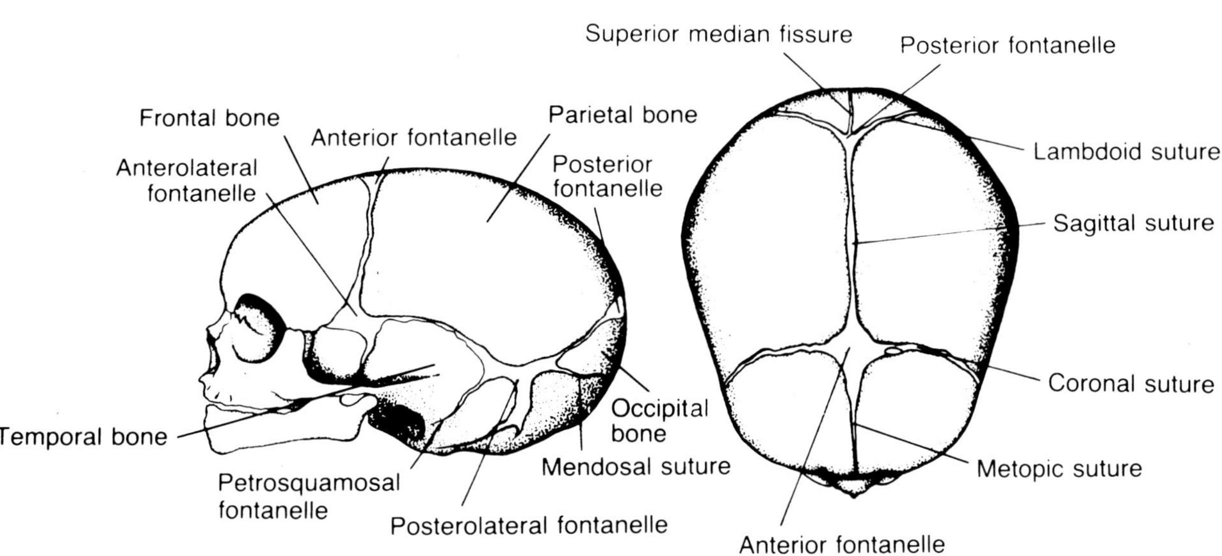

Fig. 8.1. The infant calvarium with major bones, sutures, and fontanelles

- Closure of fontanelles (average range/total range)
  - Anterior: 15–18 months/9–24 months
  - Posterior: 1–2 months/birth–3 months
- Closure of sutures (from [9])
  - Mendosal: several weeks after birth (this suture separates the interparietal and supraoccipital portions of the occipital bone)
  - Metopic: 2nd year (10% persist throughout life)
  - Coronal, sagittal, lambdoidal: about age 30
- Appearance of paranasal sinuses (great deal of variation) (from [1])
  - Ethmoid sinuses; rudimentary air cells at birth but usually no air seen radiographically until 3–6 months
  - Maxillary sinuses: rudimentary air cells at birth but usually no air seen radiographically until 3–6 months
  - Sphenoidal sinuses: 1–3 years
  - Frontal sinuses: 4–10 years

Figure 8.2 shows the multiple views necessary to evaluate the various portions of the skull. It is advisable to know these projections so that optimal visualization of particular sections of the calvarium can be obtained. The calvarium changes dramatically with age as the sutures and fontanelles close. Figure 8.3 shows the maturation process of the skull. The sutures become less obvious and the paranasal (maxillary, ethmoid and sphenoid) and mastoid sinuses aerate.

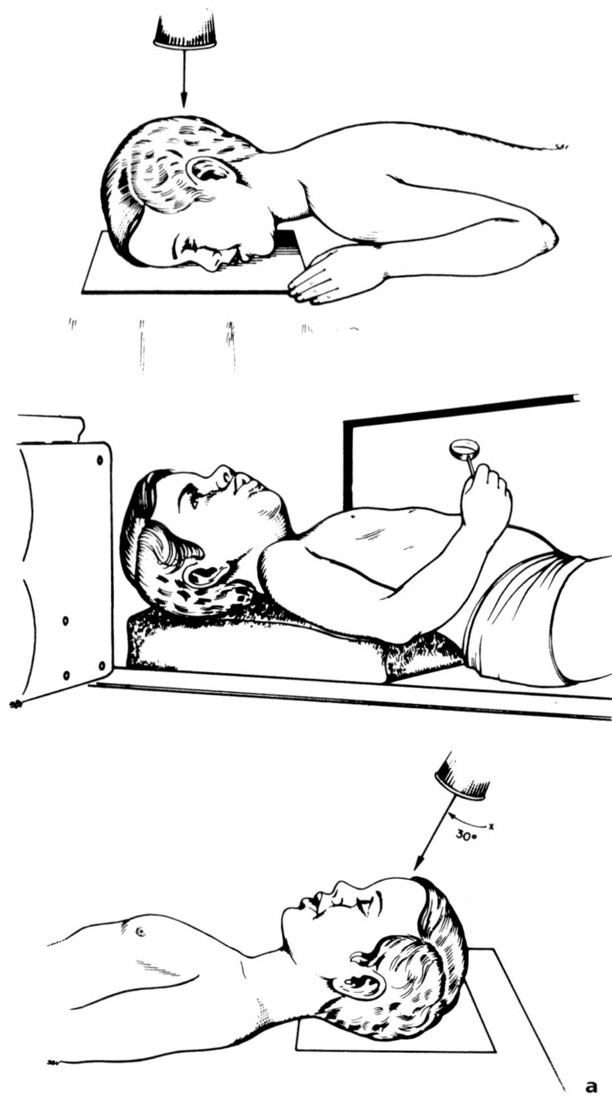

Fig. 8.2. Line drawings (**a**) and radiographs (**b–d**)of the various views of the skull. In the PA view (**a**, *above*; **b**); the beam enters the back of the child's head on a line perpendicular to the film, allowing visualization of the petrous pyramids (*p*), which are projected through the orbits. In the cross-table lateral view (**a**, *middle*; **c**) the beam enters one side of the child's head while the film is on the other. In this way a horizontal lateral is achieved. This method allows the child to remain comfortable during the procedure, and the entire calvarium and the sella turcica (*arrow*) are nicely displayed. In Towne's view (**a**, *below*; **d**). The beam is directed toward the back of the patient's head at a 30° angle. This view is designed to demonstrate the occipital bone (*o*) and the foramen magnum. Basal skull fractures are often seen best in this view

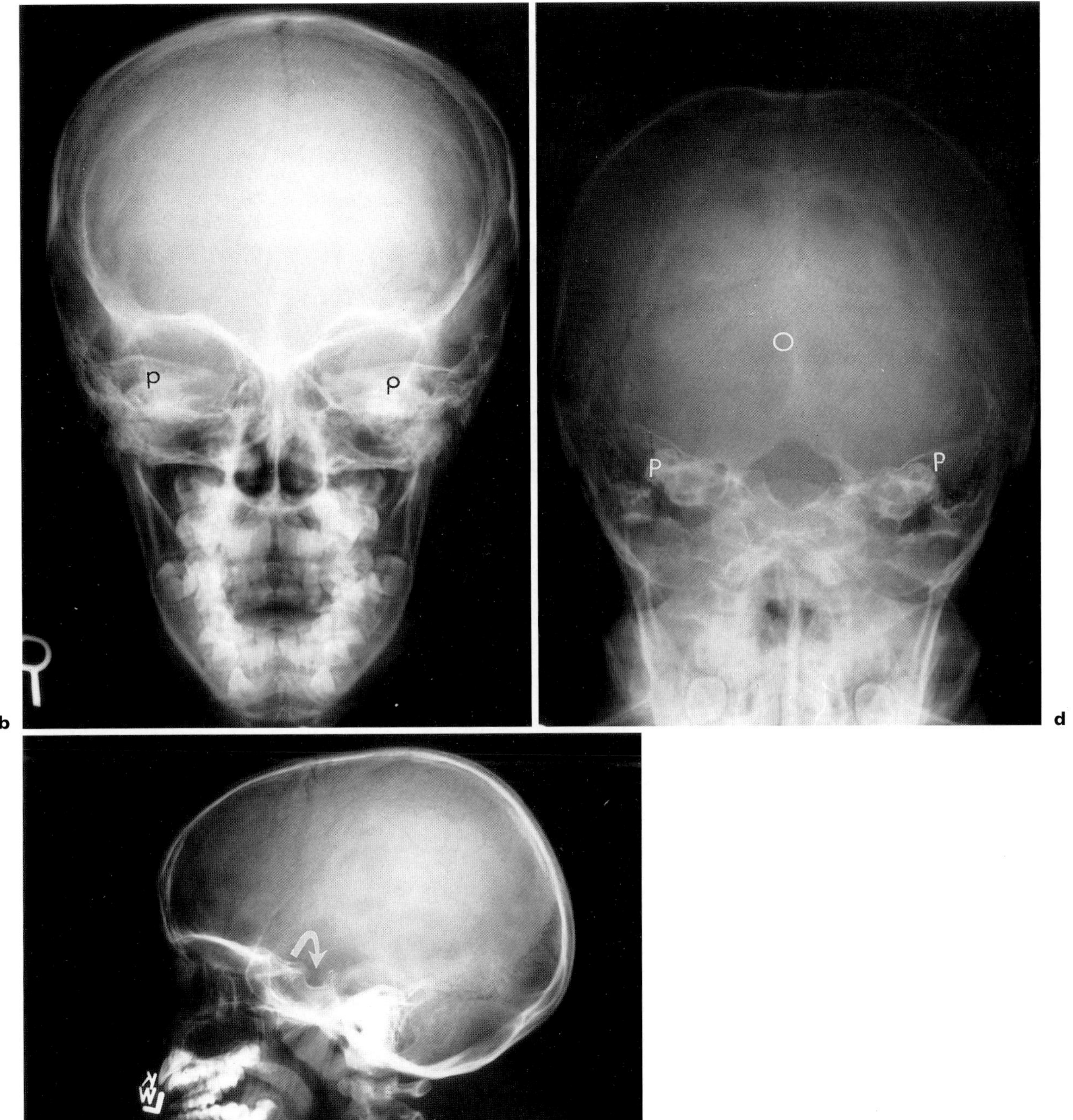
P
P
O
P
P
b
d
c

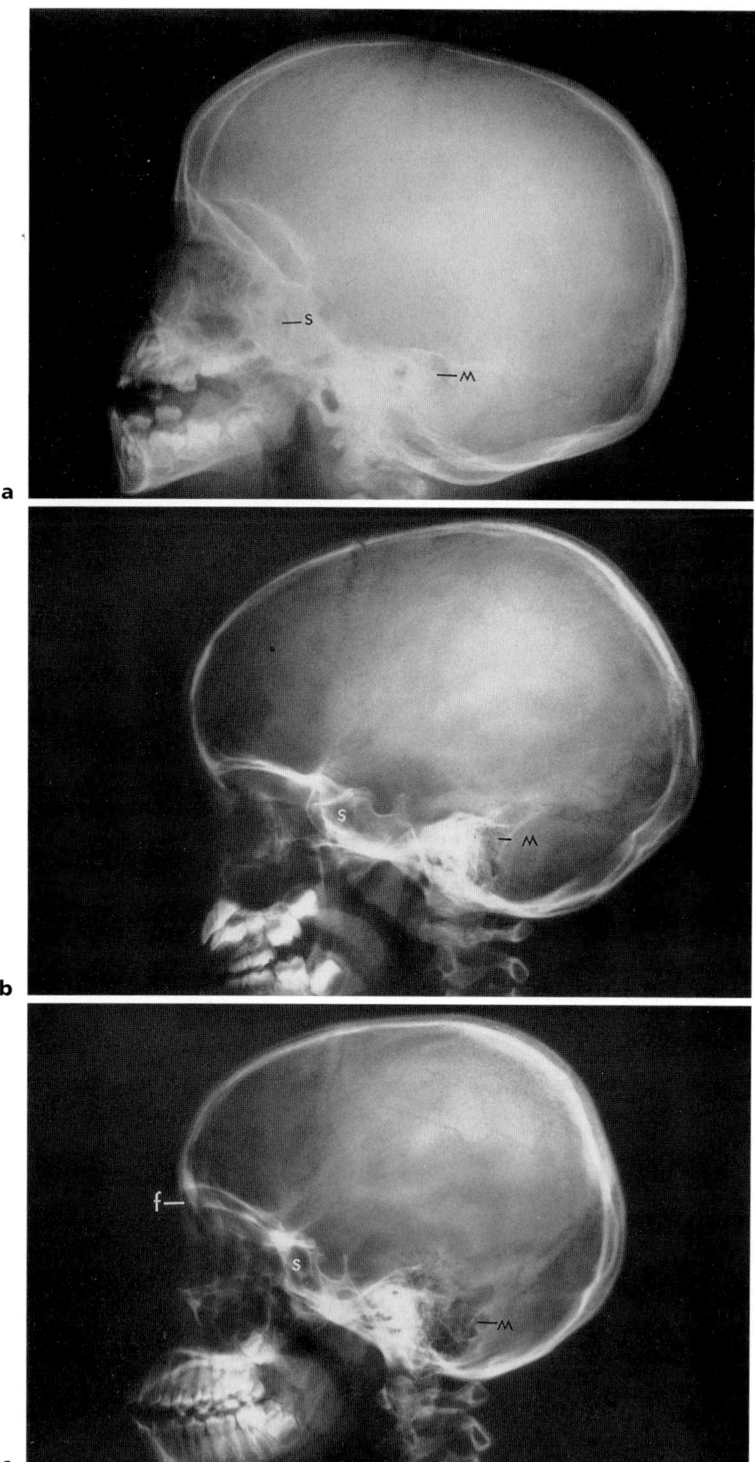

Fig. 8.3 a–c. Comparative views of the skull from early childhood through adolescence (**a**, 2 years; **b**, 6 years; **c**, 14 years). Note how the sutures become less obvious, and the paranasal sinuses aerate. *s*, Sphenoid; *m*, mastoid; *f*, frontal

Approach to the Plain Skull Film

A systematic approach for examining the skull is to begin from the external surface and work through the calvarium and down into the face and spine in all views.

The Soft Tissues

Any bulge or enlargement of the soft tissues should be noted. This may be the site of trauma (we suggest looking harder in this region for a fracture) or protuberance of intracranial contents – an encephalocele – or, if at the fontanelle, evidence of increased intracranial pressure.

The Three Bony Tables

Outer Table. This is the extreme bony margin of the skull. Irregularities or disruption of this cortex denote abnormality. Cephalohematoma, osteomyelitis, metastasis, and histiocytosis all affect this portion of the skull (Fig. 8.4 a).

Diploe. This is the middle table and contains the bone marrow. Severe hemolytic anemia can cause proliferation of bone marrow and enlargement of the diploe, giving a "hair-on-end" appearance (e.g., thalassemia; Fig. 8.4 b).

Inner Table. This portion of the bony calvarium is frequently affected by lesions within the cranial vault. The most common "erosion" is normal pacchionian granulation (Fig. 8.4 c, d).

Calvarium

Now we are looking through the bone as well as at the generalized bony covering. Pay close attention to the cranial sutures and search for possible fractures or intracranial calcifications. While common in adults, "normal calcifications" of the pineal, habenular commissure, choroid plexus, or dura are not usually seen in childhood (under the age of 15 years) on plain films; these calcifications can be frequently seen, however, on CT.

Sella Turcica

This is a site commonly affected by increased intracranial pressure. It is also an area affected by one of the pediatric tumors – the craniopharyngioma.

The Frontal Film

When viewing the skull from the front (see Fig. 8.5), the easiest way to detect an abnormality is to look for asymmetry. This body is, for the most part, symmetric, and a line drawn down the middle of the frontal skull film should result in mirror images of one side of the skull as compared to the other.

The Neck

The soft tissues of the neck and nasopharynx, as well as the cervical spine, are clearly visible. Look for displacement of the air column by a mass (this will be a mass effect) or any bony destruction.

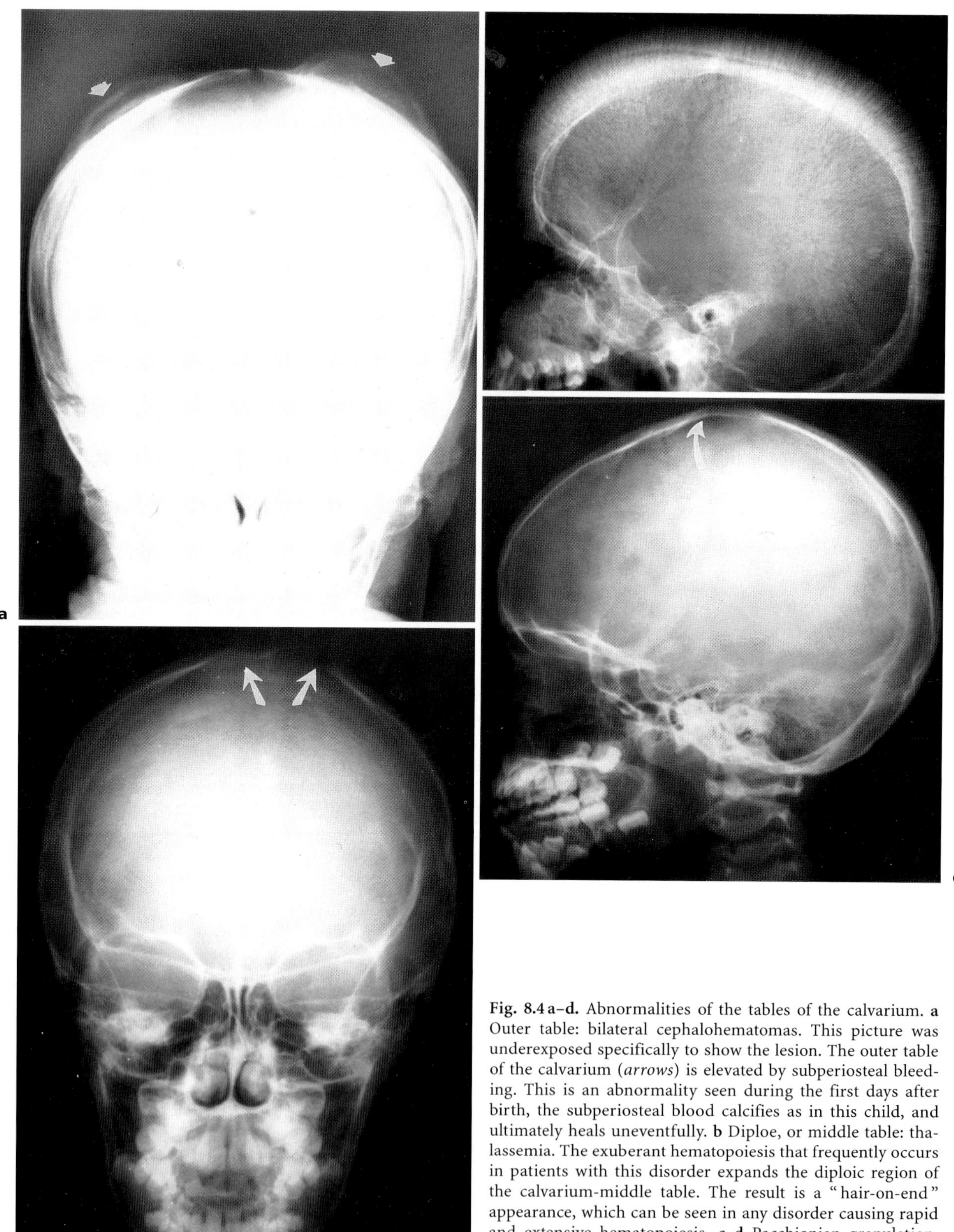

Fig. 8.4 a–d. Abnormalities of the tables of the calvarium. **a** Outer table: bilateral cephalohematomas. This picture was underexposed specifically to show the lesion. The outer table of the calvarium (*arrows*) is elevated by subperiosteal bleeding. This is an abnormality seen during the first days after birth, the subperiosteal blood calcifies as in this child, and ultimately heals uneventfully. **b** Diploe, or middle table: thalassemia. The exuberant hematopoiesis that frequently occurs in patients with this disorder expands the diploic region of the calvarium-middle table. The result is a "hair-on-end" appearance, which can be seen in any disorder causing rapid and extensive hematopoiesis. **c, d** Pacchionian granulation. The inner table (*arrow*) is bowed toward the diploe by rather abundant pacchionian granulation. These are arachnoid extensions that aid in spinal fluid resorption

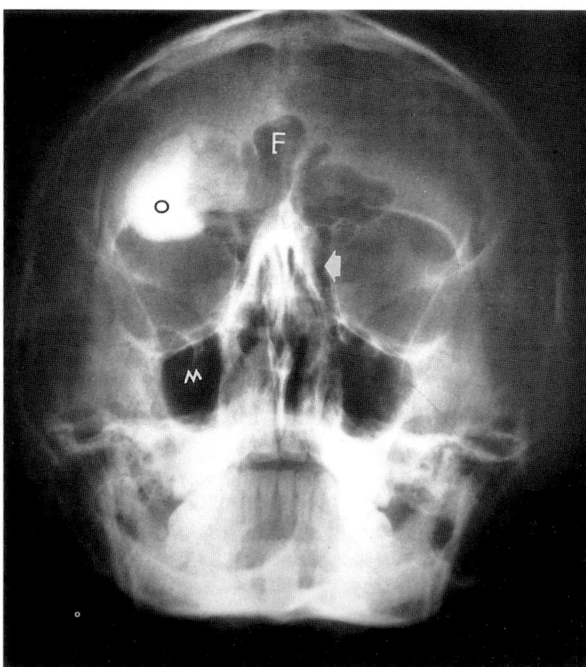

Fig. 8.5. Waters' view of the calvarium. Careful attention to symmetry of the face allows one to detect the large, bony benign tumor (*O*) of the frontal sinus. It is an osteoma. Note the well aerated maxillary (*M*), ethmoid (*arrow*), and frontal sinuses (*F*)

Intracranial Contents

In the neonate and young infant, the brain and its meninges are easily identified with ultrasound viewed through the anterior fontanel. The two standard projections are the coronal and sagittal (Fig. 8.6). These views are limited by the fontanelle so they are always angled, i.e., paracoronal and parasagittal. The ventricles are used as landmarks, but the real key is seeing the parenchyma. Extra-axial fluid is easily seen (extra-axial = between brain and bone, outside of brain). The more premature the child was, the less sulci and the more obvious the extra axial space. At term, there is little extra axial fluid, but from 2 months to 2–3 years a small amount of extra axial fluid may be seen (Fig. 8.7).

A more precise view of the parenchyma and meninges can be obtained with CT. These images are usually in the axial plane (a horizontal plane, approximately 20° above the orbital-meatal line, sparing the lens; Fig. 8.8). These anatomical sections can be as thin as 1 mm. For most intracranial imaging, 5- to 10-mm sections are performed. CT is superb for showing the bony structures, calcium, and the supratentorial brain. It is less optimal for showing the posterior fossa, brain stem, distinguishing gray-white matter differentiation, and defining white matter abnormalities. Computerized reconstruction in multiple planes can be performed, but these images are less optimal than MR.

MR is the most exquisite method of viewing brain parenchyma. It can be portrayed in any plane, has excellent tissue differentiation, and superbly defines the spine (Fig. 8.9). MR, however, is less advantageous than CT in showing bony abnormalities. An excellent text for learning the anatomy demonstrated by these modalities is that by Hayman and Hinck [2]. A comparison of modalities is found in Chap. 1 and in Table 8.1.

Table 8.1. Comparison of modalities

Modality	Time	Sedation	Contrast	Cost
Ultrasound	Very fast	No	No	Least expensive
CT	Fast	Sometimes	Yes	Middle range
MR	Slowest	Frequently	Yes	Most expensive

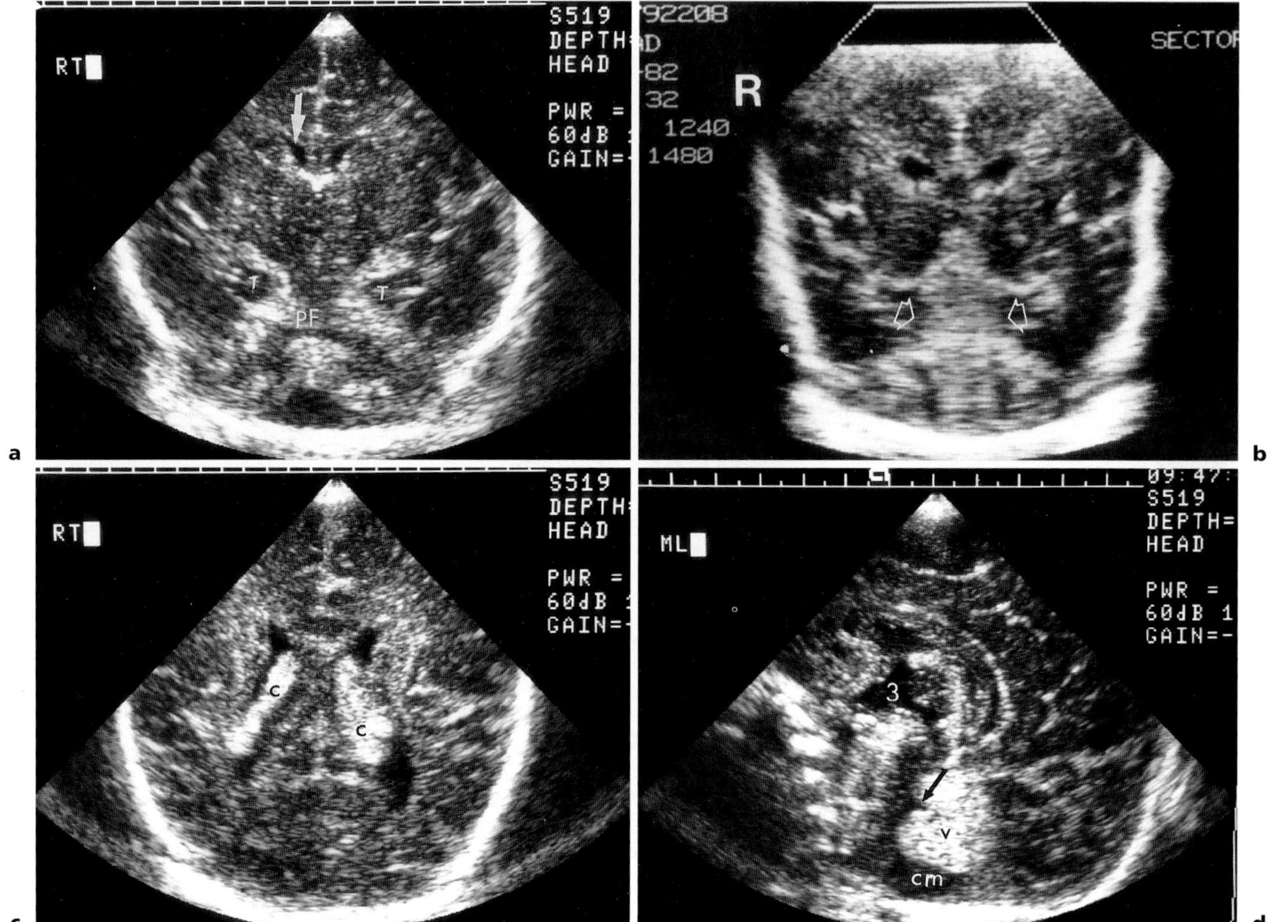
S519
DEPTH
HEAD
PWR =
60dB
GAIN=
RT
T
PF
T
92208
82
32
1240
1480
R
SECTOR
C
C
ML
3
V
cm
S519
DEPTH=
HEAD
PWR =
60dB 1
GAIN=-
a
b
c
d

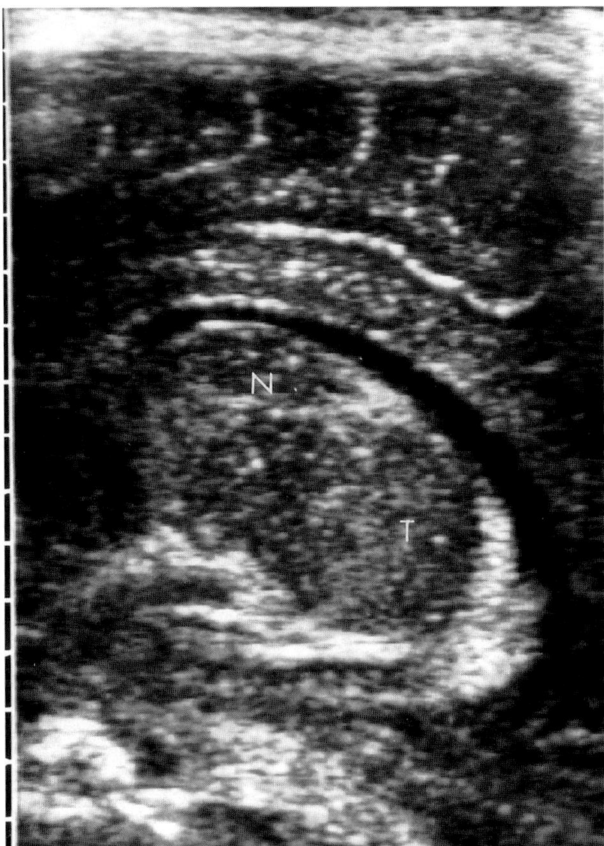

Fig. 8.6 a–e. Ultrasound of the neonate through the anterior fontanelle. **a** Coronal section through the anterior horns of the frontal ventricles (*arrow*) shows the echogenic (*white*) choroid in the floor of the ventricles. The temporal lobes (*T*) are seen as is the posterior fossa (*PF*). **b** Coronal view slightly posterior to A reveals the tentorium (*arrows*) and the bodies of the lateral ventricles. **c** Coronal section through the atria of the lateral ventricles shows the ventricular fluid (*black*) enclosing the choroid (*c*; *echogenic/white*). **d** Sagittal midline section shows the third ventricle (*3*), the echogenic vermis of the cerebellum (*V*), and the cisterna magna (*CM*). Anterior to the vermis is the fourth ventricle (*arrow*) and the brainstem. **e** Sagittal section off to one side shows the thalamus (*T*) and the caudate nucleus (*N*). The lateral ventricle is black

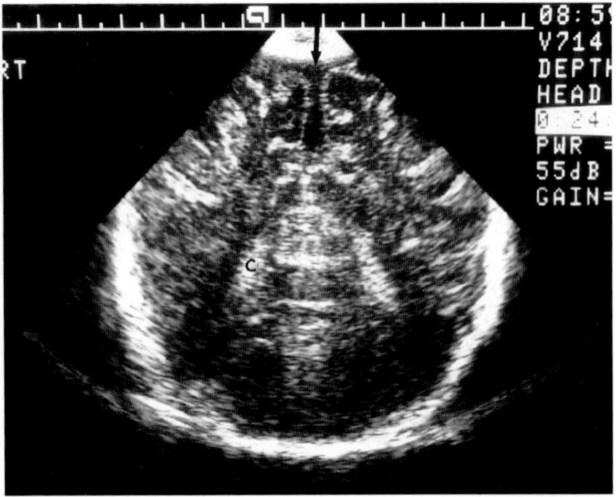

Fig. 8.7. Coronal scan at the level of the atria (see echogenic choroid, *C*) shows the black, echo-free intrahemispheric fluid (*arrow*) between the right and left frontal horns and going over the convexity. This is not a premature infant but an older infant in whom this amount of extra-axial fluid is normal

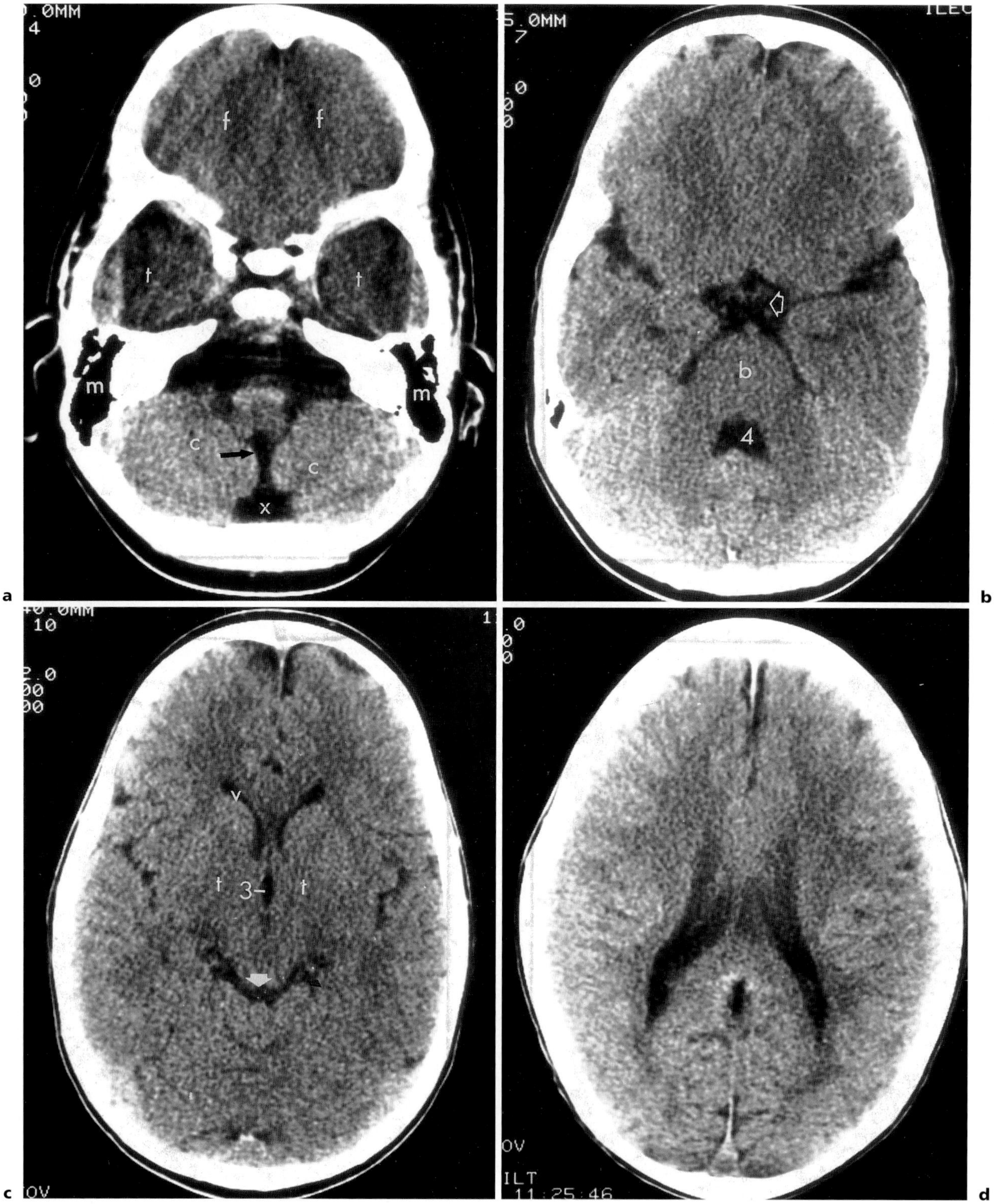

Fig. 8.8 a–h. Legend see page 186

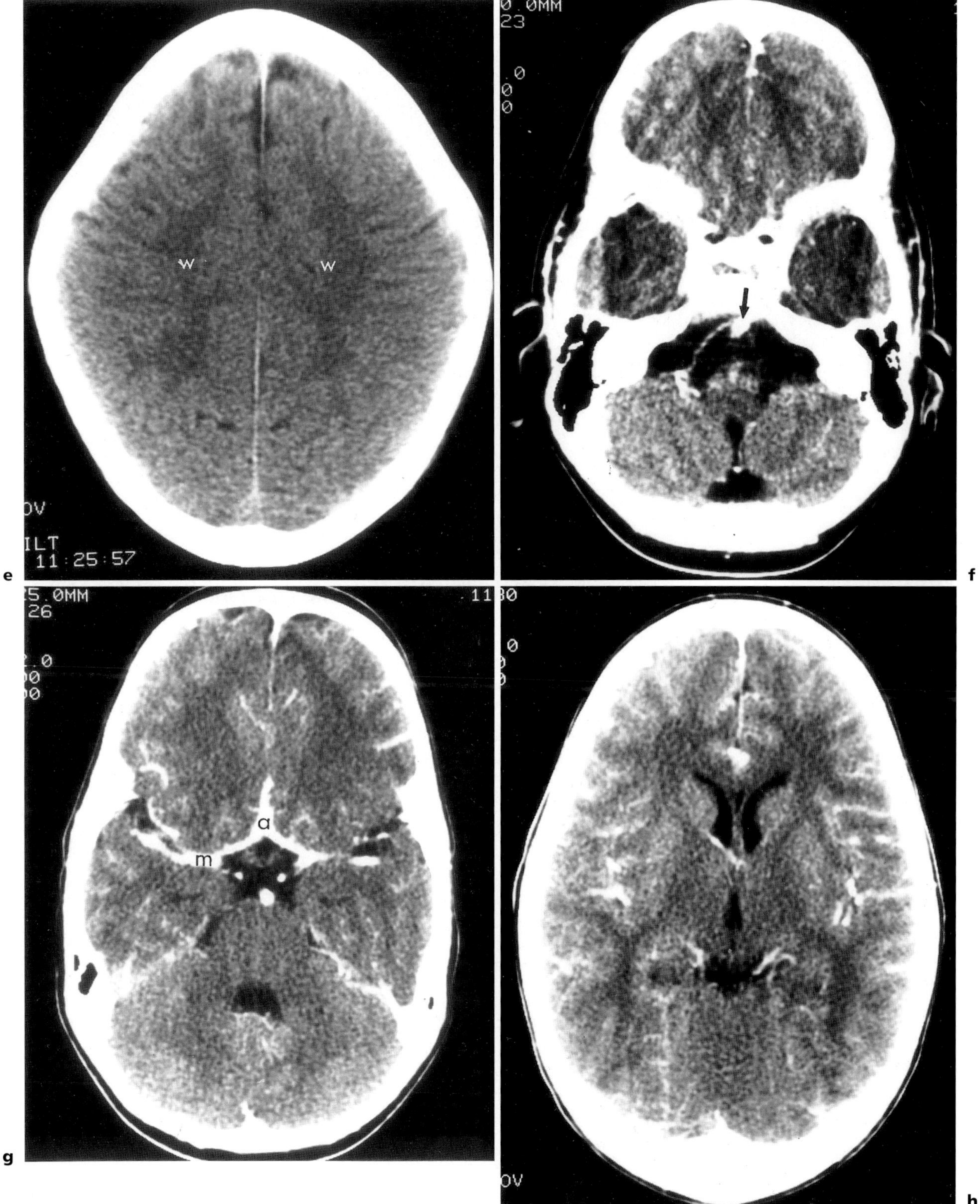

e f g h

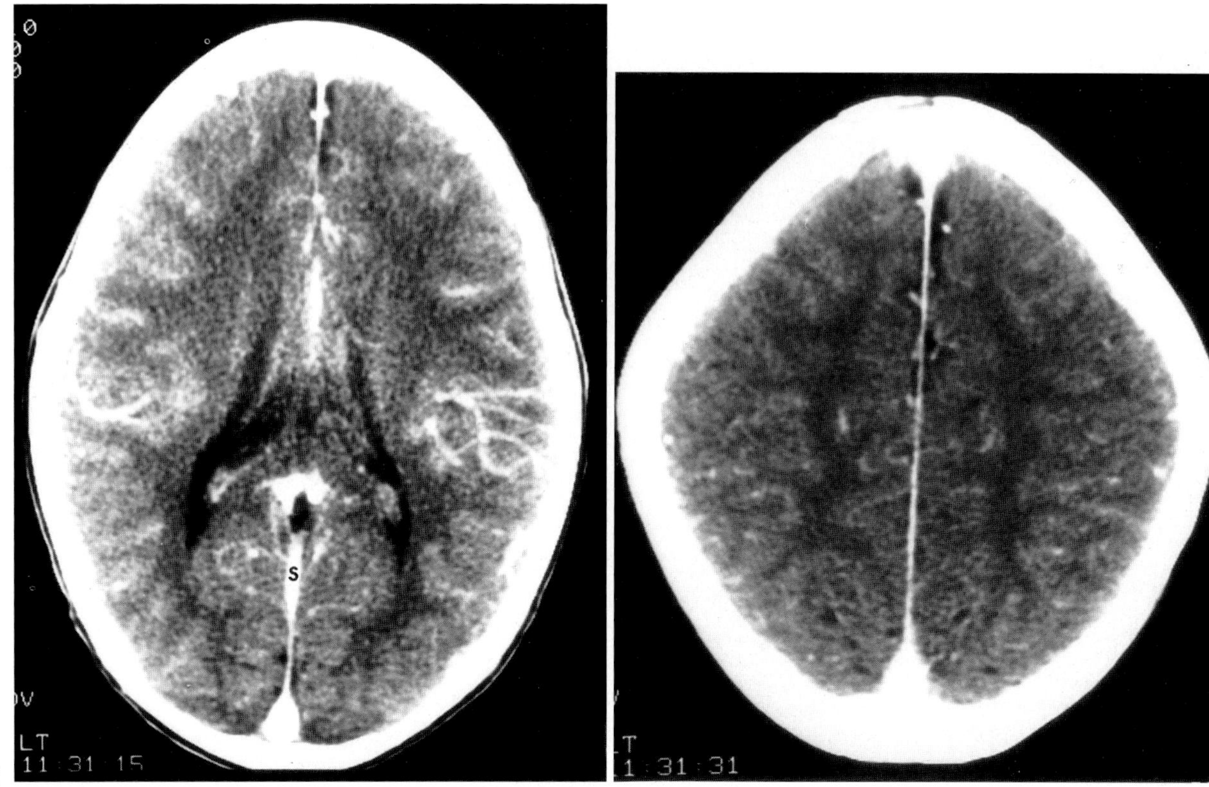

Fig. 8.8 a–j. Normal CT scan of the brain. **a–e** Unenhanced scans, that is, no IV contrast. **f–j** Comparable images with intravenous enhancement. The most inferior (lowest caudad) section (**a** without enhancement, **f** with enhancement) reveals the mastoid air cells (*m*), the temporal lobes (*t*), and frontal lobes (*f*). The posterior fossa is seen with a normal fourth ventricle (*arrow*), vallecula, and cisterna magna (*x*). The cerebellar hemispheres are noted (*c*). With intravenous enhancement (Fig. 8.8 f), note visualization of the basilar artery (*arrow*). **b, g** The next superior cuts. The suprasellar cistern (*arrow*) is seen as well as the fourth ventricle (*4*) and brainstem (*b*). With enhancement the entire circle of Willis is noted. *m*, Middle cerebral artery; *a*, anterior cerebral arteries. **c, h** The next higher sections. The frontal horns of the lateral ventricle (*v*) and the third ventricle (*3*) are noted. The thalamus is along side the third ventricle (*t*) and the quadrigeminal plate cistern is seen (*arrow*). **d, i** The next higher sections, showing the lateral ventricles. With enhancement the straight sinus (*s*) is noted draining into the torcula. **e, j** The highest sections. Gray and white matter (*w*) differentiation can be seen and there is enhancement of the falx (*midline white*)

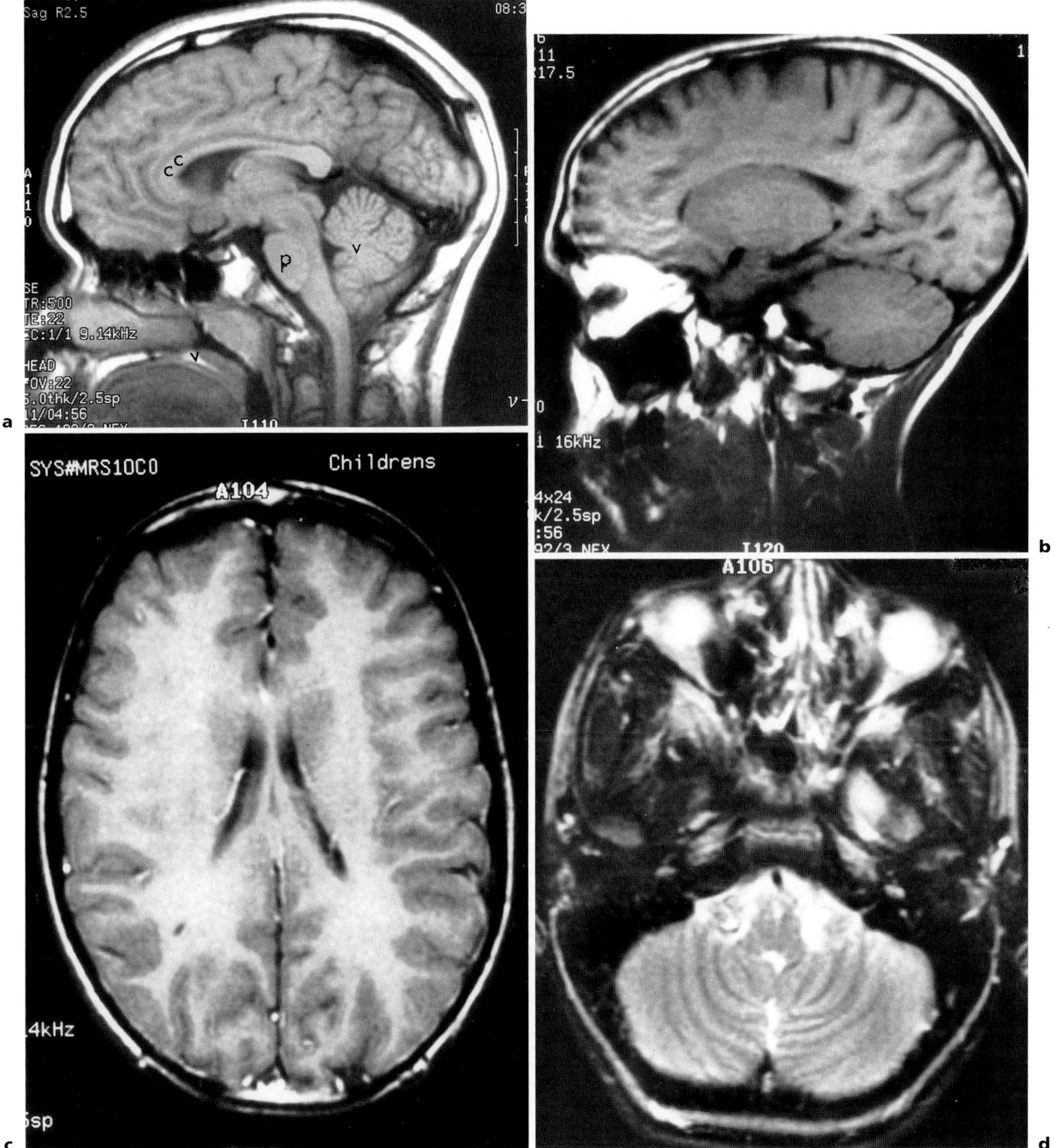

Fig. 8.9 a–d. Legend see page 189

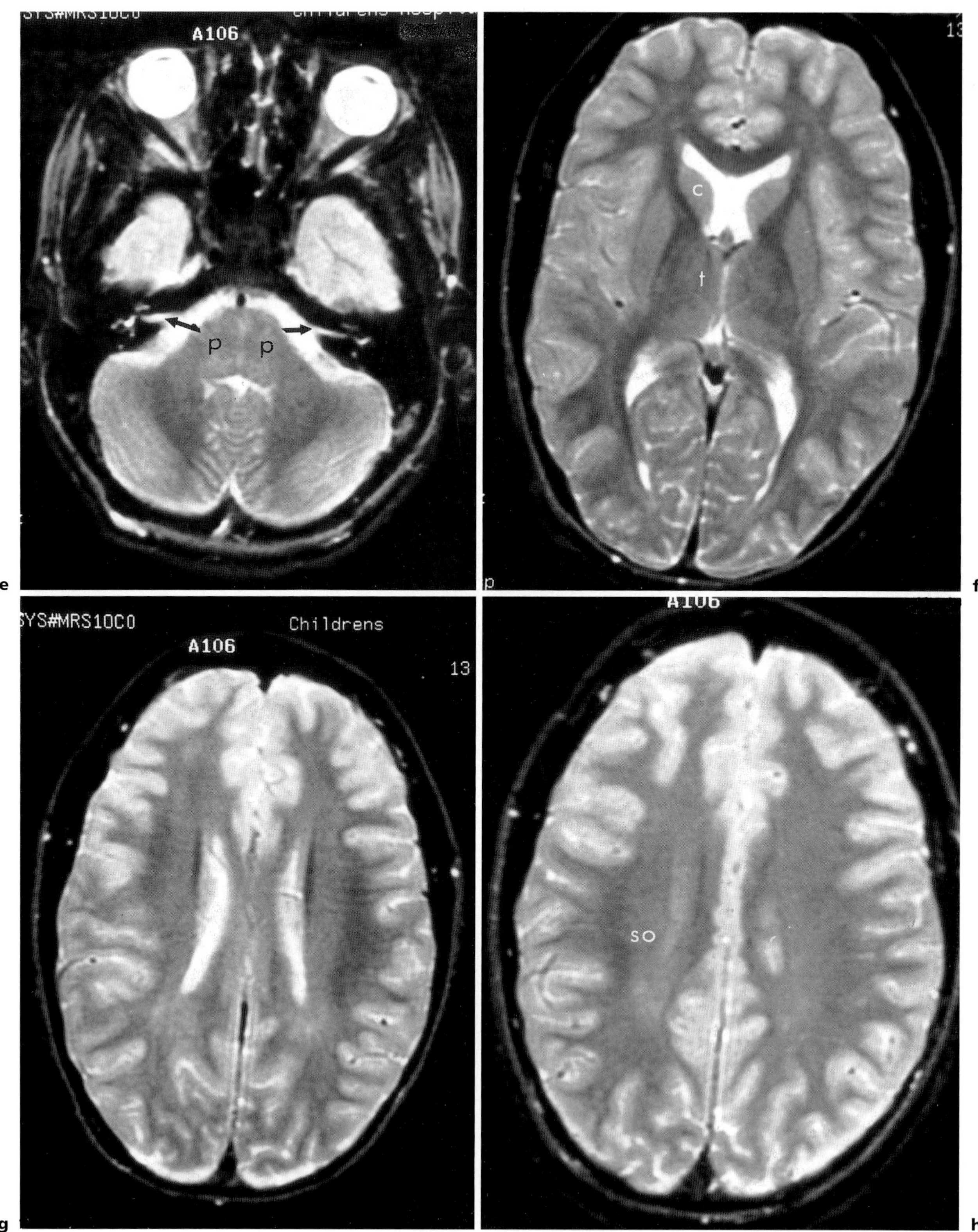
A106
p
p
c
t
SYS#MRS10C0
Childrens
A106
13
A106
so
e
f
g
h

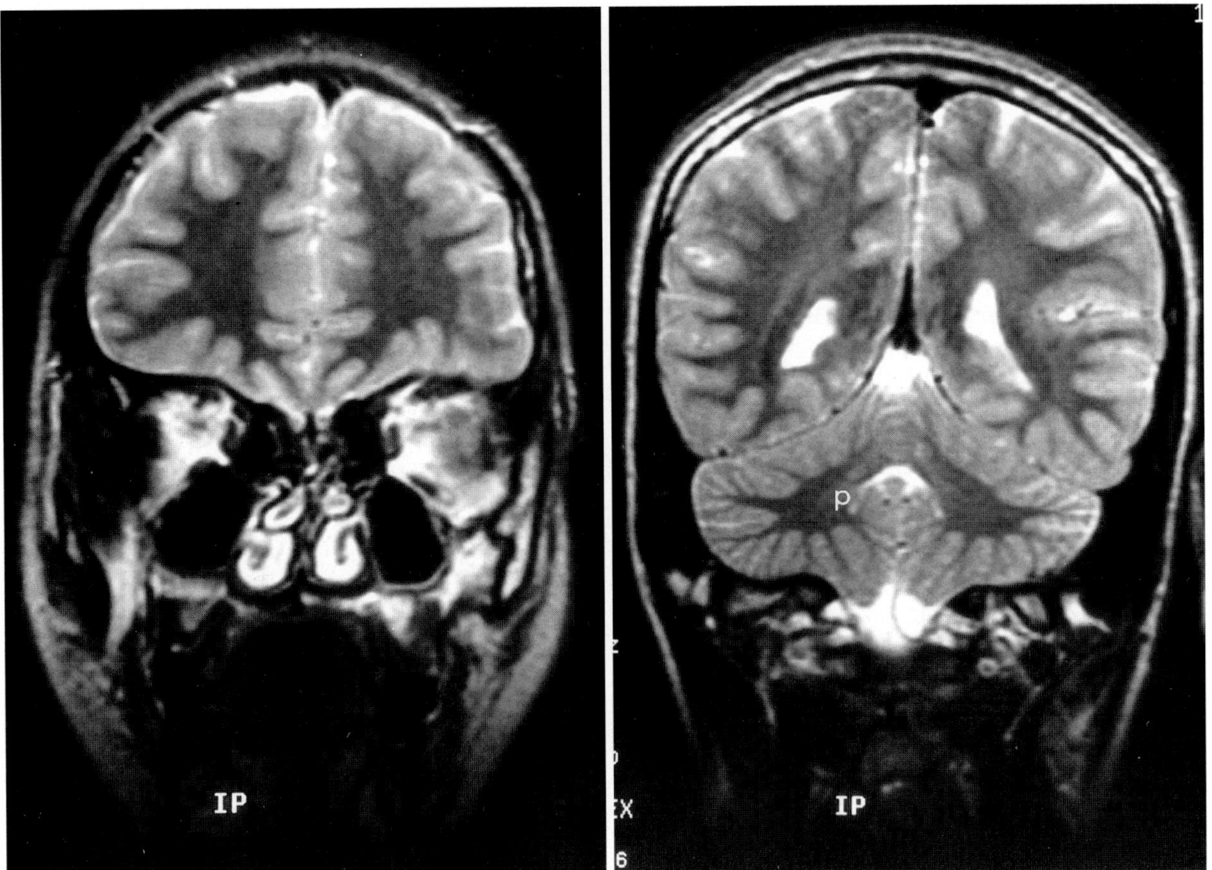

Fig. 8.9 a–j. Normal MR. **a** Sagittal section T1 imaging in the midline. This section is most valuable for evaluation of the anatomical structures including the corpus callosum (*cc*), the pons (*p*), the cerebellar vermis (*v*), the cranial cervical junction and proximal cervical spine. **b** Sagittal section T1 imaging off the midline shows the lateral ventricles. Note ventricular fluid is black on T1 imaging. **c** Axial T1 section through the lateral ventricles. All CSF is black. **d** Axial T2 image at the level of the petrous bones shows the bony structures to be black (compare this to Fig. 8.8 a). The cerebellar hemispheres are seen to advantage. **e** Axial T2 imaging at the level of the seventh and eighth nerves. Note that the sections (slices/cuts) of this MR are at a slightly different angle than the CT. The seventh and eighth nerves are easily seen (*arrow*) and one can evaluate the middle cerebellar peduncle (*p*). In addition, the orbits are well seen. **f** Axial T2 image at the level of the frontal horns (compare to Fig. 8.9 b). Note that in T2 imaging, ventricular fluid is white. The caudate nucleus (*c*), thalamus (*t*), and the cortex are all seen well. **g** Axial T2 images comparable to Fig. 8.9 d at the level of the lateral ventricles. Again note that on T2 images the ventricular fluid is white. There is superb gray-white differentiation. **h** Axial T2 image comparable to Fig. 8.9 e in an area described as the centrum semiovale (*So*). Here again, superb gray-white differentiation is noted. **i** Coronal T2 section anteriorly showing the anterior portion of the frontal lobes and the air-filled ethmoid and maxillary sinuses. **j** Coronal T2 image posteriorly showing the posterior fossa. Note that the middle cerebellar peduncles (*p*) are well delineated against the gray matter of the cerebellum

Indications for Imaging Evaluation

Trauma

Over 50% of young children with epidural and subdural hematomas do not have changes in the bony skull, i.e., do not have skull fractures [3]. Thus, absence of fracture does not rule out damage to the brain. It is apparent, then, how useful seeing the intracranial contents really is. Similarly, not all children who have had trauma need imaging evaluation. However, the unconscious patient, the child with neurological findings and changing sensorium, and the patient with a history of severe central nervous system trauma should be evaluated by CT for damage to the intracranial contents. As in all imaging evaluations, the patient should have stable vital signs before beginning this procedure. The goal of this evaluation is to detect parenchymal abnormalities or shifts of intracranial contents by either parenchymal or extra axial lesions and changes in ventricular size or contour.

If a child is brought to the emergency room after trauma and is alert and apparently well *without* a history of unconsciousness, retrograde amnesia, or physical findings suggestive of central nervous system alteration (palpable bony malalignment, CSF discharge from either the ear or nose, tympanic membrane discoloration, absence of neurological findings), the chances of a significant fracture or the need for intracranial imaging are extremely small [2, 3]. However, there is still a role for limited and selective use of skull films, especially in cases of possible child abuse or unusual skull fractures. The latter include: (a) depressed fracture, where a fragment of bone is pushed in on intracranial contents; (b) diastatic fracture, in which the meninges may become entrapped and cause, by the vascular pulsations of CSF, bone erosion and enlargement of the fracture; (c) fracture through the sinuses; and (d) fractures crossing the path of the middle meningeal artery. If these lesions are seen, CT may be ordered to rule out the complications of these fractures. Remember: we are looking at the brain primarily for evidence of bleeding. Fresh blood appears white on a CT scan, and we therefore do not want to inject contrast because it too appears white and may obscure the findings. On CT of the head we routinely obtain three types of images: one that concentrates on the bony calvarium (bone windows), one that concentrates on the brain (brain windows), and one that emphasizes the extra-axial spaces so we may see less dense subdural and extradural collections (Fig. 8.10).

One of the indications mentioned above for skull films is that of child abuse. The skull examination is merely the first of a series of skeletal examinations for detecting radiographic evidence of child abuse (see Chap. 7).

When looking for fractures on plain films, remember these rules:

- Soft tissue swelling often accompanies acute fractures.
- An acute fracture line is sharp, does not branch, and does not have sclerotic margins.
- With rare exceptions, there are no sutures within the parietal bone; therefore, any sharp, linear lucency in this region is a fracture until proven otherwise.
- There are so many vascular grooves and normal variants, that it is important to have available one of the standard references for normal skull roentgen variants (see “ References ”).

Seizures

An imaging procedure is usually not necessary for a child with febrile seizure. In most instances the major consideration is meningitis for which a spinal tap is diagnostic. However, the work-up of a child with a nonfebrile seizure is a different matter. Yet the probability is quite low of finding neurological changes or abnormalities on plain radiographs or laboratory evaluation (glucose, calcium, sodium, or magnesium). Here the major concern is an intracranial mass lesion (tumor, subdural, etc.) causing the seizure. One of the best (although nonspecific) tests is the EEG. This detects superficial masses as well as generalized electrical abnormalities. The most sensitive imaging test for detecting a mass lesion is MR. The yield of an MR on all nonfebrile seizure patients without other neurological findings is certainly very low for demonstrating a treatable condition. However, the clinical standard for a child with nonfebrile seizures is to have one imaging procedure during the work-up (not acutely if seizure is the only symptom or sign), and MR appears to be best modality. Remember: tumors and infections (both of which cause seizures) disrupt the blood-brain barrier. These abnormalities allow contrast to penetrate and enhance the areas of inflammation or tumor. Therefore, if you do order a CT examination, make sure that it is a contrast-enhanced study to demonstrate the disrupted blood-brain barrier.

The role of nuclear medicine SPECT and PET for uncontrolled seizures is being investigated. However, these procedures are for the most severe and difficult patients.

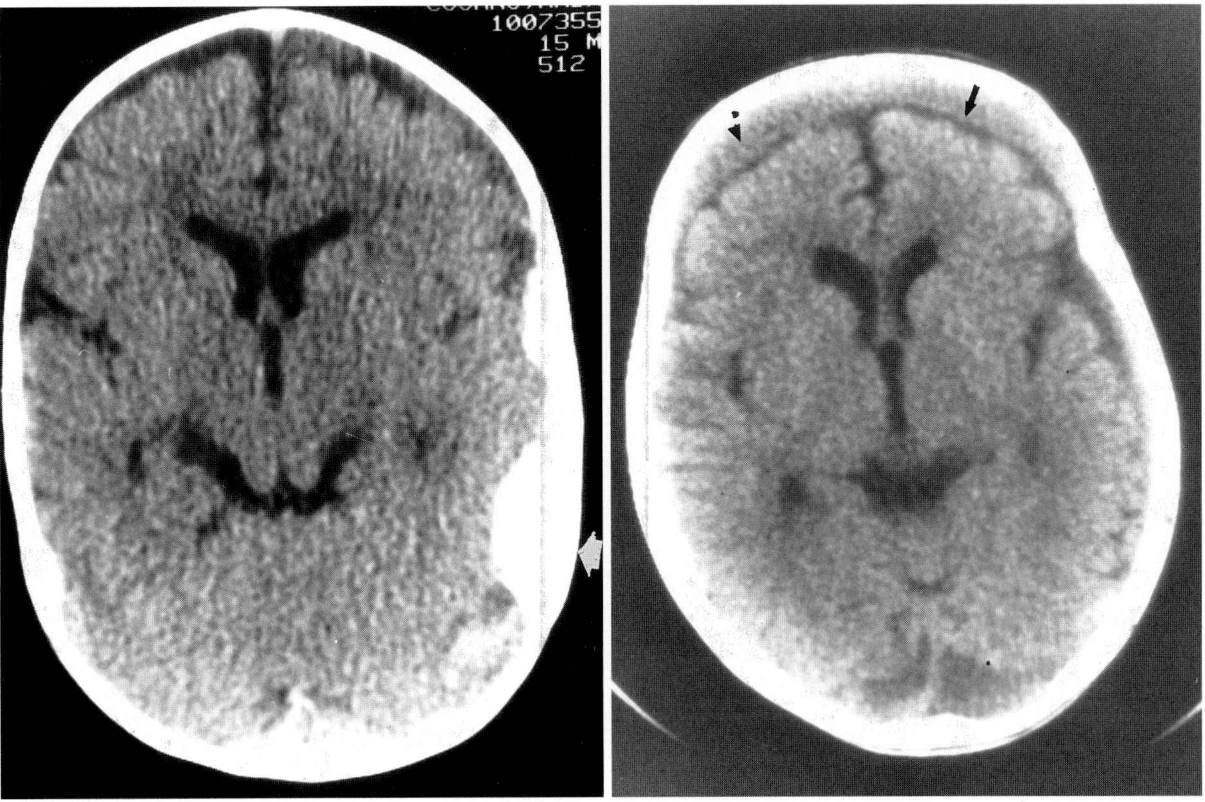

Fig. 8.10 a, b. Subdural and epidural bleeds. **a** Bright white blood is seen on the left lateral aspect of the temporal parietal region (*arrow*). Its medial border (facing the brain) is convex suggesting this represents epidural bleeding. **b** Another child with bilateral frontal collections of increased density (*arrow*) compared to the CSF (see ventricle and subarachnoid space). There are subdural collections which contain old blood. After 7–10 days blood is no longer bright white on CT

Increased Intracranial Pressure or Enlarging Head Circumference

It is easy to evaluate a child with an open fontanelle for increasing intracranial pressure. The fontanelle bulges when the child is in a sitting position, and the child may also exhibit a high-pitched cry and irritability. Prior to fontanelle closure ultrasound evaluation detects ventricular enlargement. Once the fontanelle closes, the sutures may spread before the patient exhibits some of the clinical signs of increased pressure, such as papilledema. Because radiographic signs often precede the clinical clues, you should be familiar with the major plain film radiographic signs of increased intracranial pressure. Remember, however, that a skull film is not the kind of imaging most appropriate to solve this clinical problem.

Spreading of the Cranial Sutures

The coronal suture widens first (due to increased intracranial pressure), but this is often difficult to interpret if it is the only finding. It is important to see all of the sutures widened to accurately diagnose increased intracranial pressure. The lateral view is *not* the best

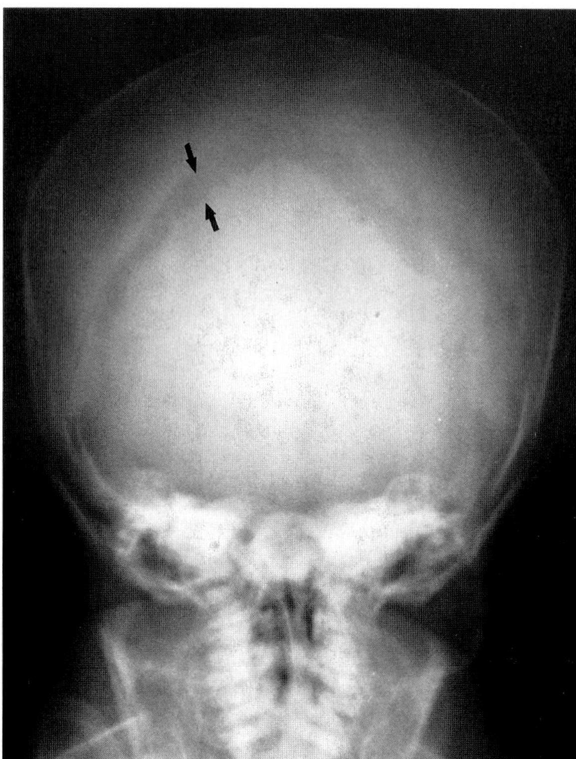

Fig. 8.11. Increased intracranial pressure: spread sutures. Towne's view of the skull shows widening in the region of the sutures (*arrows*). The interdigitations are attempts by the calvarium to bridge the sutural gap. Chronicity of the increased pressure can be judged by the length of the interdigitations

view to determine suture spread, as there may be superimposition of right and left sides; rather, the frontal projections – Towne's or PA – are best (Fig. 8.11). Children with increased intracranial pressure may have spread sutures before papilledema – up to the age of 10–12 years (Bell and McCormick [5] say 12 years, while du Boulay [7] says 10). Remember that in neglected or nutritionally starved children there may be a rebound growth with suture spread as the child recovers. In this instance the sutures are spread, but there is no increased intracranial pressure.

Alterations of the Sella Turcica

The cortical outline of the dorsum sellae may become thinned. This leads to eventual erosion of the dorsum, and it becomes truncated and sharpened. Such changes reflect increased intracranial pressure and are not specific for lesions about the sellae.

Why is there increased intracranial pressure? The differential diagnoses in children include diverse etiologies not considered in adults such as lead encephalopathy, congenitally obstructive hydrocephalus, and congenital arteriovenous malformations such as a vein of Galen malformation. Increased intracranial pressure is of course a major presenting sign in a child with a brain tumor.

The skull film, however, is not the most efficacious imaging test in a child suspected of having increased intracranial pressure; CT or MR (whichever can be obtained more quickly) should be performed to detect the etiology of the increased pressure. Unfortunately, one of the more common causes of increased intracranial pressure is subdural hematoma secondary to child abuse. Not all subdural hematomas are bright on CT (see Fig. 8.10); for this reason, if abuse is suspected, an MR should be obtained at some point to date the hemorrhage (blood and hemosiderin appear differently).

Congenital Abnormalities, Including Congenital Infections

The neonate with an abnormal configuration of the head should be examined radiographically for premature closure of a suture (craniosynostosis, craniostenosis; Fig. 8.12). We are more concerned about the cranial vault than the intracranial contents. The most common suture to close prematurely is the sagittal suture, giving the patient an elongated head from front to back with a palpable bony ridge over the top. Radiographically only a portion of a suture needs to be closed to result in an abnormal cranial configuration (because functionally the entire suture is closed).

In the child with an enlarging head, skull films are not specific. In the young infant ultrasound of the intracranial contents detects congenital anomalies and hydrocephalus (Fig. 8.13), while computerized tomographic studies provide the answer in older children.

The child with a small head may well have one of the congenital infections – the TORCH disease (TO =

Fig. 8.12 a–d. Craniosynostosis (craniostenosis). **a** Lateral view of the skull shows a very long head (scaphocephaly) caused by premature closure of the sagittal suture. **b** Towne's view shows the sagittal suture to be closed (*arrow*). Remember that the suture need not be closed in its entirety but only in one place to cause abnormal head growth. **c** Frontal view in another child reviews asymmetric orbital rims. There is a harlequin eye present on the left (*arrow*) caused by elevation of the greater wing of the sphenoid. This is a manifestation of coronal synostosis. **d** Three-dimensional reconstruction in a child with left coronal synostosis shows that the right coronal suture and sagittal and metopic sutures are open but the left coronal suture is clearly closed. Note again the harlequin eye ▶

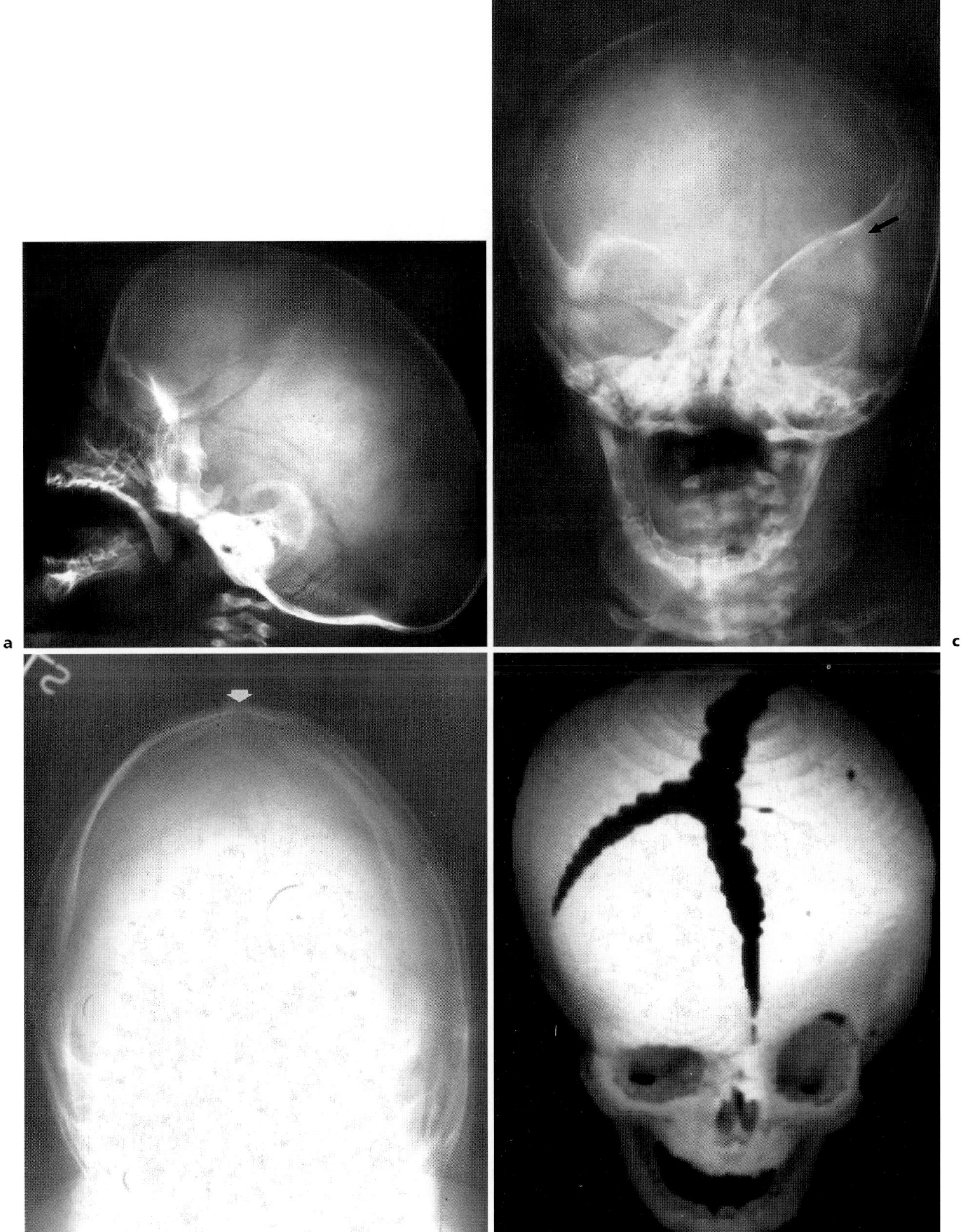
a
b
c
d

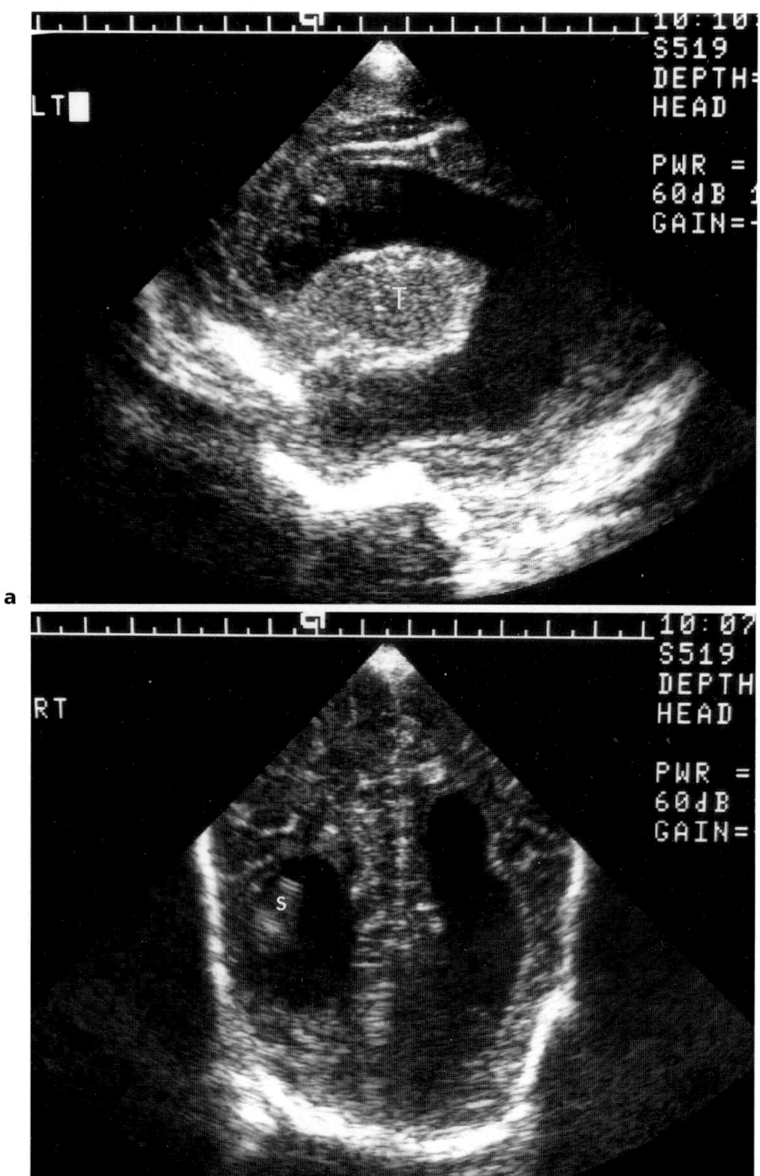

Fig. 8.13 a, b. Ventriculomegaly. **a** Sagittal view of the ventricles shows the thalamus (*T*) and the large lateral ventricles including the frontal, body and temporal horn. The occipital horn is not fully visualized. **b** Coronal scan posterior to the atria shows the large lateral ventricles with a shunt (*S*) present but not functioning

toxoplasmosis, R = rubella, C = cytomegalovirus, H = herpes). While gross calcifications are easy to detect on plain skull films, more subtle calcific deposits are best detected by CT. Contrast is not used when looking for intracranial calcium because calcium is white on CT, and contrast would therefore obscure the findings.

Other Indications for Imaging Evaluation of CNS

These include: (a) new or progressive neurological findings – with CT or MR; (b) work-up of metastatic disease – with both skull films (if this is a primary tumor that commonly goes to bone) and CT or MR (if intracranial metastasis is sought).

Supplementary Procedures in Evaluating the Central Nervous System

Arteriography. One performs arteriography by passing a catheter via the femoral artery to the carotid and/or vertebral arteries (see Chap. 9). The procedure helps map precise arterial anatomy before surgery and is frequently used in tumors to clarify and supplement CT/MR studies for delineating vascular malformations.

MR Angiography. As discussed above, the computer (provided with the correct software) can provide images by MR of the cranial blood vessels (Fig. 8.14).

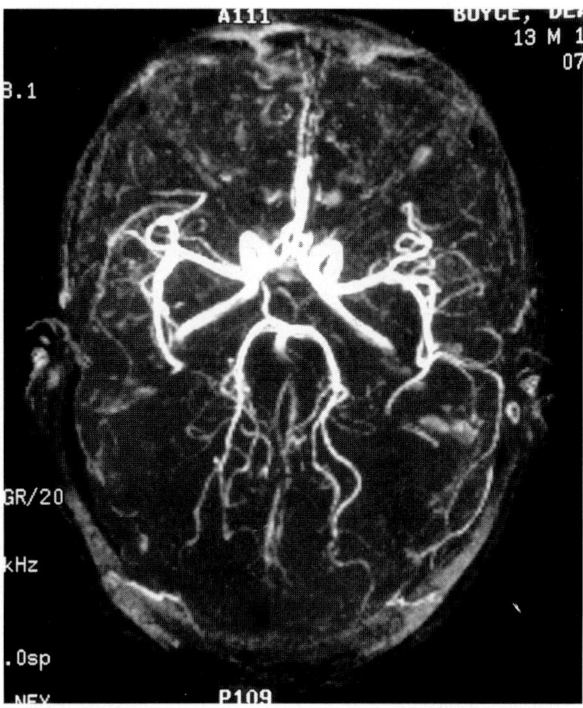

Fig. 8.14. Magnetic resonance angiography. Without the addition of contrast, computer manipulation provided this image showing the anterior cerebral, middle cerebral, and posterior cerebral vessels. This technique is excellent for large vessels but less satisfactory for the smaller vessels

Imaging the Paranasal Sinuses and Neck

The most common head and neck lesions in childhood are those related to infection – paranasal sinusitis, orbital cellulitis, and cervical adenitis. Plain films of the paranasal sinus are notoriously unreliable for diagnosing sinus involvement, except when there is an air fluid level present – a clear sign of sinusitis (Fig. 8.15).

Coronal CT is the best test for evaluating the paranasal sinuses and specifically the osteomeatal complex – the opening of the maxillary sinuses into the nose (Fig. 8.15). Orbital cellulitis most often comes from adjacent paranasal sinus infection. The inflammation may be in front of the attachment of the tarsal plate of the eyelid (preseptal) or behind this attachment (postseptal; Fig. 8.16).

Both CT and MR are excellent for evaluating masses of the neck. When it is important to detect bone involvement, CT should be carried out. The most common mass is lymphadenopathy, while the most common malignant soft tissue tumor of the neck in childhood is rhabdomyosarcoma.

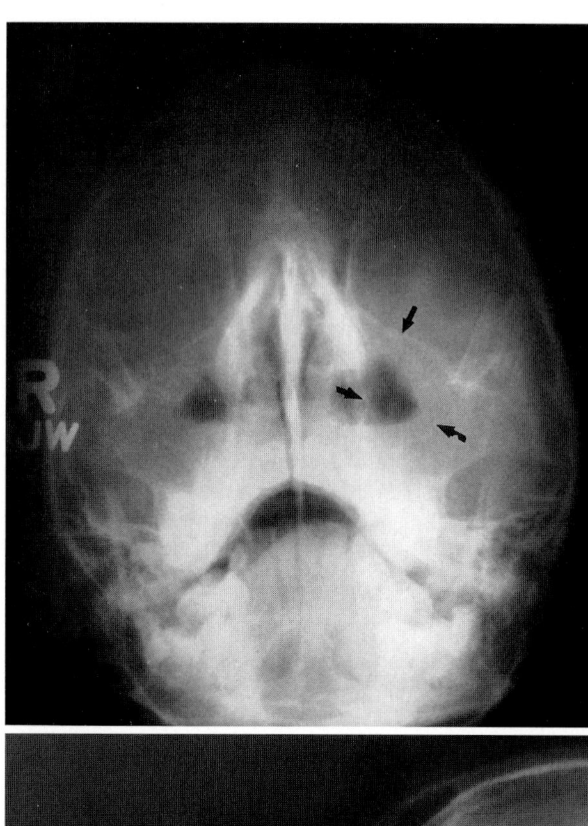

a

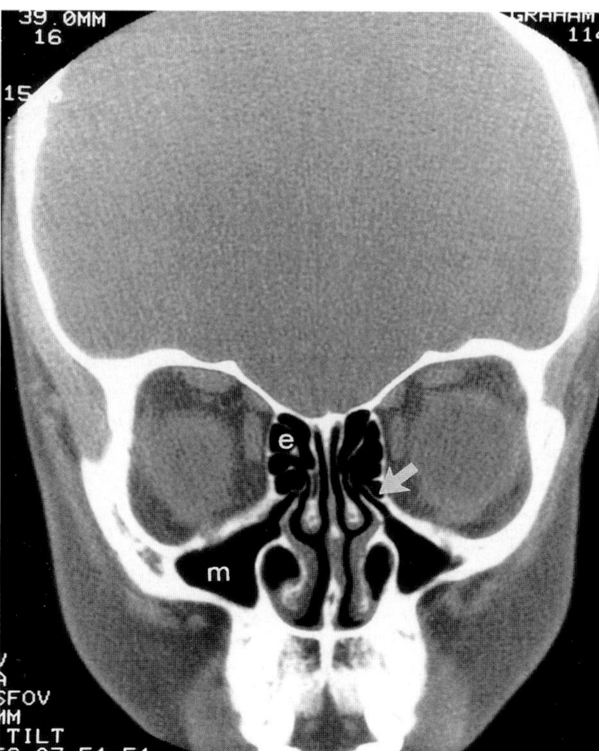

c

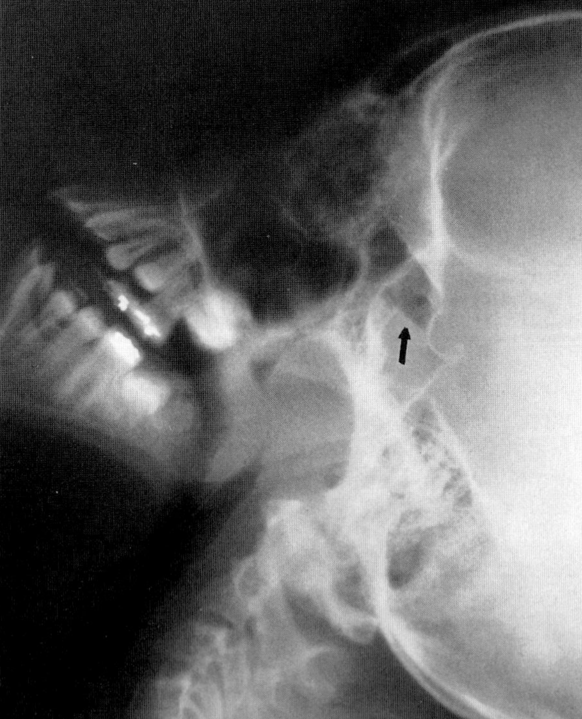

b

Fig. 8.15 a–c. Acute sinusitis on plain films. **a** Waters' view in the erect position shows bilateral air-fluid levels in the maxillary sinus. Note the walls of the maxillary sinus (*arrows*) and how much of the sinus is filled with fluid. The black areas are the residual air (compare to Fig. 8.5). **b** Sphenoid sinus air-fluid level (*arrow*) in this erect lateral film. What other abnormalities do you see? There is a large amount of adenoid tissue present obscuring the nasopharyngeal air passage. **c** Coronal CT for the paranasal sinuses (technique includes bone windows, 3 mm thick, low kilovoltage) shows the maxillary (*m*) and ethmoid (*e*) sinuses to advantage. Other views show the frontal and sphenoid sinuses. The osteomeatal complex is composed of the opening (the ostia, *arrow*) and the passage into the middle naris (infundibulum and hiatus semilunaris)

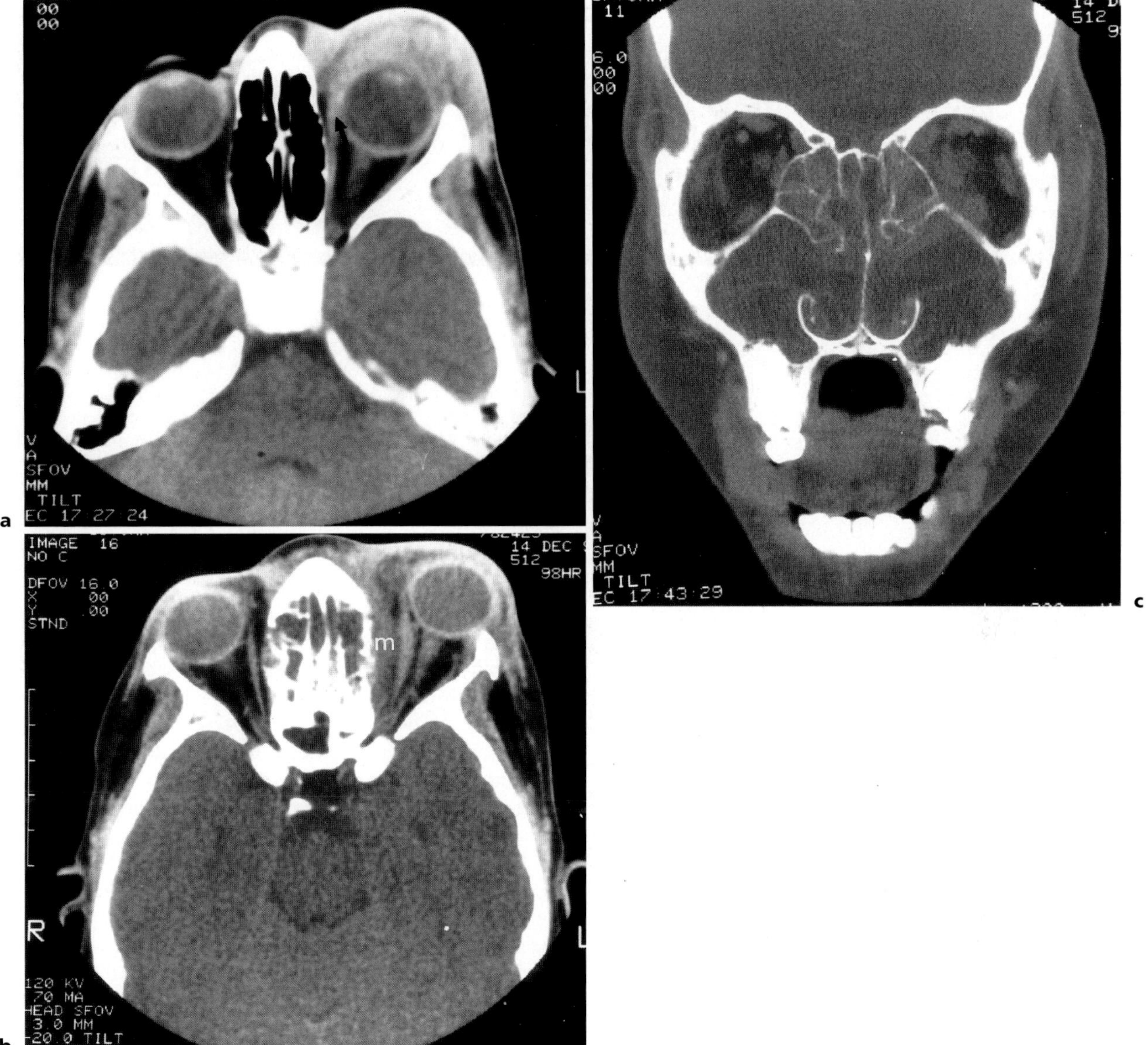

Fig. 8.16 a–c. Orbital cellulitis. **a** Left preseptal cellulitis with soft tissue swelling anterior to the tarsal plate (*arrow*). **b** Left postseptal cellulitis with debris deviating the medial rectus (*m*) laterally. There is soft tissue density between the nose and the medial rectus which is the inflammatory process. Note that the eye is pushed forward (proptosis). The ethmoid air cells are opacified. **c** Coronal CT of the sinuses in the same child as in **b**. There is complete opacification of the maxillary and ethmoidal sinuses. On other views sphenoidal and frontal sinuses were also opacified. Compare this figure to Fig. 8.15

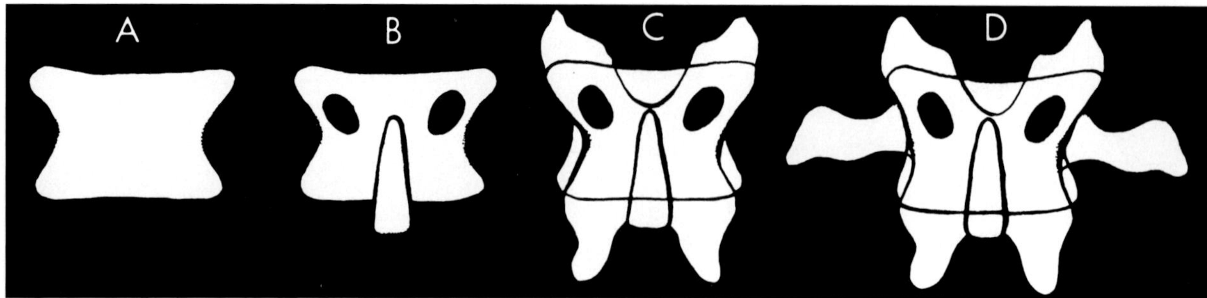

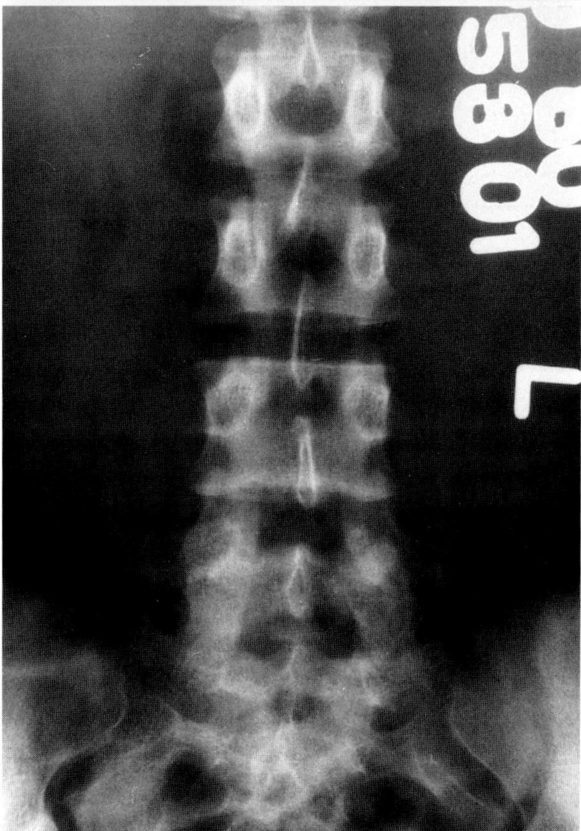

Fig. 8.17. a Schematic diagram explains the various structures and how they contribute to the final product. *A*, Vertebral body; *B*, vertebral body plus pedicles in black and spinous process; *C*, superior-inferior articulating facets have been added; *D*, transverse process. **b** Frontal view of the lumbar spine. What is wrong with L5? (See "Appendix 2")

Fig. 8.18 a–d. Lateral cervical spine. **a** Normal lateral cervical spine. *Dots*, normal spinal curve. **b–d** Can you identify the abnormalities? (see "Appendix 2")

Spine

Anatomy

The complexities of and differences among the cervical, thoracic, lumbar, and sacral segments are beyond the scope of this text; but knowledge of the general configuration of the bony anatomy is crucial (Fig. 8.17). The two major views of the spine are the frontal and lateral. It is important to identify (a) the vertebral bodies, (b) the disc spaces between vertebral bodies, (c) the posterior elements, and (d) the spinous processes. The vertebral bodies become larger in a cephalic-to-caudal direction. The ring epiphyses are best seen at the corner of the vertebral bodies on the lateral view.

The alignment of the bony spine is crucial in the radiographic diagnosis of trauma or scoliosis. This is especially true with the cervical spine; lines drawn from C1 through C7 along the anterior aspects of the vertebral bodies, posterior aspects of the vertebral bodies, and anterior aspects of the spinous processes should slope gently without sharp disruption (Fig. 8.18). Any abnormality in these lines suggests displacement. The exception is the pseudosubluxation of C2 and C3 due to the generalized laxity of ligaments in the infant. On the frontal projection, look for disruption of the vertebral bodies, transverse processes or pedicles, as well as paraspinal masses. The vertebral bodies are most frequently disrupted by infection or tumor, while the pedicles are disrupted by intraspinal processes. The pedicle is that portion of bone that borders the lateral aspect of the spinal cord and subarachnoid space. The medial aspects of the pedicles are convex; straightening of concavity of these pedicles denotes a lesion within the subarachnoid space or spinal cord. The transverse processes are most frequently affected by traumatic lesions.

We frequently ask questions about the spinal cord itself and not about the bony covering. Here MR is clearly the best test (Fig. 8.19). The entire spine can be visualized and the level of the conus medullaris demonstrated (normal T12-L2). The conus medullaris is the most inferior level of the spinal cord, with the nerve roots extending distally. Any intraspinal fluid collections (syrinx) or tumors will be seen (CT myelography currently is marginally better than MR for detecting metastasis). Swelling of the cord, traumatic lesions, and bleeding are all best detected by MR.

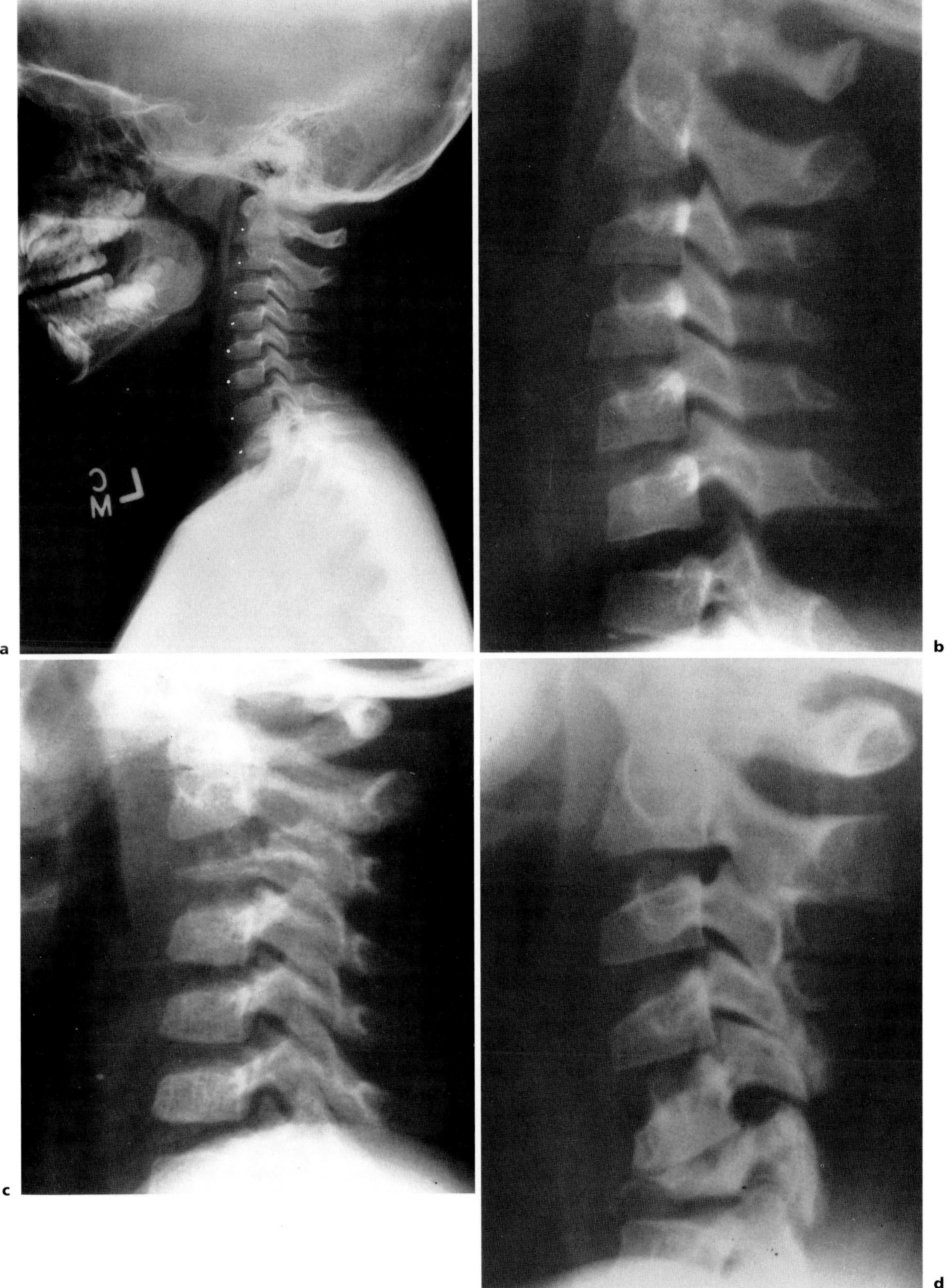

a b c d

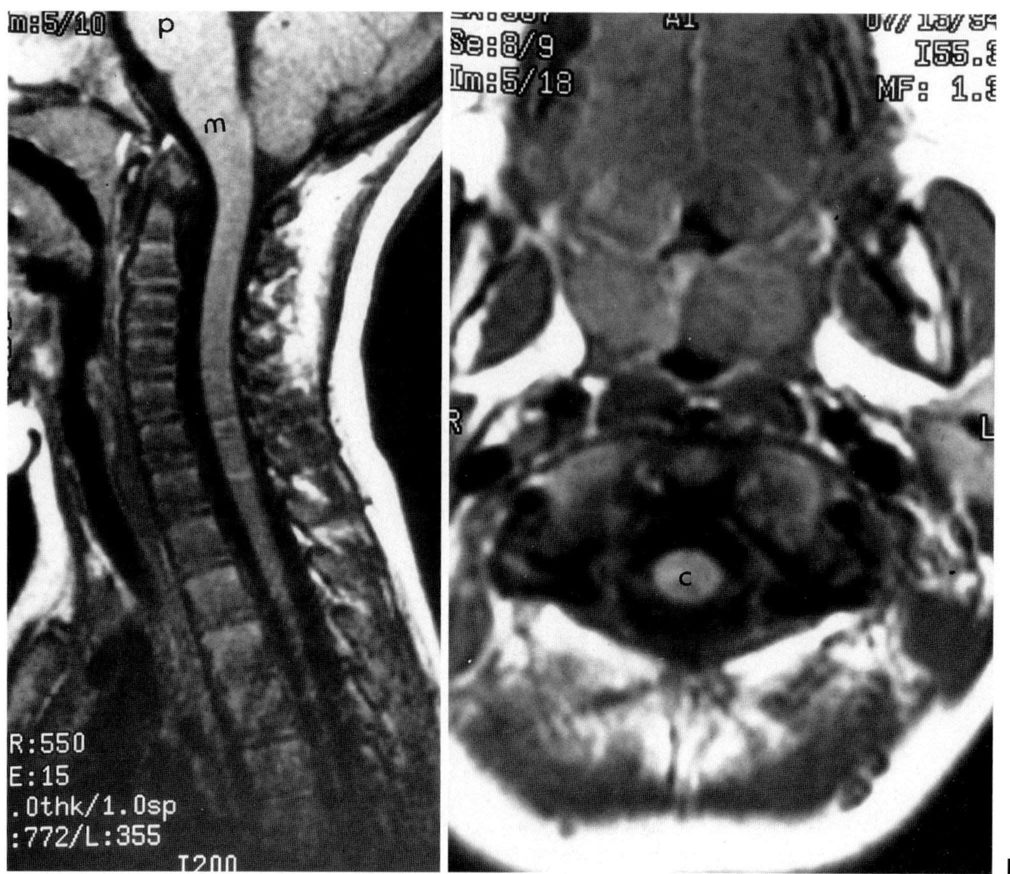

Fig. 8.19 a–f. Normal MR of the spine. **a** Lateral midline section with T1 imaging reveals the pons (*P*), the medulla (*M*), and the spinal cord. The bony vertebral bodies in this sequence are less distinct. Note that the cervical spinal cord fills less than 80% of the canal. **b** Axial section of the same child shows the cervical spinal cord (*c*) normally positioned. **c** Axial section of the thoracic spinal cord at the apex of the lung shows that the cord (*c*) is slightly smaller than that in **b** and is well positioned without mass. **d** Sagittal section of the thoracic and lumbar cord show the conus at T12-L1. The cord (*c*) is normal in position and shape. **e** Axial section at the level of the kidneys show the size of the cord relative to the vertebral bodies. *k*, Kidney. **f** Utilizing a technique called gradient imaging, sagittal section of the thoracic and lumbar spine show the disc spaces (*white*) and the vertebral bodies (*gray*). The spinal cord is less well seen on these images but the subarachnoid fluid is white, giving a myelographic effect

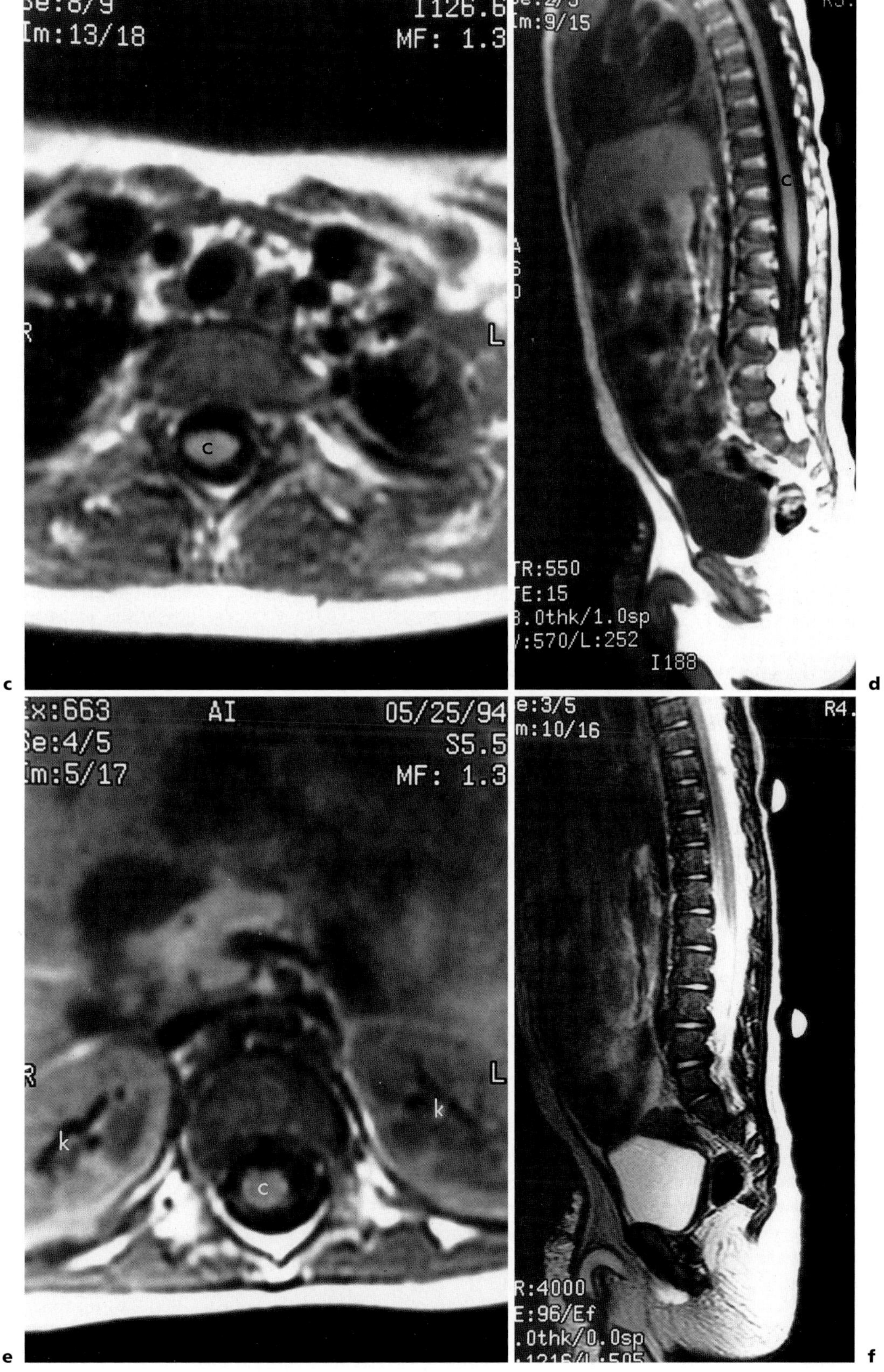
Se:8/9
Im:13/18
I126.6
MF: 1.3
R
L
C
Se:2/5
Im:9/15
R3.
C
A
S
D
TR:550
TE:15
3.0thk/1.0sp
V:570/L:252
I188
c
d
Ex:663
AI
05/25/94
Se:4/5
S5.5
Im:5/17
MF: 1.3
R
L
k
k
c
e:3/5
m:10/16
R4.
R:4000
E:96/Ef
.0thk/0.0sp
e
f

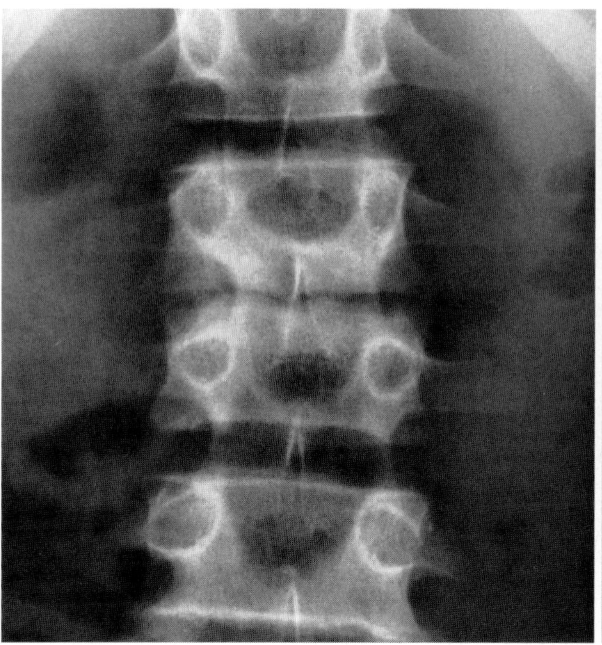

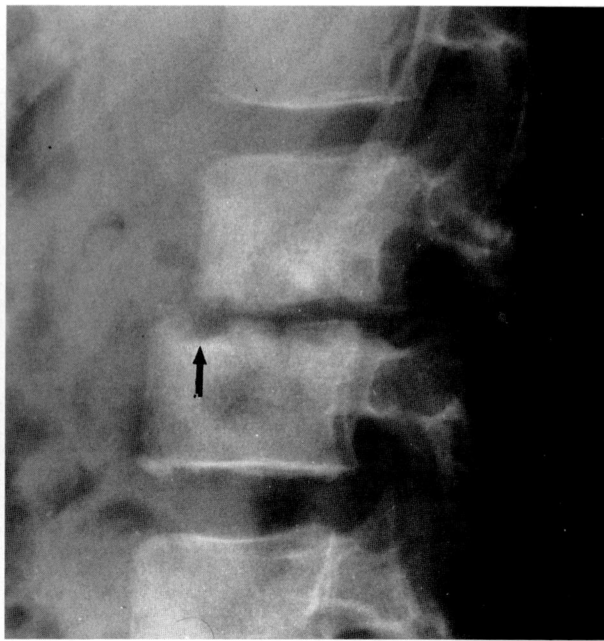

Fig. 8.20 a, b. Herniation of the nucleus pulposus: Schmorl's node. **a** Frontal view of the lumbar spine reveals narrowed disk space between L2 and L3 with irregular margins. **b** Lateral view shows the narrow disk space and the large AP diameter of L3. The anterior defect (*arrow*) is the site where the nucleus pulposus has herniated and disrupted the ring epiphysis of the vertebral body

Fig. 8.21a–e. What are these abnormalities? (See "Appendix 2") ▶

Indications for Imaging Evaluation of the Spine

The initial evaluation remains the frontal and lateral plain film, most often supplemented by oblique views and specific odontoid films if the cervical spine is to be evaluated. The major indication for this procedure is trauma. Other reasons for spinal imaging include patients with back pain (an unusual complaint in childhood), weakness of lower extremities or gait problems, unusual bladder or bowel complaints (specifically of a regressive nature), or diseases that involve metastasis to the spine. Unusual curvatures of the spine (scoliosis) and congenital anomalies of the spine (spinal dysraphism, meningomyelocele) are diseases in which the nature of the spinal cord itself is important to evaluate. In these instances, MR is necessary.

A specific abnormality seen in teenagers is herniation of the nucleus pulposus – Schmorl's node – from its normal position in the center of the disk. This herniation may occur in any direction. When anterior, it may displace the ring epiphysis of the vertebral body, leaving the corners apparently "compressed" and the disc space narrowed (Fig. 8.20). The occurrence of this at multiple levels is called Scheuermann's disease, although many children with this roentgenographic finding are asymptomatic.

What are the abnormalities in Fig. 8.21?

References

1. Silverman FN (1993) Caffey's pediatric X-ray diagnosis, 9th edn. Mosby, St. Louis
2. Hayman LA, Hinck OC (1992) Clinical brain injury. Mosby-Year Book, Chicago
3. Harwood-Nash DC, Hendrick EB, Hudson AR (1971) The significance of skull fractures in children – A study of 1,187 patients. Radiology 101:151
4. Keats TE (1992) An atlas of normal roentgen variants, 5th edn. Year Book Medical, Chicago
5. Swischuk LE (1989) Imaging of the newborn, infant and young child. 3rd edn. Williams and Wilkins, Baltimore
6. Christenson PC (1977) The radiologic study of the normal spine: cervical, thoracic, lumbar, and sacral. Radiol Clin North Am 15:133–154
7. Bell WE, McCormick WF (1978) Increased intracranial pressure in children, 2nd edn. Saunders, Philadelphia
8. du Boulay GH (1980) Principles of X-ray diagnosis of the skull, 2nd edn., Butterworth, London
9. Gooding CA (1971) Cranial sutures and fontanelles. In: Newton TM, Potts DC, (eds) Radiology of the skull and brain. Mosby, St. Louis

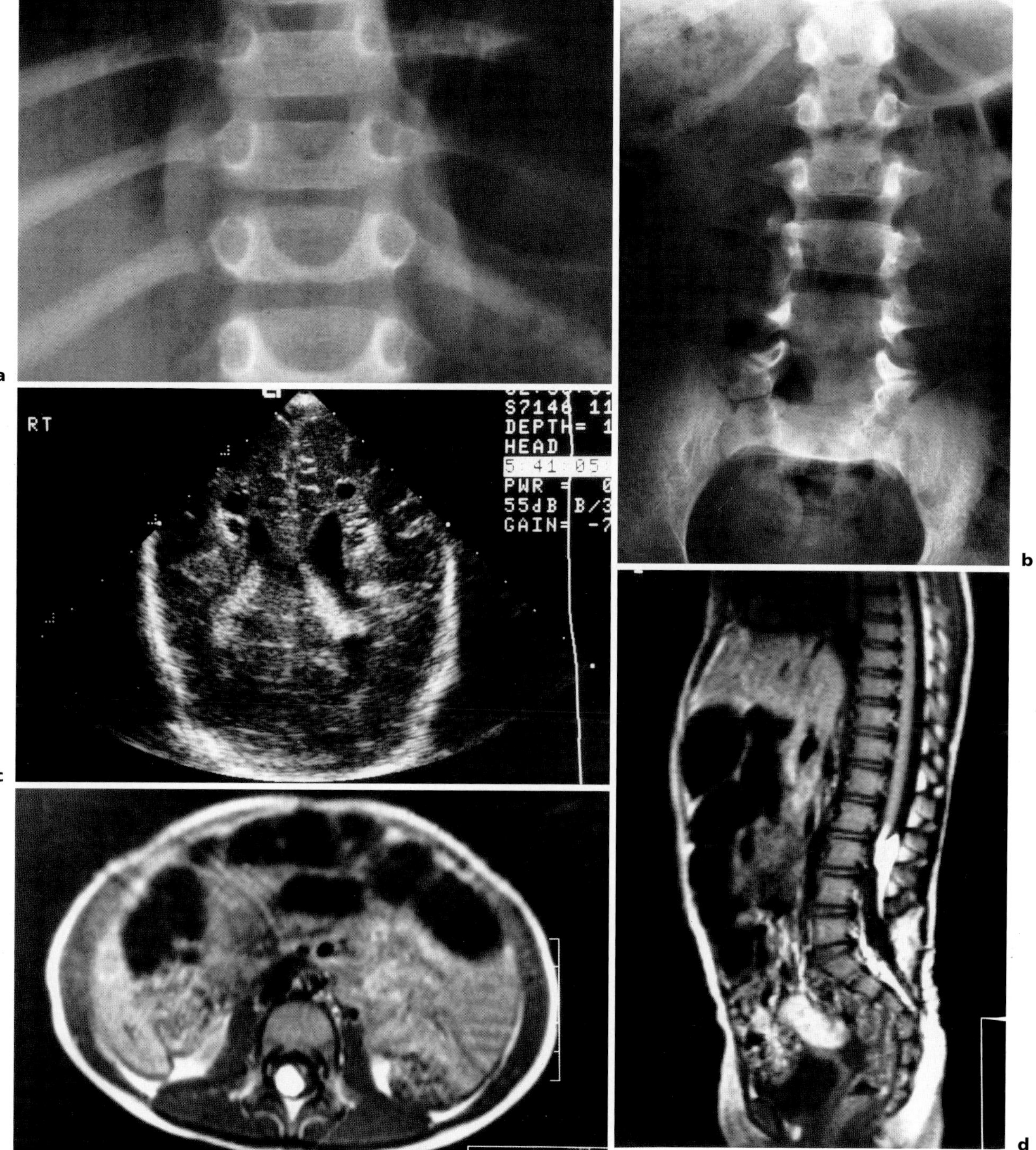
a
RT
S7146 11
DEPTH= 1
HEAD
5 41 05
PWR = 0
55dB B/3
GAIN= -7
b
c
d
e

9 Special Procedures

The first eight chapters of this volume discuss common pediatric imaging procedures. This chapter deals with the less common, frequently more invasive procedures. The more invasive the procedure is, the greater the number of people needed and the more physician-intense the environment. The pediatric imager has become very involved with sedation and monitoring practices of the child. This chapter progresses from less invasive to more invasive procedures.

Techniques to Further Evaluate the Airway

Magnification high-kilovoltage radiography is a noninvasive, useful procedure to delineate the upper airway, trachea, and major bronchi. This technique is most useful for children with stridor, choking, suspected foreign body, vascular ring, and intratracheal mass. An exquisite view is obtained (by using a Thoraeus filter to selectively screen out low-kilovoltage radiation) by increasing the kilovoltage and magnifying the child's airway. Many of the pictures of the airway shown in Chap. 2 and 3 were imaged using this technique. This technique has, for the most part, obviated the more invasive tracheogram, where contrast was instilled into the trachea and pictures obtained. The magnification high-kilovoltage technique can be used without sedation and with relatively little radiation.

CT, as shown in Chap. 2, can show the bronchi quite well. However, a bronchogram is occasionally necessary to demonstrate the more distal airways primarily for confirmation of bronchiectasis or to demonstrate obstructed or stenosed bronchus. For this procedure contrast medium is injected at the carina or selectively into one bronchus. After the contrast has been injected, the patient is tilted into various positions to fill the appropriate segmental bronchi.

Arthrography

In most instances in children MRI has replaced the need for arthrography (Fig. 9.1). However, in a child with a question of an acutely infected joint who needs to have his joint fluid cultured, arthrography is frequently performed to document that the fluid was obtained from the joint. This is done by percutaneous installation of water-soluble contrast material into the joint allowing visualization of the cartilaginous articular surfaces. This can be followed with CT if necessary. In addition to cases of acute joint infection, arthrography may be useful in evaluation of traumatic joint injury.

Sialography

Opacification of the salivary ducts and glands by injecting contrast medium into the ostium (opening) of the duct is usually performed to investigate a mass. The parotid gland is the one most often studied by this method. Injection of the duct is performed with digital subtraction images followed in certain cases by CT, as CT gives a more complete evaluation of the gland (Fig. 9.2).

Angiographic Procedures

Angiography, a contrast study of vessels, remains the gold standard against which to measure less invasive techniques, such as color-flow Doppler sonography, nuclear flow studies, magnetic resonance angiography and, now with the helical scanners, CT angiography (Figs. 9.3, 9.4). Today no more than 100–150 diagnostic angiographic procedures are performed in the course of a year in a busy children's hospital; 85% of these are of the head and neck.

Arteriography (a contrast study of the arteries) is performed by percutaneously placing a needle followed by a guidewire through the needle into the artery. The needle is removed and a catheter is placed over the guidewire. The technique is called the

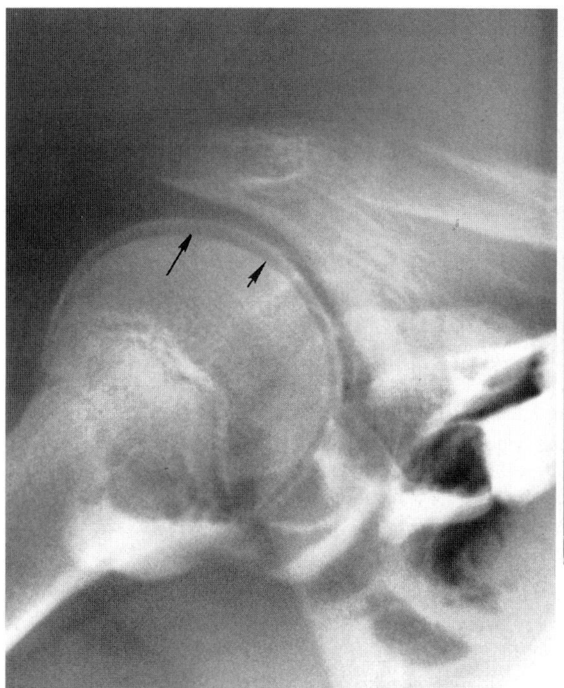

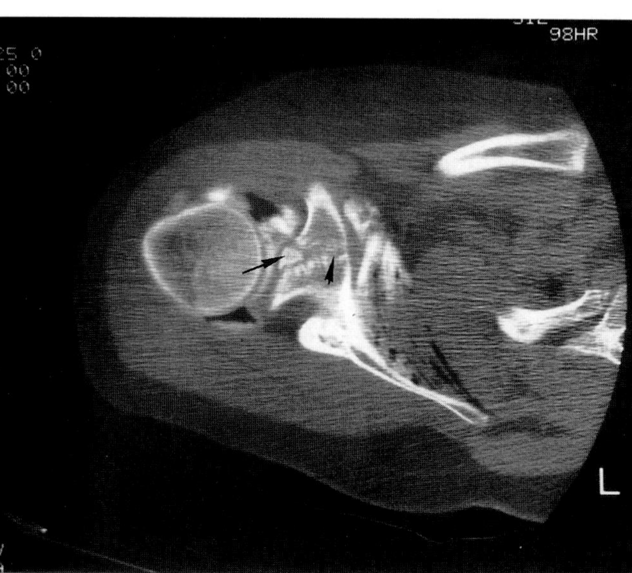

Fig. 9.1 a, b. Arthrography in a patient who sustained a traumatic shoulder injury. **a** Upright double contrast (both air and contrast were inserted) arthrogram of the right shoulder reveals normal cartilaginous covering of the humeral head (*arrows*; *black*, cartilage). However, it is difficult to evaluate the glenoid fossa on this view. Therefore CT is carried out after the arthrogram. **b** CT of the same shoulder reveals triangular fragment of bone (*arrow*) and linear fracture of the glenoid (*arrowhead*). The contrast (*white*) outlines the separation of the cartilaginous portion of the glenoid from the humeral head. Note that this glenoid fracture has not destroyed the cartilaginous cap

Seldinger method and is utilized in both arteriography and venography. Most often this occurs via the femoral artery, and the catheter is then placed in the appropriate area to be studied.

In children arteriography is used to clarify central nervous system problems and less commonly for peripheral or visceral angiography. Some of the indications for the pediatric use of peripheral angiography are:

- Trauma: evaluation of a limb secondary to an injury for vascular patency and occasionally in the abdomen to demonstrate a torn vessel or lacerated viscera. CT of the abdomen has generally replaced angiography.
- Renal hypertension: this allows for the evaluation of the main and segmental renal arteries to detect stenosis (Fig. 9.4). In addition, venography is used for renal vein sampling for renin concentration.
- In tumors where limited resection is contemplated: this occurs in children with bilateral renal masses or hepatic masses.

Currently almost all angiography is done by the digital subtraction technique mentioned in Chap. 1. This has allowed for diminished use of radiation, better resolution, and refinement of the pictures.

A major advance in the past several years has been therapeutic angiography; this is described in the next section on interventional radiography.

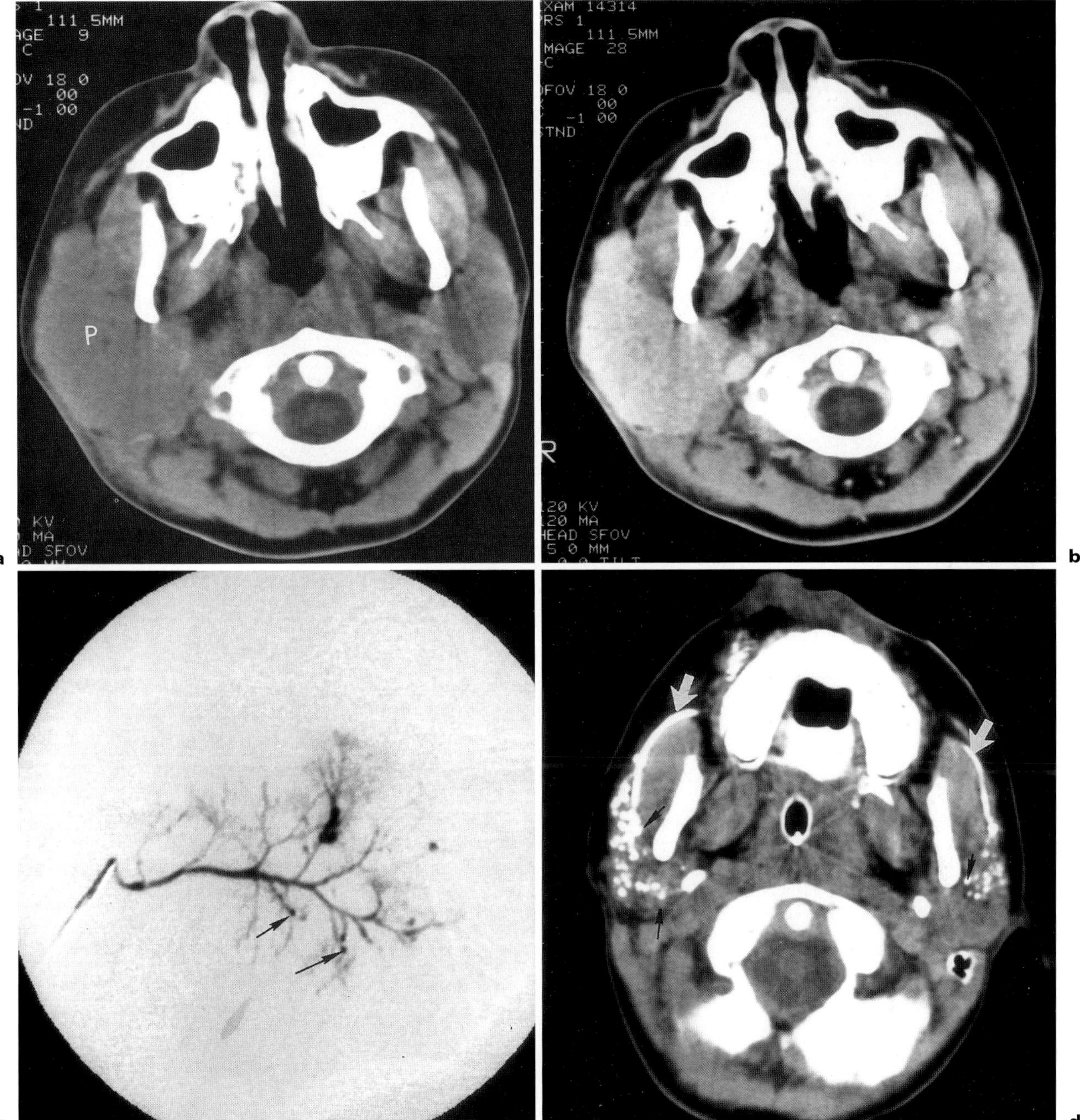

Fig. 9.2 a–d. Sialography. **a** Noncontrast CT of the parotid region shows uniformly enlarged right parotid gland (*P*) without calcification. **b** Enhanced CT (IV contrast) of the same region shows uniform enhancement of the gland similar in density to the opposite side. There is no focal region of abnormality. **c** Injection of the parotid duct on the affected side reveals no obstruction but small beaded areas of sialectasis (*arrows*). This represents chronic inflammation. **d** CT of another child after bilateral injection of Stensen's duct (the duct to the parotid gland; *white arrows*). There are multiple, small, white collections which represent sialectasis (*arrows*)

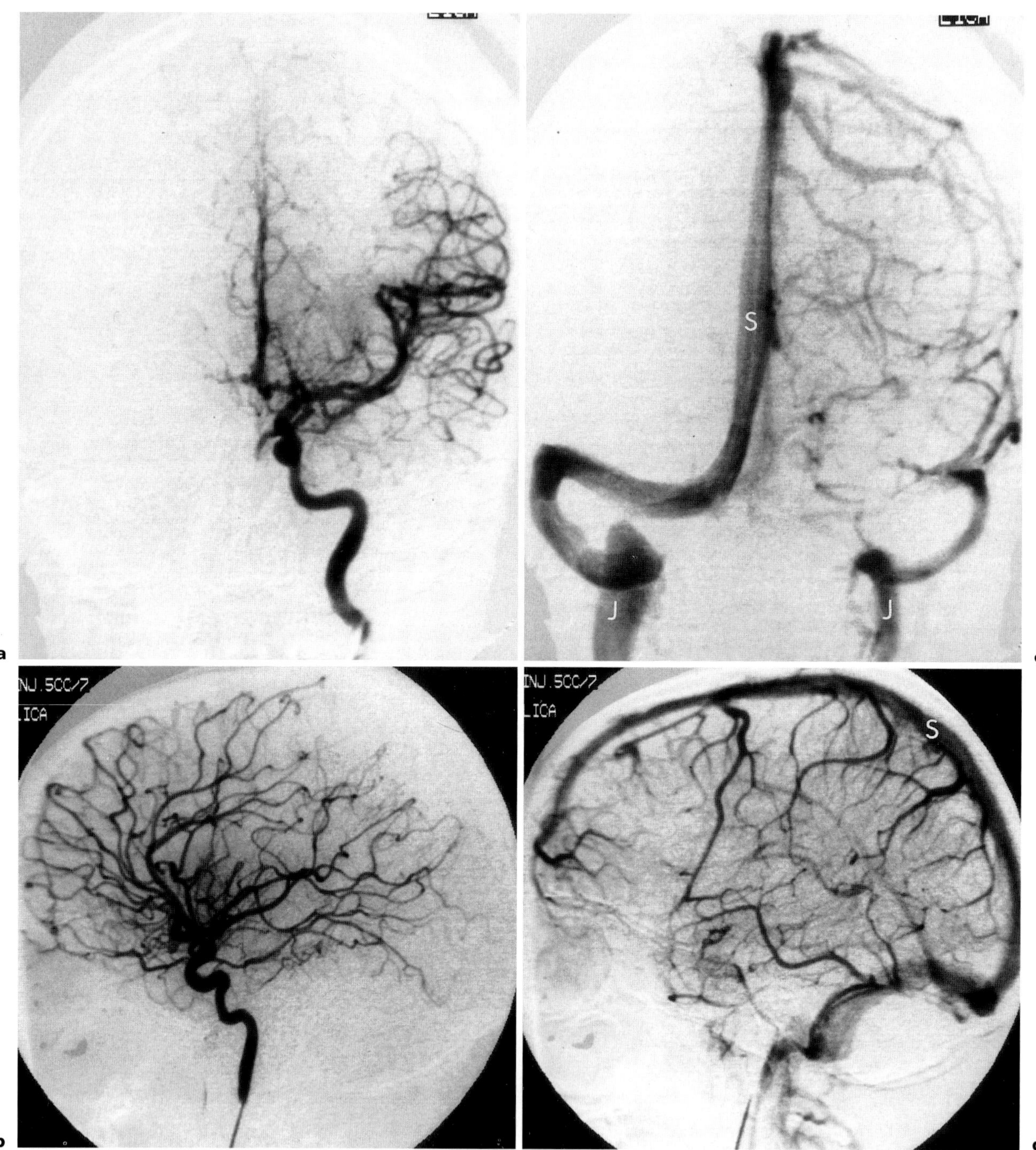

Fig. 9.3 a–d. Cerebral arteriogram. **a** Left internal carotid artery injection visualized in the AP projection reveals the middle and anterior cerebral arteries and their branches. **b** Same patient lateral view shows the normal vascular structures. **c** Venous phase of this same injection. This AP view shows contrast returning to the heart via the superior sagittal sinus (*S*) and eventually into the jugular vein (*J*). This patient demonstrates a normal variant – although we performed a left-sided injection – the predominant venous drainage is to the right. **d** Lateral view of the venous phase shows both deep and superficial venous drainage

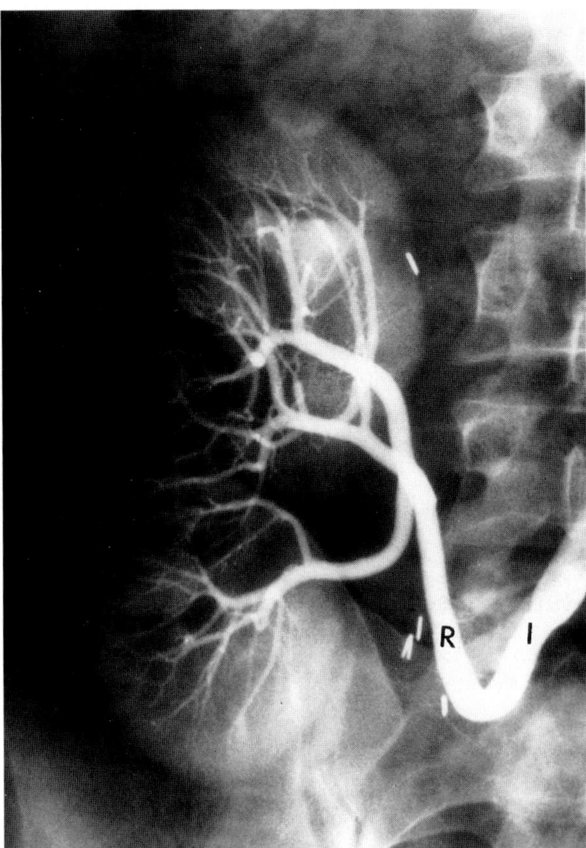

Fig. 9.4. Visceral angiogram. Arterial injection of a transplanted kidney showing the anastomosis of the renal artery (*R*) to the right iliac (*I*) artery. There is no stenosis of the major renal branches. This child was being evaluated for posttransplant hypertension

Interventional Radiography

Interventional radiography allows the radiologist to play a role in both the diagnosis and treatment of a problem. The interventional team consists of physicians, nurses, and technologists, with consultants such as the anesthesiologist and surgeon. The pediatric radiologist must become familiar with the various sedation techniques, and in most instances nonvascular intervention can be performed using intravenous sedation. Vascular intervention more frequently requires general anesthesia.

Intervention can be divided into two groups: vascular and nonvascular. "Vascular intervention is an extension of diagnostic angiography" [1]. Indications for the use of vascular interventional techniques in pediatrics are [1]:

- Embolization, neurological
  - Spinal or intracranial arteriovenous malformation
  - Cavernous carotid fistula
  - Preoperative reduction of vascularity
  - Vein of Galen malformation
  - Wada's test
  - Test occlusion prior to surgery
- Embolization, head and neck
  - Treatment of arteriovenous malformation or other vascular malformation
  - Hypervascular tumor prior to surgery, e.g., juvenile angiofibroma
  - Preoperative control of a vascular territory
  - Chemoinfusion for unresectable tumor
- Embolization, body
  - Bronchial artery, e.g., hemoptysis, unwanted collaterals
  - Upper gastrointestinal bleed
  - Postoperative or postbiopsy bleeding
  - Vascular malformation
  - Reduction in tumor vascularity, e.g., hemangioendothelioma, preoperative
  - Partial splenic bleeding
- Percutaneous transluminal angioplasty
  - Renovascular hypertension
  - Symptomatic vascular stenosis
- Fibrinolysis
  - Neonatal aortorenal occlusion
  - Access shunts
  - Miscellaneous
- Stent replacement
  - Resistent vascular stenosis
- Placement of vena caval filter
- Recurrent pulmonary emboli

Embolization procedures are performed to diminish flow to a tumor or to close off a vascular malformation. It is now possible routinely for skilled interventionalists to canalize 1- to 2-mm vessels. Percutaneous transluminal angioplasty is an endovascular approach utilized to dilate the vessel of patients with symptomatic narrowing of vessels.

Nonvascular interventional procedures include the following [1]):

- Genitourinary intervention
  - Percutaneous nephrostomy
  - Drainage of perirenal fluid collections
  - Dilation of strictures
  - Stent placement
  - Percutaneous surgical techniques: (a) stone removal, (b) pyeloplasty (endopyelotomy)
  - Renal biopsy
  - Whitaker perfusion test
  - Antegrade pyelogram
- Gastrointestional intervention
  - Esophageal foreign body removal
  - Magnetic foreign body removal
  - Balloon dilation of enteric structures: (a) esophageal, (b) colonic
  - Percutaneous gastrostomy and gastroenterostomy
  - Nasojejunostomy
  - Hydrostatic reduction of intussusception
  - Abscess drainage
  - Aspiration of fluid collections for diagnosis
  - Biopsy of abdominal and retroperitoneal masses
  - Percutaneous transhepatic cholangiography
  - Biliary drainage
  - Dilation and stenting of biliary strictures
  - Percutaneous cholecystotomy
- Thoracic intervention
  - Biopsy of pulmonary, pleural, chest wall masses, bone, and/or soft tissue lesions, etc.
  - Drainage of mediastinal, pulmonary, and loculated pleural collections
  - Balloon dilation of tracheobronchial strictures

Placement of catheters to relieve obstruction, needles to biopsy lesions so that preoperative therapy can occur, and tubes in the stomach or jejunum percutaneously to enhance nourishment are the common procedures in pediatric intervention. Once a tube has been placed, the patient may become the radiologist's patient since whenever the tube is obstructed or falls out, it needs to be replaced.

Of course, one of the more common and oldest procedures carried out by the interventionalist is abscess drainage. Nonvascular interventional techniques can be performed under sonographic, CT or fluoroscopic guidance, and this depends on the preference of the interventionalist. The use of both vascular and nonvascular interventional techniques has helped decrease hospital stay, lower patient cost, and greatly diminished the morbidity of sick children.

Reference

Towbin R (1992) Interventional procedures in pediatrics. Semin Pediatr Surg 1:296–307

Appendix 1: Reed's Rules

- ▶ 1. On every chest film, read the abdominal portion as you would read an abdominal film.
- ▶ 2. Knowledge of anatomy is the key to correct radiographic diagnosis.
- ▶ 3. The airway should be visible on all normal chest films.
- ▶ 4. A mass must be seen in two planes.
- ▶ 5. An esophagram must be performed in any child with unexplained respiratory disease.
- ▶ 6. In unilateral hyperexpansion of the lungs, you must see how the air moves. Mediastinal position is critical to this determination.
- ▶ 7. Always review all old films to properly assess the new one. Subtle findings can easily be missed when a single previous examination is reviewed.
- ▶ 8. The abdominal examination should include a minimum of three views: supine, prone and erect.
- ▶ 9. On every abdominal examination, evaluate the chest as if you were looking at a chest film.
- ▶ 10. In obstruction of the lumen, there should be proximal distention.
- ▶ 11. During intravenous urography, continue to take films as long as they provide needed information.
- ▶ 12. Try to find the effects of the mass on adjacent organs on each abdominal film. Draw the mass, if necessary.
- ▶ 13. After the mass has been defined, find the center of the lesion. Then consider all structures, gross and microscopic, near the center of the lesion as possible sources of the mass. Think skin to skin.
- ▶ 14. The periosteum is normally not seen.
- ▶ 15. When viewing an extremity, try to imagine the appearance of the patient. An excellent example is bowed legs or knock knees.

Appendix 2: Answers to Questions

Chapter 2

Fig. 2.6. The patient in **b** is rotated to the left. The heart is appreciably in the left hemithorax, and the left side of the chest is relatively elongated, as compared to the right. The reverse is true in **a**. In **b** there are basilar opacities.

Fig. 2.24. Acute epiglottitis. In **a** is a 3-year-old with respiratory distress. The chest is normal, but the lateral neck shows an enlarged epiglottis and arytenoepiglottic folds.

Fig. 2.48. Unusual pulmonary densities. Frontal radiograph of the chest reveals cardiomegaly and increased vascularity. When one looks through the gas in the right midabdomen, gallstones are seen. This patient had sickle cell disease.

Fig. 2.49. A child with onset of acute respiratory distress. Frontal (**a**) and lateral (**b**) films. Did you notice the white, linear density along the right heart border? A pin was removed from the right main stem bronchus.

Fig. 2.50. This 18-year-old male has chronic lung disease. In **a** an acute onset of right chest pain. The frontal examination shows a large pneumothorax with the inability of the lung to collapse because of the chronic lung disease. Careful attention shows cystic changes at the apex. In **b** CT of that area shows the blebs and also the chronic bronchiectatic changes throughout both right and left lungs.

Fig. 2.51. A child with a cough. In **a** frontal examination reveals a large density extending to the left paraspinal line behind the heart. Its borders are convex laterally suggesting an extrapleural mass. In **b**, on the lateral view, the mass is difficult to see. The vertebral bodies are whiter inferiorly than they are superiorly, indicating disease in the posterior aspect of the hemithorax. This was a ganglioneuroblastoma.

Fig. 2.52. A child with wheezing. In **a** the frontal radiograph shows the distal airway pushed to the left; the carina is not adjacent to the right pedicles. In **b** the lateral film reveals the airway bowed forward and slightly narrowed. In **c** the frontal view of a barium swallow shows the right and left indentations on the esophagus. In **d** the lateral views reveal a bulge behind the esophagus and some narrowing and bowing of the airway. The patient has a vascular ring, specifically a double aortic arch.

Chapter 3

Magnification of the chest occurs because of the portable technique. There is an apparent "large cardiomediastinal silhouette" because the tube-to-film distance is only 36–40 in. Since the child is supine, the vascularity of the upper and lower lungs is equal.

Chapter 4

Fig. 4.34. CT of the upper abdomen shows a large pancreas (at center of image) and a fluid-filled mass in the body. These findings are consistent with a pancreatic pseudocyst.

Fig. 4.35. An infant with abdominal distention. In **a** the supine film reveals air-filled bowel within the inguinal canals. These are bilateral inguinal hernias. (The two circles of air near the femoral necks.)

Fig. 4.36. Panel **a**, abdominal pain after trauma. A plain film of the abdomen was unremarkable. Contrast was given by mouth, and there was an abrupt change in the size and contour of the duodenum in its horizontal portion. The wall is effaced, that is, the mucosal pattern is stretched over a submucosal mass. Panel **b**, CT of the same child, shows the same portion of duodenum (see dark gray area at about 11 o'clock from vertebral body) with a low density, soft tissue mass – the duodenal hematoma.

Fig. 4.37. Two neonates with abdominal distention. In **a** there is extraluminal gas in the descending colon (linear black streaks along left lateral abdominal cavity). This is pneumatosis intestinalis or air in the wall of the bowel. In **b**, another infant with necrotizing enterocolitis has portal venous gas (look into the liver). There is abdominal distention, but the pneumatosis is not as clearly defined.

Chapter 5

Fig. 5.5. What abnormalities do you see? Panel **a**, an infant who had the bladder filled during VCU. A portion of the bladder wall has herniated into each inguinal canal (laterally). These are called "bladder ears" and are of no clinical significance. Panel **b**, an IVU in a 7.5-year-old who was in an automobile accident. The upper tracts appear normal, but the bladder is raised off the pelvic floor and pushed to the left. There is obvious disruption of the left pubic bone. Panel **c**, same patient as in **b**. A retrograde study was performed, and the catheter was removed. There is contrast in the pelvis because of disruption of the posterior urethra. Contrast in the left hip joint indicates disruption of the bones of the acetabulum as well.

Fig. 5.10. Multiple abnormal IVUs. In **a**, a 10-year-old with a left flank mass. This is a 10-min film. The right kidney appears normal, but on the left there is a large mass with linear densities. The densities represent the parenchymal tubules being pushed in a vertical direction (parenchymal rims about a more lucent, dilated, urine-filled collecting system). In **b**, a coned-down view of this kidney shows the rims to better advantage. This patient had ureteropelvic junction obstruction. In **c**, a 5-min film from a 6-year-old with repeated urinary tract infections. The left kidney is considerably smaller than the right and measures less than three vertebral bodies in height. The right kidney is larger than normal, measuring just about five vertebral bodies in height. Note how close the left upper pole calyx comes to the spine!! In **d**, a 2-year-old with fever. The excretory urogram shows the lower pole calyces overlying the spine. This was a *horseshoe kidney*, perhaps unrelated to the fever.

Chapter 7

Fig. 7.11. The medial epicondyle is displaced inferiorly due to a fracture through the apophyseal growth plate. There is marked soft tissue swelling. Sometimes subtle growth-plate injuries require comparison views of the other extremity.

Fig. 7.13. Panel **b**, there are posterior rib fractures of the left fifth, sixth, seventh, and eighth ribs and healing fractures of the ninth and tenth ribs posteriorly on the right. There is soft tissue calcification lateral to the radius. The distal humerus (left) is also fractured. Note the displaced left proximal humeral epiphysis. This is a fracture through the growth plate.

Fig. 7.33. Panel **a**, benign bone cyst of the calcaneus. It is a solitary lesion which has a clear zone of demarcation, no periosteal reaction, and a single lucency, typical of a cyst. You certainly thought this was benign, didn't you? Panel **b**, Legg-Calvé-Perthe disease, or aseptic necrosis. The child complained of left hip pain, and the left femoral head appears somewhat shallower and flatter than the right. Note the defect at the most lateral aspect of the growth plate. These findings are typical of early aseptic necrosis. Panel **c**, bone abscess. The sclerosis at the posterior aspect of the proximal tibia diaphysis is a clue. A lucency can be seen in the center, and the differential diagnoses include infections such as a chronic abscess, osteoid osteoma, and healing fracture.

Chapter 8

Fig. 8.17. Panel **b**, compare the pedicles. The left pedicle of L5 is dense when compared to the right pedicle or to either pedicle of L4. This is a common location for an osteoid osteoma, which is a benign bone lesion causing pain.

Fig. 8.18. In **b**, careful attention to the vertical lines reveals that C7, the lowest cervical vertebra, is out of position. Look at the relationship of the articulating facets. This is a dislocation of C7. Note the normal anterior inferior ring apophysis of C7 (looks like chip of bone at inferior surface). In **c**, are all the vertebral bodies the same height? C3 is a "wafer" vertebra. The joint space is intact, but the vertebral body is severely compressed. This is commonly found in eosinophilic granuloma of bone. In **d**, a compression fracture of C5 and C6. Trauma is a major cause of vertebral compression fractures and wedging.

Fig. 8.21. Panel **a**, tuberculosis: Pott's disease. Note the disk space narrowing of T11-12. There are bilateral paraspinal masses which may calcify as they heal. Panel **b**, meningomyelocele. You should have detected the absence of the spinous processes of L2 through the sacrum. Did you notice that the pedicles have lost their convex inner margin? Panel **c**, coronal ultrasound of this neonate reveals multiple cavities (black holes) surrounding the ventricle. This represents ischemic disease called periventricular leukomalacia. The ventricles are minimally enlarged. Panels **d,e**, a lipoma (fat is white on T1 imaging) within the spinal canal. T1 images of the sagittal and axial lumbar spine show fat involving the region of the conus and extending down the canal. The cord is deviated and somewhat lower than expected. This is a lipoma with a low or tethered cord.

Subject Index